Other monographs in the series, Major Problems in Clinical Pediatrics:

Altman and Schwartz: *Malignant Diseases of Infancy, Childhood and Adolescence* — 1978

Avery, Fletcher and Williams: *The Lung and Its Disorders in the Newborn Infant* — Fourth Edition, 1981

Bell and McCormick: *Increased Intracranial Pressure in Children* — Second Edition, 1978

Bell and McCormick: *Neurologic Infections in Children* — Second Edition, 1981

Brewer: *Juvenile Rheumatoid Arthritis* — 1970

Cornblath and Schwartz: *Disorders of Carbohydrate Metabolism in Infancy* — Second Edition, 1976

Dubowitz: *Muscle Disorders in Childhood* — 1978

Gryboski: *Gastrointestinal Problems in the Infant* — 1975

Hanshaw and Dudgeon: *Viral Diseases of the Fetus and Newborn* — 1978

Harrison and Harrison: *Disorders of Calcium and Phosphate Metabolism in Childhood and Adolescence* — 1979

Lubchenco: *The High Risk Infant* — 1976

Markowitz and Gordis: *Rheumatic Fever* — Second Edition, 1972

Oski and Naiman: *Hematologic Problems in the Newborn* — Second Edition, 1972

Rowe, Freedom and Mehrizi: *The Neonate with Congenital Heart Disease* — Second Edition, 1980

Royer, et al: *Pediatric Nephrology* — 1974

Scriver and Rosenberg: *Amino Acid Metabolism and Its Disorders* — 1973

Smith: *Recognizable Patterns of Human Deformation* — 1981

Smith: *Growth and Its Disorders* — 1977

Smith: *Recognizable Patterns of Human Deformations* — 1981

Solomon and Esterly: *Neonatal Dermatology* — 1973

Solomon, Esterly and Loeffel: *Adolescent Dermatology* — 1978

Volpe: *Neurology of the Newborn* — 1981

Forthcoming Monographs

Bluestone and Klein: *Otitis Media in Infants and Children*
Drash: *Juvenile Diabetes*
Glader: *Anemias in Children*
Griffin: *Children's Orthopedics*
Ingelfinger: *Pediatric Hypertension*
Kerns: *Child Abuse and Neglect*

GENITOURINARY PROBLEMS IN PEDIATRICS

by
A. Barry Belman, M.D.

Professor of Urology and Child Health and
Development, George Washington University School of
Medicine and Health Sciences; Chairman, Department
of Pediatric Urology, Children's Hospital
National Medical Center, Washington, D.C.

George W. Kaplan, M.D.

Clinical Professor of Surgery/Urology and Chief of
Pediatric Urology, School of Medicine, University of
California, San Diego, San Diego, California;
Chief of Urology, Children's Hospital of San Diego

Volume XXIII in the Series
MAJOR PROBLEMS IN
CLINICAL PEDIATRICS
ALEXANDER J. SCHAFFER
Consulting Editor
MILTON MARKOWITZ
Associate Consulting Editor

W. B. Saunders Company, Philadelphia, London, Toronto, Sydney   1981

W. B. Saunders Company: West Washington Square
Philadelphia, PA   19105

1 St. Anne's Road
Eastbourne, East Sussex BN21 3UN, England

1 Goldthorne Avenue
Toronto, Ontario M8Z 5T9, Canada

9 Waltham Street
Artarmon, N.S.W. 2064, Australia

Library of Congress Cataloging in Publication Data

Belman, A. Barry, 1938–

Genitourinary problems in pediatrics.

(Major problems in clinical pediatrics; v. 22)

1. Pediatric urology.   I. Kaplan, George W., joint author.
II. Title.   III. Series. [DNLM: 1. Urologic diseases—
In infancy and childhood. W1 MA492N v. 22 / WS 320
B451u]

RJ466.B42   618.92′6   80–53367

ISBN 0–7216–1678–X

Genitourinary Problems in Pediatrics   ISBN   0-7216-1678-X

Last digit is the print number: 9   8   7   6   5   4   3   2   1

We wish to dedicate this book to our wives, Paula and Susan, without whose support this effort would surely have been abandoned, and to Dr. John T. Grayhack, Herman C. Kretschmer Professor and Chairman, Department of Urology, Northwestern University Medical School, our teacher, who provided an example of excellence and intellectual honesty which we continuously strive to emulate.

A. BARRY BELMAN
GEORGE W. KAPLAN

Foreword

Pediatricians and other physicians who treat children frequently encounter conditions that require a urologic evaluation. Because many of these conditions are unique to infants and children, they are managed best by urologists who devote their time entirely to urologic diseases of childhood. There is now a growing number of pediatric urologists who by concentrating on children have contributed a valuable body of knowledge and have been responsible for many of the diagnostic and therapeutic advances in recent years.

Two-well-known leaders in this field have authored this monograph. Dr. George Kaplan received his medical degree and urologic training at Northwestern University. He then joined the faculty of the University of California, San Diego, where he is currently Clinical Professor of Surgery and Chief of Pediatric Urology. He is a contributing author of more than 80 papers. Dr. A. Barry Belman also obtained his medical and urologic training from Northwestern. He is at present Professor of Urology and Child Health at George Washington University and Chairman of the Department of Pediatric Urology at Children's Hospital National Medical Center in Washington, D.C. Dr. Belman has authored or coauthored more than 70 papers and books.

This book was written primarily for the generalist who cares for children. It is clinical in orientation and contains a great deal of practical information on problems ranging from, in the words of the authors, "the common—bedwetting—to the rare—exstrophy of the bladder—and from the simple—cystitis—to the overwhelmingly complex—myelomeningocele."

MILTON MARKOWITZ, M.D.

Preface

The publication of this volume as part of a series dedicated exclusively to pediatric medicine emphasizes the importance pediatric urology has achieved as a discipline over the past two decades. Largely owing to the devotion of a relatively few physicians with great foresight, it became evident in the early sixties that the urologic problems seen in children required a unique perspective and, with that perspective, a separate approach from that employed with adults. During that same period advances in pediatric imaging, anesthesia, and nephrology, as well as improved optics and miniaturization of endoscopic instruments, transformed the field. With centralization of care in major children's hospitals, the opportunity then existed for those few individuals who were devoting their efforts primarily or exclusively to the care of the genitourinary systems in children to study the approaches and treatment of problems such as urinary tract infection, vesicoureteral reflux, the obstructed urinary tract, genital abnormalities, and other major anomalies. Through these combined labors great advances were made.

Over the ensuing years a consensus has developed regarding the approach to many genitourinary problems of childhood, although by no means are all questions resolved, nor is there agreement over all approaches to diagnosis or therapy. In this volume we have attempted to present an overview of problems of the genitourinary tract that the primary physician might face in pediatric care. In this endeavor we have leaned heavily upon the experience of others and are grateful to Drs. Panayotis P. Kelalis and Lowell R. King for allowing us to use numerous illustrations from Clinical Pediatric Urology (W. B. Saunders Co., 1976) and to Drs. J. Hartwell Harrison and Alan Perlmutter for permitting the use of illustrations from the pediatric portion of the fourth edition of Campbell's Urology (W. B. Saunders Co., 1979).

We have relied upon our own clinical experience in many areas; however, particular effort has been made to provide references for problems that remain controversial. While definitive statements can be made in reference to many of the subjects addressed, significant topics of concern remain that cannot be conclusively addressed at present. These include the question of surgical versus medical management of vesicoureteral reflux, which is currently being evaluated prospectively under an international protocol. The optimal age for genital surgery is as yet unknown and awaits definitive study to ascertain the psychological and functional implications. Although great strides have been made in the treatment of certain neoplasms through national and international study groups, there are other areas in which little progress has been made. Progress can only result from pooling our limited resources, especially in instances of rarer tumors. By maintaining open communication, we can continue to improve our store of knowledge and thereby follow the example of those who have led us into this most gratifying subspecialty.

Finally, we wish to offer our appreciation to the numerous individuals who were supportive of this endeavor: Mrs. Hilary Kavanagh, Mrs. Mary Moyta, and Ms. Bette Jo Garrett for exhaustive secretarial help and Mrs. Deborah Gilbert for her untiring assistance in locating references. We are particularly grateful to Mr. Jack Hanley of W. B. Saunders Co., who originally nurtured the idea for this work, and to Mary Cowell and her associates for their editorial assistance and efforts in gathering the various borrowed illustrations.

Contents

Chapter One

UROPATHOLOGY IN THE PEDIATRIC PATIENT

Pediatric urology is a discipline that encompasses a spectrum of problems ranging from the common — bedwetting — to the rare—exstrophy, and from the simple—cystitis — to the overwhelmingly complex — myelomeningocele. Congenital anomalies of the urogenital tract affect a significant percentage of the population. Although some are inconsequential, others result in major morbidity and occasionally mortality. Additionally, urinary tract infection is one of the commonest bacterial diseases seen in the pediatric population. Despite the frequency of uropathologic conditions in children, pediatric urology is only now maturing as a separate discipline. Consequently, "the state of the art" and the progress made in this subspecialty is often poorly appreciated.

The diagnostic capabilities for evaluation of the urinary tract have recently made tremendous advances. It is, therefore, usually not difficult to arrive at the proper diagnosis of a urologic problem if one only suspects that such a problem exists. Most acute as well as the more chronic problems of the urinary tract will be associated with some symptom or readily documented sign that will lead the thoughtful observer to a correct diagnosis. Even infants with urinary tract infections usually exhibit some change in urinary habits; if not, some other sign, such as fever or failure to thrive, will become evident. It is truly unfortunate when these symptoms remain unrecognized for a protracted period of time prior to evaluation, as most serious problems of this system are amenable to treatment if the diagnosis is made promptly.

It is a truism that before being able to arrive at a diagnosis, one must first consider the existence of a disease as a possibility. This statement is particularly applicable to disorders of the urinary tract since significant information can often be obtained with simple and straightforward studies, such as history, physical examination, urinalysis, and urine culture. Because it is often a little more difficult to obtain a urine specimen in the population in question, routine urinalysis has not achieved the prominence in pediatric practice that it has in adults. With just a modicum of forethought and patience, specimens can be collected routinely, even in infants. Toilet-trained children, when reassured, will usually void on request, and infants urinate frequently when well hydrated. When the specimen obtained is collected in a sterile container, it then can also be used for culture. Urine cultures have not been used routinely as they are perceived as being costly. The recent introduction of "mini-cultures" has removed this objection. Obviously, any positive culture obtained from a voided, bagged collection in an infant should be confirmed by a second, fresh specimen or, preferably, by suprapubic aspiration or catheterization prior to treatment or radiographic evaluation.

The question often arises as to the benefit of routine urine screening in children. The term "screening" is generally applied to public health programs designed to cover large population groups, but in this context we will consider it only as it relates to well-child care. If one assumes that all infants and children receive some regular pediatric care, then sometime prior to school age, urine screening cultures are indicated. This applies most specifically to girls.

The incidence of urinary tract infection in school-age girls has been tabulated at between two and five per cent. Girls are affected 20 times more frequently than boys. Over 15 per cent of children with asymptomatic bacteriuria have radiographic changes consistent with bacterial pyelonephritis (renal scarring), and one third have vesicoureteral reflux.

The incidence of pyelographic "renal scars" in adolescents and adults is the same as that seen in children. This implies that if these findings are acquired and are secondary to infection, the causative episode was overlooked. Even in those children discovered to have bacteriuria before one year of age, pyelonephritic renal scarring was observed in one third of these cases. It is becoming increasingly apparent that the renal damage associated with vesicoureteral reflux and bacteriuria has its onset in infancy.

Urine cultures performed periodically at six-month intervals for the first two or three years of life and then annually may be the only way renal scarring can be minimized in this otherwise asymptomatic group. This recommendation assumes that (1) abnormalities detected are promptly treated, (2) that early treatment can prevent these changes, and (3) that the radiographic findings noted are not congenital but do actually result from acquired bacterial infection.

PRESENTING SYMPTOMS

Voiding symptoms, the most common and easily recognizable presenting urologic complaints, are directly referable to the urinary tract. Urinary urgency, incontinence, and dysuria are indicative of acute lower urinary tract inflammation. Pyuria also suggests an inflammatory process. Nonetheless, these symptoms, even when coupled with the finding of pyuria upon microscopy of the urinary sediment, are insufficient evidence for diagnosis of urinary tract infection.

As will become clearer in subsequent chapters, the diagnosis of urinary tract infection carries with it a responsibility to prove that the affected child does not harbor an underlying anatomic abnormality that contributed to that infection. Hence, all children other than black girls with documented urinary tract infection must, in our opinion, be studied at least by cystography and excretory urography. Radiographic evaluation is invasive, expensive, and time-consuming and should not be performed indiscriminately. However, evaluation is essential in children with proven urinary tract infection. Black girls have a significantly lower incidence of anatomic urinary abnormalities and therefore represent an exception to the recommendation for radiographic evaluation of bacteriuria responsive to treatment and not associated with fever (Chap. 4).

INCONTINENCE

One of the more frequent presenting symptoms is the involuntary loss of urine. To better understand this symptom and its etiology, several parameters must be detailed. It should be determined whether the enuresis is primary (present since birth) or of secondary onset (developing after an interval of normal control), whether it is nocturnal, diurnal, or both, and whether the child dribbles continuously or intermittently. In addition, it is important to learn whether there also are irritative symptoms, such as urgency or dysuria, and how often the child voids. The force and character of the urinary stream, as well as discovering if the child has periods of normal control, are significant.

Urinary incontinence may exhibit a certain pattern, and this will often lead to the underlying problem. Total incontinence is the inability to store any urine and indicates that the urinary sphincters are anatomically or functionally absent (as in patients with epispadias or myelomeningocele) or that they have been bypassed (such as in vesicovaginal fistula). Overflow incontinence occurs when the urinary outlet is obstructed and the patient dribbles frequently to relieve a consistently full bladder. Urge incontinence occurs when there is a sudden and uncontrollable need to void that cannot be suppressed. This implies bladder irritability. Precipitate voiding is much the same but occurs without a preceding urge to void and suggests neurologic origins. Stress incontinence occurs when intravesical pressure momentarily exceeds infravesical resistance (such as in "giggle incontinence"). Lastly, paradoxic incontinence describes the girl who is always wet and yet voids normally. This is suggestive of an ectopic ureteral orifice outside the urinary sphincter mechanism.

IRRITATIVE SYMPTOMS

Irritative symptoms, such as dysuria, frequency, and urgency, are indicative of bladder hyperactivity. Children so affected often have urinary incontinence with urgency. This is usually secondary to inflammation and may also be associated with suprapubic or perineal pain.

HEMATURIA

Hematuria is a common problem for which children are referred to the urologist or nephrologist. Since hematuria is a symptom shared by many diverse disorders (Table 1–1), it is advantageous to perform some preliminary screening studies prior to for such preliminary evaluation is found in Table 1–2.

History alone will often provide valuable clues to the pathogenesis of hematuria. Total hematuria, i.e., blood throughout the deciding the propriety of referral. A schema urinary stream, is of renal or bladder origin. Patients with urinary urgency, frequency, and dysuria along with hematuria are likely to have hemorrhagic cystitis. Urine culture will corroborate the diagnosis in most cases of bacterial infection. Confusion can result in children with viral cystitis, in which case routine bacterial cultures will be negative.

Table 1–1. Causes of Hematuria

MEDICAL	SURGICAL
Urinary tract infection	Urinary tract infection
Acute glomerulonephritis	Obstructive uropathy
Rapidly progressive glomerulonephritis	Trauma
Chronic hypocomplementemic glomerulonephritis	Neoplasm
Henoch-Schöenlein nephritis	Vascular malformation
Lupus erythematosus nephritis	congenital (AV fistula, hemangioma)
Goodpasture's syndrome	acquired (AV fistula, renal vein
Hemolytic uremic syndrome	thrombosis)
Benign hematuria	Foreign body
Familial hematuria	
Periarteritis nodosa	
Subacute bacterial endocarditis	
Sepsis	
Bleeding diathesis	
Drug toxicity	
Urethral meatal excoriation	

(Modified from Burke, R. H.: Urinalysis; The investigation of hematuria and renal biopsy. *In* Kelalis, P. P., King, L. R., and Belman, A. B.: Clinical Pediatric Urology, Vol. 1. Philadelphia, W. B. Saunders Co., 1976.)

Table 1–2. Schema for Evaluation of Pediatric Hematuria

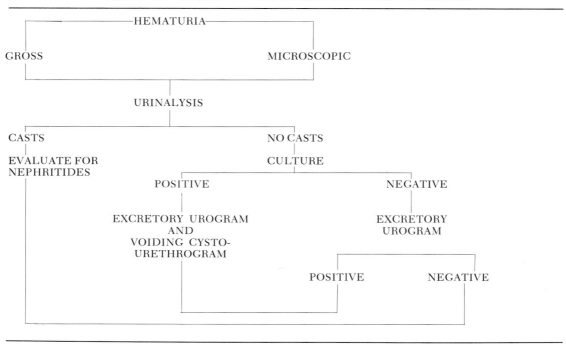

Initial or terminal hematuria suggests that the responsible lesion is at the bladder base or in the proximal urethra. Although radiographic evaluation, including voiding cystourethrography, is recommended, this type of bleeding is poorly understood and rarely is of significance in children. Blood staining of the underwear in boys without true hematuria is almost always of urethral origin and secondary to either a nonspecific and poorly understood urethritis or urethral irritation. In the absence of actual hematuria, evaluation of such problems with studies additional to urine culture and excretory urography with a film during voiding will probably contribute little.

In infant males, ammoniacal meatitis may cause blood staining on diapers. The underlying cause should be obvious, and local treatment is all that is necessary. Bright red urine, especially with clots, suggests urologic pathology, whereas tea-colored or smoky urine is more likely nephrologic in origin. It is to be emphasized that all red urine is not necessarily bloody, and microscopic or chemical confirmation of

hematuria is advisable before embarking on further studies. Causes for discoloration of the urine are listed in Table 1–3.

A history of recent upper respiratory tract illness or streptococcal infection suggests post-streptococcal glomerulonephritis, particularly in younger children. Such children, who also have edema, hypertension, and fever, do not constitute a diagnostic dilemma. Those children found to have red blood cell casts on microscopic urinalysis require no further urologic evaluation but should have appropriate studies to elucidate the cause of the nephritis. Appropriate laboratory studies, including a throat culture, serum complement level, and anti-streptolysin-O (ASO) titer or streptozyme reactivity, are in order prior to further evaluation in all children presenting with asymptomatic gross or microscopic hematuria.

A history of trauma can often be obtained when dealing with children since their level of activity is so high. However, urinary obstruction with a dilated, tense system proximal to the site of obstruction becomes very susceptible to injury. There-

Table 1–3. Causes of Urinary Discoloration

CAUSES OF ABNORMAL URINE COLOR

Colorless:
Diabetes mellitus, diabetes insipidus, dilution of urine.
Milky:
Chyluria, pyuria.
Yellow:
Normal, phenacetin, quinacrine, riboflavin.
Red:
Hemoglobinuria, myoglobinuria, hematuria, chronic lead and mercury poisoning; eosin, acetophenetidin, diphenylhydantoin, phenindione, emodin, anisindione, phenolphthalein, phenothiazines, phensuximide, rifampin; anthocyanin.
Blue, Blue-green to Green:
Biliverdin, indicanuria; amitriptyline, anthraquinone, arbutin, flavin derivatives, indigo blue, indigo carmine, methylene blue, tetrahydronaphthalene, thymol, phenol, resorcinol, salol, toluidine blue, triamterene.
Orange:
Dehydration; santonin, cryptophanic acid, salicylazosulfapyridine, phenazopyridine.
Brown:
Porphyria, presence of urobilinogen; nitrofurantoin, primaquine, chloroquine, furazolidone, metronidazole, argyrol; fava beans, aloe.
Brown black:
Hemorrhage, melanin, homogentisic acid (alcaptonuria), p-hydroxyphenylpyruvic acid (tyrosinosis); methyldopa, cascara, pyrogallol, iron sorbitol, methocarbamol, senna, phenylhydrazine; rhubarb.

Note: Malingerers sometimes color their urine with blood, food coloring, or colored crepe paper; or by ingesting food or substances that will color it.

(From Elkins, M., and Kabat, H.: Causes of urinary discoloration. Am. J. Hosp. Pharmacol., 25:489–519, 1968.)

fore, hematuria, even when associated with mild trauma, requires radiographic evaluation.

FEVER

Otherwise unexplained fever should direct one's attention to the urinary tract as a possible etiologic source. When fever accompanies urinary tract infection, there is an increased likelihood that one is dealing with bacterial pyelonephritis rather than cystitis. Govan and colleagues (1975) found that 60 per cent of children with febrile urinary tract infection had demonstrable vesicoureteral reflux and, hence, presumed pyelonephritis. Since bacterial pyelonephritis can lead to renal scarring, it is desir-

able to recognize this problem so that it can be treated as rapidly as possible.

PAIN

Abdominal pain is a very common symptom in children. However, it is rarely due to anatomic pathology of the urinary tract. Pain following high fluid intake may be the result of acute dilatation of the urinary tract behind an obstruction (ureteropelvic junction obstruction). Ultrasonographic screening is a reasonable, noninvasive means to rule out long-standing obstruction as a cause for pain. Occasionally excretory urography must be performed to insure that the urinary tract is not the underlying cause. Lower abdominal discomfort may also be attributable to cystitis. If questioned closely, such children often have a history of squatting and pressing the perineum with a heel at the time of these pains to prevent incontinence. This complex is only seen in girls and is explained by a very irritable bladder usually brought about by chronic cystitis (Chap. 3).

Back pain in children is rarely caused by urinary tract pathology. Musculoskeletal problems are a much more common cause. Children localize abdominal pain poorly. Even when unilateral ureteral obstruction is the cause, the pain is frequently perceived periumbilically. Acute obstruction is more likely to cause pain than is the chronically dilated urinary tract.

Flank pain is an uncommon symptom in children, although children with acute pyelonephritis may localize pain to the ipsilateral kidney. Occasionally, children with severe vesicoureteral reflux complain of flank discomfort associated with voiding that disappears shortly after completion of that act. Acute distension of the upper urinary tract from large volume reflux is the cause.

PHYSICAL EXAMINATION

Inspection of the patient may suggest certain diagnoses. Microcephaly can be seen in association with obstructive urop-athy, and hydrocephalus suggests neuro-genic bladder disease (in association with myelomeningocele).The recognition of Pot-ter's facies will lead to a prompt diagnosis of renal agenesis or severe obstruction. Many of the chromosomal abnormalities are also manifested by physical appearance.

Bladder or cloacal exstrophy, myelo-meningocele, imperforate anus, and siren-omelia are easily recognizable at birth, and all suggest the need for further urologic assessment. The blueberry muffin syndrome (cutaneous neurofibromata and café au lait spots) are related to various neural crest tumors.

Low-set and malformed ears also sug-gest renal abnormalities. Webbing of the neck is found in Turner's syndrome. Later-ally placed nipples occur in Turner's and Noonan's syndromes. Pneumomediastinum and pneumothorax are occasionally seen in newborn males with obstructive uropathy.

Urologic abnormalities in childhood may also be completely asymptomatic but offer the opportunity to be discovered in the course of routine physical examination. The first such opportunity is the initial newborn examination, but many others present dur-ing the child's first several years of life. We have chosen to discuss findings in the order in which they may be discovered rather than in order of frequency or importance. In addition, certain organ system abnormali-ties or constellations of abnormalities often have associated developmental urinary tract abnormalities. Awareness of such associa-tions will lead the astute clinician to an early diagnosis.

HYPERTENSION

An often neglected part of the child's physical examination is measurement of

Table 1–4. Differential Diagnosis of Abdominal Masses Referable to the Genitourinary Tract

Hydronephrosis
   Ureteropelvic junction obstruction (may be bilateral)
   Ureterovesical obstruction (may be bilateral)
   Posterior urethral valves (hydronephrosis may be unequal)
   Ectopic ureter with obstruction
   Ureterocele (almost always associated with duplication)
Cystic dysplasia (multicystic kidney)
Polycystic disease
   Infantile (autosomal recessive)
   Adult (autosomal dominant)
Wilms' tumor
Mesoblastic nephroma (neonate)
Neuroblastoma
Idiopathic adrenal hemorrhage of newborn
Renal vein thrombosis
Renal ectopia
Horseshoe kidney (palpable isthmus)
Hamartoma (associated with tuberous sclerosis)
Renal cell carcinoma (rare in children)
Retroperitoneal sarcoma or teratoma
Distended bladder
   Posterior urethral valves
   Neurogenic bladder
Hydrometrocolpos
Lower genitourinary rhabdomyosarcoma

blood pressure. This is probably a reflection of the low incidence of blood pressure ele-vation in the pediatric population. Never-theless, hypertension can be a serious prob-lem in children, and its recognition demands a thorough search for an underly-ing, reversible cause.

ABDOMINAL EXAMINATION

Careful abdominal palpation, particu-larly in infants, can be rewarding (Table 1–4). The art of medicine implies a certain skill and patience that separates the novice from the master. This especially applies to

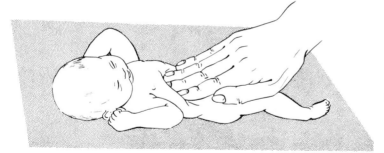

Figure 1–1. Method of ab-dominal palpation in an infant. Note that the flat portion of the fingers is used rather than the tips. (From Ke-lalis, P. P., King, L. R., and Belman, A. B.: Clinical Pediatric Urology, Vol. 1. Philadelphia, W. B. Saunders Co., 1976, p. 110.)

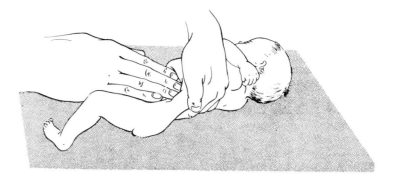

Figure 1–2. Method of left renal palpation in an infant. The examiner's right hand lifts while the left hand explores the left upper quadrant and flank. (From Kelalis, P. P., King, L. R., and Belman, A. B.: Clinical Pediatric Urology, Vol. 1. Philadelphia, W. B. Saunders Co., 1976, p. 111.)

the abdominal examination. Recently we have had occasion to see two patients, one with a Wilms' tumor and another with a neuroblastoma. Early diagnosis resulting in complete resection of a localized lesion was accomplished in each instance because the primary physician in each case refused to allow children to leave his office until an adequate abdominal examination had been performed.

Initially, examination of the abdomen should be carried out with the patient supine, thoroughly palpating all four abdominal quadrants. Ectopic and horseshoe kidneys may be found easily. Abdominal relaxation is usually required to satisfactorily feel normally sized and positioned kidneys and to detect small renal or suprarenal masses. Such relaxation can often be produced by having the older child breathe in and out deeply while probing, especially during the expiratory phase. In infants and younger children it may be helpful to use a pacifier rather than a bottle. A full stomach often prevents adequate examination. Counterpressure in the flank region aids considerably in "trapping" the

kidney after inspiration, allowing for better palpation (Figs. 1–1 to 1–3).

Abdominal masses in the newborn period arise within the urogenital systems in more than two thirds of those with this finding. The incidence of hydronephrosis and multicystic kidneys in infants in this group is approximately equal. Other less common causes include renal vein thrombosis, polycystic kidneys, and solid renal tumors.

The sudden discovery of an abdominal mass, often of mammoth proportions, can be a most startling finding in infants and children. In the toddler and older children, tumors of the kidney, the adrenal, or the sympathetic chain should be suspected. However, unrecognized hydronephrosis is also a definite consideration. Evaluation should be immediately pursued starting with either excretory urography or ultrasonography.

A distended bladder may be the result of voluntary urinary retention brought about by dysuria. It is not uncommon for children to refrain from urinating for 18 hours voluntarily because of pain. Catheterization

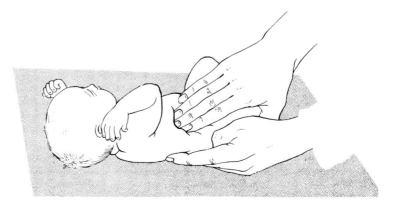

Figure 1–3. Method of right renal palpation in an infant. The examiner's left hand lifts while the right hand explores the right upper quadrant and flank. (From Kelalis, P. P., King, L. R., and Belman, A. B.: Clinical Pediatric Urology, Vol. 1. Philadelphia, W. B. Saunders Co., 1976, p. 111.)

should not be carried out. Instead, the child should be placed in a warm tub to stimulate voiding. In infant males, congenital urethral obstruction is a cause of vesical distension. In the female with a pelvic mass, likely possibilities include an obstructed, dilated vagina or uterus. If the girl's external genitalia are abnormal, a urogenital sinus anomaly should be considered. If only a single perineal opening is present, a cloacal abnormality in which urinary, fecal, and internal genital tracts join is most likely. A mobile lower abdominal mass in a girl may be ovarian in origin.

Frequently, examination of the lower abdomen will reveal what is at first thought to be an abdominal mass but what subsequently is proved to be stool in the colon. A repeat examination following voiding helps in differentiating stool from a distended bladder. However, rectal examination should always be carried out in any child with unexplained abdominal symptoms or findings and will often eliminate this source of diagnostic error. Sarcomas of the lower genitourinary tract are palpable rectally as well as abdominally and hence will not be overlooked if considered in the differential diagnosis.

GENITAL EXAMINATION

Genital abnormalities as a rule are rare in girls. In most males such problems are usually obvious and do not pose a diagnostic dilemma. Hypospadias should be obvious. An incompletely formed prepuce is a clue to hypospadias and can direct one's attention to more mild forms. If hypospadias is identified, circumcision should not be performed until the child has been evaluated by a surgeon accustomed to dealing with this problem frequently. The evaluation of the newborn with ambiguous genitalia is discussed more fully in subsequent chapters. The presence or absence of testes should be documented on initial examination.

When examining the newborn's penis, it is unrealistic to expect to separate the foreskin from the glans without force. This finding should not be termed "phimosis" but rather failure of separation of the tissue

Table 1–5.   More Common Hereditary Diseases Due to Single Mutant Genes

DISEASE	GENETIC TRANSMISSION	GU EFFECT
Hereditary nephritis with deafness (Alport's syndrome)	Autosomal dominant	Renal failure
Benign familial hematuria	Autosomal dominant	Hematuria
Adult polycystic disease	Autosomal dominant	Renal cystic disease
Infantile polycystic disease	Autosomal recessive	Renal cystic disease
Medullary cystic disease (juvenile nephronophthisis)	Autosomal recessive	Renal failure
Diabetes insipidus, nephrogenic	X-linked	Polyuria, dilated collecting system
Ehlers-Danlos syndrome	Autosomal dominant	Ureteropelvic junction obstruction
Sickle cell disease	Autosomal recessive	Priapism, hematuria
Sickle cell trait	Autosomal recessive	Hematuria, papillary necrosis
Nail-patella syndrome (hereditary onychoosteodysplasia)	Autosomal dominant	Renal insufficiency hydroureteronephrosis
Von Hippel Lindau syndrome	Autosomal dominant	Wilms' tumor
Tuberous sclerosis	Autosomal dominant	Renal hamartoma and cystic disease
Cystic fibrosis	Autosomal recessive	Atresia of vas deferens
Laurence-Moon-Biedl syndrome	Autosomal recessive	Hypogonadism
Noonan's syndrome	Autosomal dominant	Cryptorchidism, renal anomalies
Testicular feminization	X-linked recessive	⎤
Reifenstein's syndrome	X-linked recessive	⎟ Spectrum of genital abnormalities
Adrenogenital syndrome	Autosomal recessive	⎟
Kallman's syndrome	Autosomal recessive	⎦

(Modified from Burger, R. H., and Burger, S. E.: Genetic determinants of urologic disease. Urol. Clin. North Am., *1*:419, 1974.)

Table 1–6. Chromosomal Anomalies

Klinefelter's syndrome	47, XXY	Eunuchoid appearance, small gonads, infertility
Turner's syndrome	45, XO	Infertility, renal anomalies
Mixed gonadal dysgenesis	45, XO-46, XY mosaicism	Ambiguous genitalia, wolffian and mullerian structures present, gonadal neoplasia
XYY syndrome	47, XYY	Cryptorchidism, small penis, hypospadias
XXXXY syndrome	49, XXXXY	Cryptorchidism, small penis
Down's syndrome (Trisomy 21)		Genital abnormalities, horseshoe or cystic kidneys
Trisomy 13		Cystic kidneys, bicornuate uterus, cryptorchidism
18q deletion syndrome		Hypoplastic genitalia

(Modified from Burger, R. H., and Burger, S. E.: Genetic determinants of urologic disease. Urol. Clin. North Am., *1*:419, 1974.)

planes, an entirely normal phenomenon. It is not uncommon to see incomplete separation of these layers lasting until three to five years of age or longer.

NEUROLOGIC EXAMINATION

Finally, some degree of attention should be paid to the spine and neurologic systems. The most common malformation affecting the innervation of the lower urinary tract is myelomeningocele and is recognizable at birth in almost all affected children. Less dramatic but potentially serious midline closure defects may be suspected by tufts of hair or hemangiomata overlying the lower sacral spine. Physical examination should include evaluation of anal reflexes, sensation, and sphincter tone.

INHERITED DISEASES

Hereditary diseases due to a single mutant gene are determined by simple mendelian laws of inheritance. Those problems are relatively easily categorized and have been well studied. The most common of those that involve the genitourinary tract are listed in Table 1–5.

CHROMOSOMAL ABNORMALITIES

There are many problems of urologic interest that are recognized as being secondary to noninherited chromosomal abnormalities. Common examples that involve

the X and Y chromosomes include Klinefelter's syndrome (47, XXY) and Turner's syndrome (45, XO). Chromosomal nondysjunction results in a number of trisomy syndromes that also have genitourinary implications (Table 1–6).

DEVELOPMENTAL ABNORMALITIES

There are also developmental abnormalities that may or may not have some underlying inherited basis that are often associated with genitourinary abnormalities (Table 1–7). The relationship of many of these problems, e.g., congenital, nonfamilial aniridia or hemihypertrophy, with Wilms' tumor are well documented though difficult to explain. Others, such as the high incidence of urinary abnormalities with abnormal sacral development and imperforate

Table 1–7. Developmental Anomalies Associated With a High Incidence of Genitourinary Abnormalities (Radiographic Evaluation Recommended)

Hemihypertrophy	Wilms' and adrenal tumors
Congenital, non-familial aniridia	Wilms' and adrenal tumors
Vaginal agenesis	Pelvic kidney, solitary kidney
Congenital scoliosis	Renal ectopia
Sacral agenesis	Neurogenic bladder
Imperforate anus	Unilateral renal agenesis, renal ectopia
Tracheoesophageal fistula	Imperforate anus (see above)
Myelomeningocele	Neurogenic bladder
Malformed ears	Renal agenesis
Potter facies	Oligohydramnios, renal agenesis
Prune belly syndrome	Dilatation of renal collecting system, megalourethra, undescended testes

anus, can be related to embryogenic timing as well as their physical proximity at the time of probable fetal insult. The awareness of these relationships is so significant that evaluation of the urinary system becomes mandatory when certain problems, such as sacral agenesis or imperforate anus, are discovered.

REFERENCES

These references are intended to supplement the general information in this chapter.

URINARY TRACT INFECTION

Bergström, T., Larson, H., Lincoln, K., et al.: Studies of urinary tract infections in infancy and childhood. J. Pediatr., 80:858, 1972.

Cardiff-Oxford Bacteriuria Study Group: Sequelae of covert bacteriuria in school girls. Lancet, April 29, 1978, p. 799.

Govan, D. E., Fair, W. R., Friedland, G. W., and Filly, R. A.: Management of children with urinary tract infections. Urology, 6:273, 1975.

Kunin, C. M.: Detection, Prevention and Management of Urinary Tract Infections, 2nd ed. Philadelphia, Lea and Febiger, 1974.

Kunin, C. M., Deutscher, R., and Paquin, A., Jr.: Urinary tract infections in school children: An epidemiologic, clinical and laboratory study. Medicine, 43:91, 1964.

Randolph, M. F., and Majors, F.: Office screening for bacteria in early infancy: Collection of a suitable urine specimen. J. Pediatr., 76:934, 1970.

Smellie, J. M., Hodson, C. J., Edwards, D., and Normand, I. C. S.: Clinical and radiological features of urinary infection in children. Br. Med. J. 2:1222, 1964.

Timmons, J. W., and Perlmutter, A. D.: Renal abscess: A changing concept. J. Urol., 115:299, 1976.

Winberg, J., Anderson, H. J., Bergström, T., et al.: Epidemiology of symptomatic urinary tract infections in childhood. Acta Pediatr. Scand. Suppl., 252:1, 1974.

URINARY CONTROL

Osborne, J.: Bladder emptying in neonates. Arch. Dis. Child., 52:896, 1977.

Vincent, S. A.: Postural control of urinary incontinence. Lancet, 2:631, 1966.

HEMATURIA

Burke, R. H.: Urinalysis: The investigation of hematuria and renal biopsy. In Kelalis, P. P., King, L. R., and Belman, A. B.: Clinical Pediatric Urology, Vol. 1. Philadelphia, W. B. Saunders Co., 1976.

Chan, J. C. M.: Hematuria and proteinuria in pediatric patients: Diagnostic approach. Urology, 11:205, 1978.

Emanuel, B., and Aronson, N.: Neonatal hematuria. Am. J. Dis. Child., 128:204, 1974.

Hubbard, J. G., and Amin, M.: Pseudohematuria. Urology, 10:190, 1977.

Ingelfinger, J. R., Davis, A. E., and Grupe, W. E.: Frequency and etiology of gross hematuria in a general pediatric setting. Pediatrics, 59:557, 1977.

Wyatt, R. J., McRoberts, J. W., and Holland, N. H.: Hematuria in childhood: Significance and management. J. Urol., 117:366, 1977.

ABDOMINAL MASSES

Emanuel, B., and White, H.: Intravenous pyelography in the differential diagnosis of renal masses in the neonatal period. Clin. Pediatr., 7:529, 1968.

Longino, L. A., and Martin, L. W.: Abdominal masses in the newborn infant. Pediatrics, 21:596, 1958.

Melicow, M. M., and Uson, A. C.: Palpable abdominal masses in infants and children: A report based on a review of 653 cases. J. Urol., 81:705, 1959.

Perlman, M., and Williams, J.: Detection of renal anomalies by abdominal palpation in newborn infants. Br. Med. J., 2:347, 1976.

Raffensperger, J. G., and Abousleiman, A.: Abdominal masses in children under one year of age. Surgery, 63:514, 1968.

Sherwood, D. W., Smith, R. C., Lemmon, R. H., and Vrabel, I.: Abnormalities of the genitourinary tract discovered by palpation of the abdomen of the newborn. Pediatrics, 18:782, 1956.

Wedge, J. J., Grosfeld, J. L., and Smith, J. P.: Abdominal masses in the newborn. J. Urol., 106:770, 1971.

GENITAL ABNORMALITIES

Fallon, B., Devine, C. J. Jr., and Horton, C. E.: Congenital anomalies associated with hypospadias. J. Urol., 116:585, 1976.

Farrington, G. H.: The position and retractibility of the normal testis in childhood in reference to the diagnosis and treatment of cryptorchidism. J. Pediatr. Surg., 3:53, 1968.

Farrington, G. H., and Kerr, I. H.: Abnormalities of the upper urinary tract in cryptorchidism. Br. J. Urol., 41:77, 1969.

Hendron, W. H.: Surgical management of urogenital sinus abnormalities. J. Pediatr. Surg., 12:339, 1977.

Johnston, J. H.: The undescended testis. Arch. Dis. Child., 40:113, 1965.

Leduc, B., Van Campenjout, J., and Simard, R.: Congenital absence of the vagina. Observations on 25 cases. Am. J. Obstet. Gynecol., 100:512, 1968.

Levitt, S. B., Kogan, S. J., Schneider, K. M., et al.: Endocrine tests in phenotypic children with bilateral impalpable testes can reliably predict "congenital" anorchism. Urology, 11:11, 1978.

Øster, J.: Further fate of the foreskin. Arch. Dis. Child., 43:200, 1968.

Raffensperger, J. G.: Anomalies of the female genitalia. In Kelalis, P. P., King, L. R., and Belman, A. B.: Clinical Pediatric Urology. Philadelphia, W. B. Saunders Co., 1976.

Ramenofsky, M. L., and Raffensperger, J. G.: An abdomino-perineal-vaginal pull through for definitive treatment of hydrometrocolpos. J. Pediatr. Surg., 6:381, 1971.

Scorer, C. G.: The descent of the testis. Arch. Dis. Child., 39:605, 1964.

Scorer, C. G., and Farrington, G. H.: Congen' ' Deformities of the Testis and Epididymis. London, Appleton-Century-Crofts, 1971.

ASSOCIATED ANOMALIES

Bergsma, D. (Ed.): Birth Defects Atlas and Compendium. Baltimore, Williams and Wilkins Co., 1973. The National Foundation March of Dimes.

Bjorklund, S. E.: Hemihypertrophy and Wilms' tumor. Acta Pediatr. Scand., 44:287, 1955.

Bourne, G. L., and Benirschke, K.: Absent umibilical artery: A review of 113 cases. Arch. Dis. Child., 35:534, 1960.

Burger, R. H., and Burger, S. E.: Genetic determinants of urologic disease. Urol. Clin. North Am., 1:419, 1974.

Carlton, C. E., Jr., and Scott, R., Jr.: Incidence of urological anomalies in association with major neurological anomalies. J. Urol., 84:43, 1960.

Curran, A. S., and Curran, A. P.: Associated sacral and renal malformations: A new syndrome. J. Pediatr., 49:716, 1972.

Duhamel, B.: From the mermaid to anal imperforation: The syndrome of caudal regression. Arch. Dis. Child., 36:152, 1961.

Feingold, M., Fine, R. N., and Ingall, D.: Intravenous pyelography in infants with single umbilical artery. N. Engl. J. Med., 270:1178, 1964.

Froelich, L. A., and Fujikura, T.: Follow up on infants with single umbilical artery. Pediatrics, 52:6, 1973.

Gryboski, J. (Ed.): The peritoneum, abdominal wall and omphalomesenteric duct. In Gastrointestinal Problems in the Infant. Philadelphia, W. B. Saunders Co., 1975.

Hilson, D.: Malformations of ears as a sign of malformation of the genitourinary tract. Br. Med. J., 2:785, 1957.

Miller, R. W., Fraumeni, J. F., Jr., and Maiing, M. D.: Association of Wilms' tumor with aniridia, hemihypertrophy and other congenital malformations. N. Engl. J. Med., 270:922, 1964.

Newman, H., Molthan, M. E., and Osborn, W. F.: Urinary tract anomalies in children with congenital heart disease. Am. J. Roentgenol., Rad. Ther. Nucl. Med., 106:52, 1969.

Persky, L., and Owens, R.: Genitourinary tract abnormalities in Turner's syndrome. Trans. Am. Assoc. Genitourin. Surg., 62:135, 1970.

Potter, E. L.: Facial characteristics of infants with bilateral renal agenesis. Am. J. Obstet. Gynecol., 51:885, 1946.

Potter, E. L.: Oligohydramnios: Further comment. J. Pediatr., 84:931, 1971.

Rubenstein, M. M., and Stickler, G. B.: Familial onycho-osteodysplasia. Am. J. Dis. Child., 107:640, 1964.

Smith, D. W.: Recognizable Patterns of Human Malformation, 2nd ed. Philadelphia, W. B. Saunders Co., 1976.

Taylor, W. C.: Deformity of ears and kidneys. Can. Med. Assoc. J., 93:107, 1965.

Thomas, I. T., and Smith, D. W.: Oligohydramnios: Cause of the non renal features of Potter's syndrome including pulmonary hypoplasia. J. Pediatr., 84:881, 1974.

Vitko, R. J., Cass, A. S., and Winter, R. B.: Anomalies of the genitourinary tract associated with congenital scoliosis and congenital kyphosis. J. Urol., 108:655, 1972.

Warkany, J. (Ed.): Malformations of the urogenital system. In Congenital Malformations. Chicago, Year Book Med. Publ., Inc., 1971.

Williams, D. I., and Nixon, H. H.: Agenesis of the sacrum. Surg. Gynecol. Obstet., 105:84, 1957.

Winter, J. S. D.: A familial syndrome of renal, genital and middle ear anomalies. J. Pediatr., 72:88, 1968.

HYPERTENSION

Belman, A. B., and Lewy, P.: Acute transient renin-mediated hypertension in children following urinary diversion. Urology, 3:693, 1974.

Fay, R., and Kaufman, J. J.: Renal hypertension in children. Urology, 3:149, 1974.

Londe, S.: Blood pressure in children as determined under office conditions. Clin. Pediatr., 5:71, 1966.

Shapiro, S. S., Adelman, R. D., and Tesluk, H.: Non-renovascular renal hypertension in children. Urology, 10:517, 1977.

Chapter Two

DIAGNOSTIC
EVALUATION

EXAMINATION OF THE URINE

COLLECTION OF THE SPECIMEN

There is increasing recognition of the importance of routine testing of the urine as part of the general care of the pediatric population. Implicit in this statement is the need for recommendation as to the manner of collection of the urine and the time of day that provides the best sample for examination. Urinalysis and urine culture will more accurately reflect the bladder urine if the external genitalia in girls are cleansed prior to collection of the specimen. A simple soap and water wash followed by a thorough rinse is adequate; in boys, retraction of the foreskin (if present) and collection of a midstream specimen are all that is necessary. Collection of a clean urine sample is less complicated in prepubertal girls than in women since the vaginal and introital contamination is of a lesser degree. If the toilet-trained girl is asked to sit well back on the standard-sized toilet seat, her legs will, by necessity, separate, virtually guaranteeing a straightforward urinary stream in all but the minority (Fig. 2–1). Children who are markedly obese or cannot abduct their hips may present a challenge in collecting a clean specimen. Toilet-trained boys can void on request at almost any time if the atmosphere is re-

laxed. Of course, situational anxiety often interferes with this ability. One may conclude that in the toilet-trained child, a combination of hydration and patience will assure the collection of an adequate specimen.

Collection of urine in infants by noninvasive techniques requires application of an

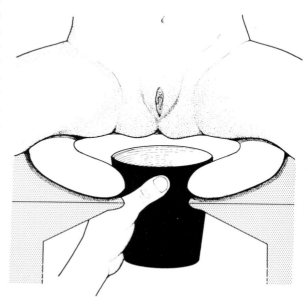

Figure 2–1. A midstream urine collection can be facilitated by having the small girl sit far back on the toilet seat, requiring her to spread her legs and separate her labia. (From Kelalis, P. P., King, L. R., and Belman, A. B.: Clinical Pediatric Urology, Vol. 1. Philadelphia, W. B. Saunders Co., 1976, p. 189.)

12

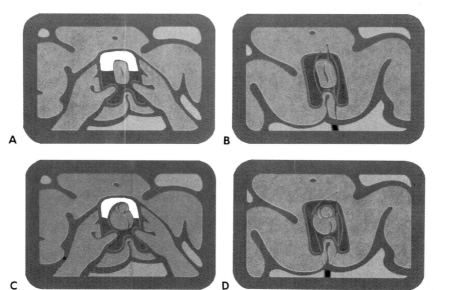

Figure 2–2. Application of Hollister U-Bag.® *A,* In girls, stretch the perineum to separate skin folds and expose the vagina. When applying adhesive to the skin, be sure to start at the narrow bridge of skin separating the vagina from the anus. Work outward from this point. *B,* Press the adhesive firmly against the skin and avoid wrinkles. When the bottom part is in place, remove the paper from the upper portion of the adhesive. Work upward to complete application, pressing the adhesive all around the vagina. *C,* in boys, when pressing adhesive to the skin, be sure to start at the narrow bridge of skin between the anus and the base of the scrotum. Work outward from this point. Be sure the skin is dry before applying the collector. *D,* Continue to press the adhesive firmly against the skin, avoiding wrinkles. When the bottom part is in place, remove the paper from the upper portion of the adhesive patch. Work upward to complete application.

external device. After a soap and water wash and adequate drying, a sterile plastic collection bag (U-Bag) is applied (Fig. 2–2). Application of the plastic bag at home by the parent prior to a visit to the primary physician with its immediate removal at the office is an acceptable screening method if the urine collected is sterile on culture. If significant bacterial growth is reported, a confirmatory culture carried out on a fresh specimen is mandatory prior to treatment. A less redundant alternative is to apply the U-Bag to the well-hydrated baby immediately upon arrival at the office (Randolph and Majors, 1970). Additional fluids are offered, and the parent is informed to notify the nurse or receptionist as soon as voiding is observed. The specimen is then plated or refrigerated at once to limit growth of contaminants after an aliquot is removed for analysis.

In the older, pretoilet-trained group, spontaneous voiding becomes more infrequent, and obtaining a urine specimen often constitutes a real challenge. For routine urine cultures done at regular intervals it may be necessary to bring the specimen from home. To ensure a meaningful culture, that specimen should be refrigerated immediately upon collection and should be kept cold on the way to the office by placing the sealed, sterile container in a plastic kitchen bag filled with ice. Upon its receipt, the specimen should be either maintained on ice or immediately plated. Meaningful culture results are obtainable for up to 48 hours when urine is kept refrigerated (Kass, 1956), although cellular breakdown after a few hours limits the interpretability of formed elements.

In those voided specimens of questionable significance or in the ill child in whom urinary tract infection is suspected and a voiding specimen is not readily attainable, more invasive means of urine collection may be necessary. The practicing physician should not be reluctant to perform the following maneuvers when they are indicated. Repeated trips to the office, prescription of unnecessary medication, or unindicated urologic evaluation based on an inaccurate culture result may be prevented by culturing urine obtained by more aggressive collection techniques.

CATHETERIZATION

Urethral catheterization carries the stigma of being a primitive, painful procedure likely to cause urinary infection when it does not already exist. Unfortunately, this is probably true in some circumstances, depending upon the method and the catheter size employed. In actuality, catheterization should be a simple, quick procedure in children. After explanation to the child, insertion of a small, well-lubricated straight catheter or feeding tube (8–10 French) should not constitute a problem. Catheterization can be done with a sterile instrument (Fig. 2–3) or with the gloved hand. In girls the major difficulty often surrounds visualization of the urethral meatus. In those in whom the meatus cannot be seen, the catheter is slid under the clitoris, where it will, by virtue of its position, invariably enter the urethra. The exception will be the

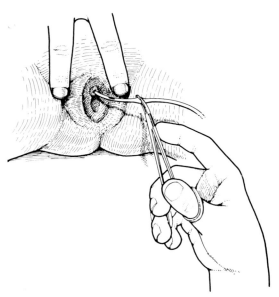

Figure 2–3. Urethral catheterization is an acceptable means of verifying urinary tract infection. (From Kelalis, P. P., King, L. R., and Belman, A. B.: Clinical Pediatric Urology, Vol. 1. Philadelphia, W. B. Saunders Co., 1976, p. 189.)

child with female hypospadias, which occurs occasionally.*

In boys the two problems most often encountered in catheterization include an inability to visualize the meatus in an uncircumcised child and hang-up of the catheter tip at the external urinary sphincter (urogenital diaphragm). The former can be overcome by simply retracting the redundant distal foreskin as far as possible (without tearing the skin) and inserting the catheter. It will generally pass directly into the urethral meatus even if that orifice itself is not visible. External sphincter spasm sometimes stops the catheter short of its goal. Since no urine returns, the inexperienced observer may interpret this as evidence of an empty bladder. Constant but gentle pressure upon the catheter will prevail, however, and as that voluntary muscle fatigues (or often when the child relaxes or stops crying to take a deep breath), the catheter slips in the remaining few centimeters and urine returns. One generally need not be concerned about urethral trauma if a soft, straight catheter or feeding tube is employed. Filling a Foley balloon inadvertently lying in the urethra, on the other hand, may cause bleeding and carries the risk of partial urethral disruption.

SUPRAPUBIC ASPIRATION

Suprapubic aspiration (SPA) as a means of collection of urine for culture has justifiably become very popular in the hands of the pediatrician. No special equipment is required that is not normally present in an office milieu. Culture accuracy is excellent, and its usefulness, particularly in the nursery, cannot be overstated. Although the theoretical likelihood of bleeding from a lacerated pelvic vein is real, and bacteremia

---

*One of us (ABB) had the occasion to be asked to pass a urethral catheter in a patient who was to have a craniotomy for a possible subdural hematoma. Attempts at localization of the urethra, which was apparently located more cranial than expected, frustrated the effort. The "patient" was a six-week-old gorilla whose mother had dropped her on her head in a fit of rage, and the "hypospadiac" position was normally located for that species.

related to bowel aspiration has been reported; there have been few significant complications (Rockoff, 1976; Mandell and Stevens, 1978; Pass and Waldo, 1979).

The bladder must be partially distended for successful aspiration; one should not attempt aspiration of a nonpalpable bladder. We have learned that prior to aspiration it is advisable to place a U-Bag over the child's cleansed genitalia, as urination upon preparation or needle insertion is not uncommon. If the child urinates prior to aspiration, the attempt should be abandoned, and the voided urine should be immediately refrigerated or plated for culture. This fresh voided specimen, if handled appropriately, represents a highly accurate collection.

The lower abdomen is dabbed with antiseptic solution (Betadine), and a small, standard needle (21–22 gauge) attached to an 8 ml syringe is used. Insertion of the needle 2 cm above the symphysis perpendicular to the horizontal axis of the supine child is recommended (Fig. 2–4). We have observed attempts at SPA with the needle angled toward the child's anus. One must be aware that the bladder in the child is an abdominal organ, and inferior angulation of the needle may result in its inadvertent insertion in the bladder neck or urethral area; no urine is then obtained. If urine is not obtained after two attempts, the effort should be abandoned. The septic child who is somewhat dehydrated and requires rapid institution of antibiotic therapy should then be catheterized for collection of a specimen for culture, and treatment should be instituted. In other situations, a repeated attempt at a later time may be justifiable; however, with equal or less effort, a clean bagged or catheterized specimen can be obtained.

Although some blood in the urine is common, postaspiration hematuria is rarely severe and should not be expected to persist for over 24 hours. Prevesical hematomas are probably more common than appreciated (Fig. 2–5), but in any case, bleeding stops spontaneously and is rarely so great as to require transfusion in the normal individual. Persistent or severe bleeding suggests a coagulopathy or anomalous pelvic vessels,

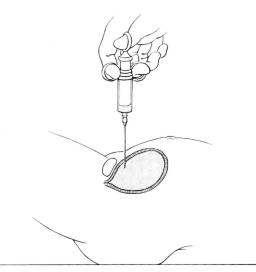

Figure 2–4. Suprapubic aspiration is a safe means of collecting bladder urine when the bladder is full. The needle is inserted 2 cm cephalad to the symphysis perpendicular to the axis of the child. (From Kelalis, P. P., King, L. R., and Belman, A. B.: Clinical Pediatric Urology, Vol. 1. Philadelphia, W. B. Saunders Co., 1976, p. 189.)

and an underlying cause should immediately be sought.

URINALYSIS

When suspicion of renal parenchymal disease exists, it is often advantageous to examine the first voided morning specimen. This particular sample is most helpful in determination of specific gravity, which represents the kidneys' concentrating ability. This function may be destroyed with significant structural pathologic conditions affecting the medulla (obstruction, inflammation, and scarring) or as a consequence of decreased glomerular filtration. Although urine osmolality more accurately measures renal concentrating ability, specific gravity correlates well with this function and can usually substitute, particularly in the office situation. As renal function falls to the level at which routine blood chemistries become abnormal (20 to 40 per cent of total renal function), concentrating ability is also affected, limiting the specific gravity to no higher than 1.010. Loss of concentrating ability is an early sign of medullary disease and may imply serious damage.

Standard dipstick urinalysis is valuable in the determination of the presence of protein, glucose, or hemoglobin-myoglobin. (These tests are relatively insensitive to the intact red blood cell.) Myoglobinuria may occur following trauma (including child abuse). The standard dipstick also incorporates a pH indicator. One might consider the diagnosis of renal tubular acidosis in the child with persistently alkaline urine. More commonly, the child with persistently alkaline urine has a urea splitting bacterial infection. This is best confirmed by urine culture.

Proteinuria is a nonspecific finding. A small amount of protein is present in all urine. Generally, this does not exceed 10 to 20 mg per ml; the amount becomes abnormal when it exceeds 150 mg per 24 hours. Before elaborate work-up and nephrologic

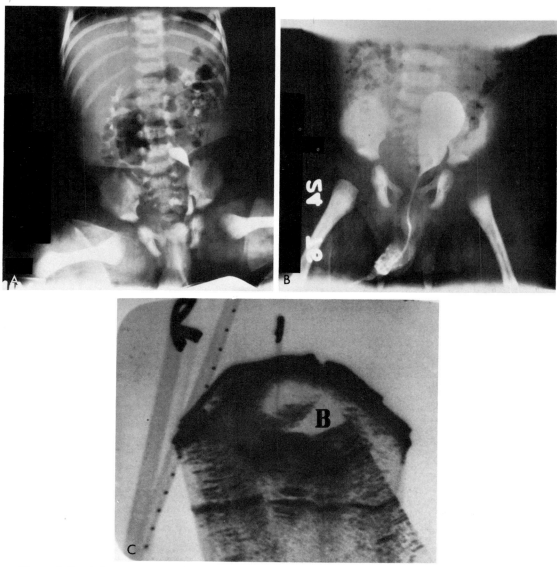

Figure 2–5. A, Intravenous pyelogram shows normal upper tracts with the bladder displaced to the left. B, Static cystogram reveals left lateral displacement of the bladder. C, Pelvic sonogram shows a cystic mass anterior to the bladder (B). (From Mandell, J., and Stevens, P. S.: Suparavesical hematoma following suprapubic urine aspiration. J. Urol., *119*:286, 1978.)

or urologic consultation is sought, it is important to separate those patients with isolated proteinuria from others with more significant pathologic conditions. Proteinuria may be increased during febrile illnesses, as a result of urine concentration due to relative dehydration. This is not in itself of any significance. Additionally, increased protein levels may be noted in association with hematuria in response to red cell breakdown. When associated with hematuria, proteinuria less than 3 to 4+ (by dipstick evaluation) is generally of no consequence. Finally, one must be aware that a segment of the population has orthostatic proteinuria. The healthy child noted to have protein in a random urine sample should have this confirmed with the first-voided specimen collected after being supine during the night. Proteinuria is not found on this first-voided specimen in those with orthostatic proteinuria. However, in the same group, protein loss may be as high as 5 to 10 gm per l (4+ on dipstick) when in the upright position. The total 24-hour urine protein output, taking the supine and upright periods into account, is rarely greater than 1.5 gm. The prognosis in this group is an optimistic one, and no further evaluation is necessary (Royer et al., 1974).

Glycosuria, although rare in children, may explain urinary frequency and enuresis. Routine urinalysis for sugar should be carried out in all children with voiding complaints, particularly if they have a family history of diabetes mellitus. This may also represent tubular dysfunction — renal glycosuria.

The sudden onset of gross hematuria in an otherwise healthy-appearing child generally results in medical consultation. Ingelfinger and colleagues (1977) reported the incidence of gross hematuria in an unselected outpatient population to be 1.3 per 1000 visits. The majority had obvious extrinsic causes (such as meatitis, trauma, or coagulopathy); however, 26 per cent had urinary infections, and 9 per cent had glomerular disease. Wyatt, on the other hand, found that in a group of 164 children referred for gross or microscopic hematuria (in other words, the obvious causes were removed),

68 per cent of cases were thought to be of glomerular origin while 15 per cent were of extraglomerular origin. The etiology was not determined in 17 per cent. In the pediatric population, the likelihood of an unrecognized preceding streptococcal infection leading to glomerulonephritis is a real one, with hematuria often persisting for several weeks or months. Additionally, it is generally not appreciated that these patients may have recurrent gross or microscopic hematuria following supervening upper respiratory infections. As noted in Chapter 1, the history plays a significant role in determining the etiology of hematuria. A scheme for the evaluation of hematuria is presented in Table 1-1.

Sickle hemoglobin is a leading cause of gross hematuria in blacks, accounting for about one third of all cases (Chapman et al., 1955). It occurs in both the trait and disease and apparently is more common in adults than children and in males more than females (Alfrey, 1976). It should be kept in mind in the differential diagnosis when dealing with a black child who presents with hematuria.

The need for cystoscopy in the child with unexplained hematuria and otherwise normal radiographic evaluation has recently come under discussion in urologic circles (Walker, 1977); (Walther and Kaplan, 1979). Because of the relative absence of epithelial tumors in children, endoscopic evaluation with its inherent trauma and anesthetic risk (minimal as it may be with competent pediatric anesthesiologists) is probably not justified in a child with microscopic hematuria alone. In those with gross hematuria, one may very rarely find a lesion that is not demonstrated by the urinary radiographs. Whether the incidence is high enough to justify endoscopy in all patients with gross hematuria is as yet unanswered. It is likely that cystoscopy is probably also not indicated in this group.

The various causes of hematuria in children are listed in Table 1-1. The extent of the evaluation that may be carried out includes consideration for angiography in patients with suspected tumors or arteriovenous malformations or percutaneous biopsy

Table 2–1. Work-Up for Hematuria

Gross Hematuria°
  Urinalysis
    RBC casts (see microscopic hematuria)
  Urine culture
    Positive
      Urography in 4 to 6 weeks with IVP† and cysto-
      gram with VCU‡ in boys
    Negative
      IVP and cystogram with VCU in boys
        Normal radiographs
          Consider cystoscopy
          See microscopic hematuria
          Consider arteriography
        Abnormal radiographs — urologic evaluation
Microscopic Hematuria°
  Urinalysis
    RBC casts, proteinuria
      Creatinine clearance
      Serum complement
      ASO titer
      L.E. preparation
      Sedimentation rate
      Serum and urine electrophoresis
      24-hour urine sample for protein
      Consider renal biopsy
  Urine Culture
    Positive
      See gross hematuria
    Negative
      IVP
      Cystogram with VCU in boys
      Urologic evaluation if radiographs abnormal

°A sickle cell index should be carried out in all black children with hematuria.
†IVP — intravenous pyelography
‡VCU — voiding cystourethrography

in those in whom an etiology cannot be determined or in whom a glomerulopathy requires assessment (Table 2–1).

Terminal hematuria or a few drops of blood noted on the underwear of preadolescent males is a common complaint which, in the absence of urinary infection or findings on physical examination (including rectal examination), does not justify evaluation beyond a voiding cystourethrogram (Kaplan and Brock, 1980). This may be carried out as part of an excretory urogram with a voiding film taken after the contrast medium has filled the bladder. To ensure adequate concentration of contrast medium, the child should fast for 12 hours before the study.

MICROSCOPY

Microscopic analysis of the urine appears to be a dying art, but it should not be.

Although it is helpful in recognizing the likelihood of urinary tract infection, confirming the presence of blood, and in differentiating upper tract (renal) from lower tract pathology, more sophisticated and definitive studies have lessened its importance. Nevertheless, the configuration of the renal tubules as outlined by precipitated Tamm-Horsfall mucoprotein and the formed elements captured in these casts may be diagnostic. If red blood cell casts are seen, one must suspect acute nephritis. White blood cell casts are suggestive of pyelonephritis. The presence of mucous casts is a nonspecific finding often seen in the dehydrated state.

Pyuria is the response to inflammation of the urinary tract. Since urination in the female often results in vaginal washout, the presence of epithelial cells and white blood cells may be misleading if the specimen is not collected properly. This applies also in the uncircumcised male who fails to or cannot retract his foreskin when collecting the specimen.

The number of white cells seen on urinalysis does not correlate well with the presence of infection. It is not adequate to rely on urinalysis as the sole means of determining the presence or absence of urinary infection. Pyuria is generally defined as more than five white blood cells per high powered field (WBC/HPF) of a centrifuged sample; however, fewer cells do not rule out associated bacteriuria. Pryles and Eliot (1965) found that 50 per cent of children with culture-confirmed bacteriuria have fewer than five WBC/HPF while 76 per cent of those with more than five WBC/HPF have positive cultures. The child who has a microscopically clear urine but is still having lower urinary tract symptoms (primarily enuresis, frequency, urgency, or urgency incontinence) deserves a urine culture.

Seeing gram-negative rods on urinalysis is highly suggestive of urinary tract infection. Nevertheless, even with adjunctive gram staining, the incidence of false negative results is 20 per cent (Kass, 1956). Without staining, infection was missed in about one third, as reported by Winter in 1975. The incidence of false positive reports by urinalysis is about 20 per cent. Confusion often results when amorphous crystals are present, which the inexperienced observer may report as bacteria.

Historically, pyuria in the absence of a positive routine urine culture implies tuberculous urinary infection. In children this is most unlikely, and other uncommon causes, such as stone disease, parasitic infestation, or, more likely, infection with an atypical organism that will not grow with standard plating techniques, should be considered (Chap. 3). Other microscopic findings, such as the presence of renal tubular epithelial cells and crystals, have little practical applicability in the pediatric evaluation.

URINE CULTURE

Developmental abnormalities of the urinary tract are generally heralded by urinary tract infection. Early detection of infection, for the present, remains the primary means of preventing morbidity. Unfortunately, according to a survey performed in 1973 by Dolan and Meyers, objective substantiation of urinary tract infection with culture is carried out by only half of those responsible for pediatric health care (pediatricians and family practitioners).

The bacteriology laboratory's calibrated loop culture techniques are being supplemented by less complicated and less expensive methods applicable to standard office use. *No matter the method of culture, the most significant determinant as to interpretability of the findings on that culture is the time between collection of the specimen and inoculation into the culture medium.* If it is anticipated that inoculation is to be delayed for more than 10 minutes, the specimen should be immediately refrigerated or placed in an ice bath. Urine transported from the patient's home to the office or from the office to the laboratory should be kept in a cold environment.

Interpretation of significance of bacterial growth based on the colony count has withstood the test of time. It is apparent that the growth of more than 100,000 colonies of a single bacterium is the rule when infection is present, and fewer colonies are most likely to represent contaminants (Kass, 1956). There are exceptions, although these are most unusual. In infants who void frequently because the bladder is uninhibited or in the very well hydrated child who voids frequently, numbers of colonies may be reduced. Repeatedly questionable colony counts (50,000–100,000) should be confirmed by suprapubic aspiration or urethral catheterization. Although the growth of any bacteria obtained by direct means (suprapubic aspiration, catheterization, or urine collected at cystoscopy) has been suggested as being absolute confirmation of infection, it is doubtful that this is a wholly justifiable conclusion. Nelson and Peters (1965) consistently noted more than 100,000 col/ml in those specimens collected by aspiration in a study comparing voided urine cultures to those obtained by suprapubic aspiration in an infected group. The authors reported that infants with urinary infection have more than 100,000 col/ml in urine collected by aspiration and that those without infection had either no growth of bacteria at all or only an occasional colony. None presented with intermediate counts (around 50,000). This, coupled with our own experience, suggests that the bladder bacteria are rapidly multiplying and are present in large numbers in infants and children as well as in adults. *Questionable culture results, regardless of the means of collection, should be an indication for a repeated culture.*

In the past few years, a number of commercial preparations have been introduced that have made office bacteriology both simple and economical. Means of both direct and indirect detection of bacteriuria exist. The popular indirect measurement employs the Griess test. Reagent paper is impregnated with sulfanilic acid and alpha-naphthylamine. Nitrite diazotizes the sulfanilic acid, which then reacts with the alpha-naphthylamine to form a red azo dye. Given adequate contact, bacteria convert nitrate, normally present in the urine, to nitrite. Thus, a positive colorometric reaction implies the presence of bacteria in the bladder. However, a relatively long incubation period (four hours) is required for conversion of nitrate to nitrite. For this reason, the first morning urine is really the only reliable specimen for this test. This study might serve as a means of home evaluation for patients being followed with chronic or recurrent cystitis (Kunin and DeGroot, 1977) but is probably not a reliable office screening test when used alone (Marr and Traisman, 1975).

The direct tests for bacteriuria involve urine culture. Two basic types are available. Microstix Reagent Strips employ both the direct and indirect approach. A strip of filter paper is impregnated with nitrite-sensitive dye with two other areas impregnated with culture media. One of these two media supports only the growth of gram-negative organisms, making it possible to delineate false positives based on gram-positive contaminants. A semiquantitative colony count is achieved by comparison at 24 to 48 hours to a set of standards. This method correlates fairly accurately in the presence of infection (80 to 90 per cent) and has a low incidence of false negatives (Winter, 1975; Craig et al., 1973; Gillenwater et al., 1976).

Numerous dip slide methods are also available that allow for subculturing if antibiotic sensitivities are indicated. A distinction can also be made between gram-negative and gram-positive organisms with the presence of a different medium on each side of the slide. The accuracy of the slide method is comparable to the dipstick method, again with few false negative results. As in all culture techniques, accuracy depends on rapidity of inoculation and experience in interpretation (Fig. 2–6).

It is apparent that office screening for urinary tract infection is now simple and available at low cost. Most of the techniques described require no special storage, and incubation of the inoculated media can be done at room temperature for some, although use of an inexpensive incubator will give earlier results. If it is highly likely that urinary tract infection is present based on the child's symptoms and results of microscopic analysis, antibacterial therapy can be instituted immediately after inoculation of the fresh urine on the culture medium. In

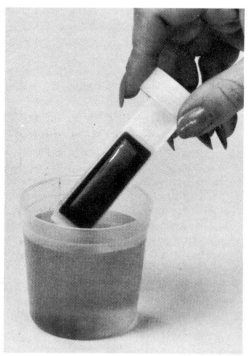
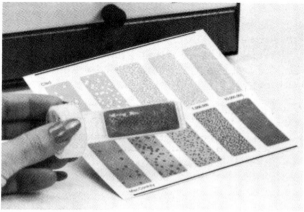

A   **B**

Figure 2–6. A, Inoculation of the dip slide in urine is demonstrated. B, Interpretation of the density of bacterial colonies on the dip slide. (From Schaeffer, A. J.: The office laboratory. Urol. Clin. North Am., 7:29, 1980.)

less obviously infected children, treatment should be withheld until the definitive diagnosis is made. If results of the culture are negative in those started on therapy, treatment should not be continued, and the culture should be repeated at the follow-up visit.

BLOOD CHEMISTRIES

AZOTEMIA

Blood chemistries are of little value in the usual urologic situation. Since renal functional impairment must be severe before the BUN or serum creatinine levels rise, the finding of azotemia in a child suggests advanced, long-standing congenital or acquired disease. In the normal course of events, then, little is to be gained by ordering serum chemistries unless a serious pathologic condition is suspected. Biochemical determinations should be saved for those children who are hypertensive, fail to grow or gain weight as expected, or are found to be chronically anemic.

Once a child becomes azotemic, renal functional status can be followed by serially measuring serum creatinine concentration. Careful monitoring of calcium and phosphorus levels along with awareness of the likelihood for metabolic acidosis, anemia, and hypertension must also be kept in mind. Dietary regulation, particularly in terms of restriction of phosphorus absorption either by reduction of intake or the use of phosphate-binding gels, is essential to prevent renal osteodystrophy (Lewy, 1976). Significant hyperkalemia in children is rarely a problem until the stage requiring chronic dialysis or renal transplantation is reached. Dietary and biochemical management in these children becomes so complex that it is our practice to leave this in the hands of the pediatric nephrologist.

HEMOGRAM

Chronic renal insufficiency should be considered in the differential diagnosis in all children noted to be anemic. The degree of anemia is proportional to the loss of renal function, with hemoglobin levels as low as 4.5 to 6.5 g per dl at serum creatinine levels of 8 to 12 mg per dl (Lewy, 1976). Anemia does not generally appear until the creatinine clearance drops below 15 to 25 ml per min per 1.73 m^2 (Royer et al., 1974).

RADIOGRAPHIC EVALUATION

The ease and availability of visualization of the urinary tract by the various radiographic techniques developed over the past several years would appear to be one of the most significant contributions to pediatric urology. Rapid and safe studies allow for ease of diagnosis and the ability to formulate a therapeutic plan within hours in all but the most perplexing situations. More recently, the introduction of various isotopic scintiscanning techniques that offer sensitive blood flow-function studies at a reduced radiation exposure as well as the noninvasive ultrasonographic means of evaluating masses have added significantly to our diagnostic capabilities.

EXCRETORY (INTRAVENOUS) UROGRAPHY

The mainstay in the uroradiographic armamentarium continues to be the excretory urogram. Tested through the years and, in children at least, virtually free of life-threatening risks and adverse reactions, its usefulness in determining the presence of urinary pathologic conditions cannot be overstated. Indications for excretory urography include culture-proven urinary infection, hematuria, the presence or suspicion of an abdominal mass, significant abdominal trauma even if unaccompanied by hematuria, unexplained abdominal pain or vomiting, hypertension, and, in some situations, enuresis. Routine urographic evaluation is also indicated when certain syndromes or developmental anomalies are recognized that are associated with a known high risk for a urinary abnormality, such as imperforate anus.

Although many radiologists do not feel that bowel preparation is necessary in children, cleansing of the bowel the evening before the examination often aids in visual clarification by decreasing overlying stool. Whether a preparation is given only by mouth or in association with an enema is inconsequential. An enema immediately prior to the study, however, is worse than no preparation at all since the air introduced into the colon makes visualization more difficult. In children less than two years old, bowel cleansing is generally not pursued, although offering a carbonated beverage immediately following the injection of medium not only helps soothe the unhappy infant but also contributes to renal visualization by virtue of the air-filled stomach pushing the intestines away (Fig. 2–7). However, as this air enters the small bowel, visualization can become impaired later in the study. Along with bowel cleansing, fluid deprivation two to four hours before the study in the otherwise normal child contributes to the quality of the examination by increasing the concentration of contrast medium in the renal collecting system as well as obviating the concerns about vomiting

and potential aspiration at the time of the study.

Concern regarding toxicity of iodinated medium is generally unfounded in children, although injection of excessive amounts can produce profound electrolyte imbalance in ill infants, particularly when the sodium salts are used. It is important not to withhold fluids in newborns, seriously ill infants, or any child unable to concentrate urine. These children should be maintained on supplemental intravenous fluids while NPO or, to avoid the risk of a high solute load entirely, should be considered for radioisotopic evaluation rather than standard radiographic studies.

The dose of contrast medium recommended varies; however, volumes up to 4 ml per kg of 50 per cent diatrizoate (Hypaque) or its equivalent have been noted to be safe (Martin et al., 1975). Many centers use a standard dose based on age groups or weight ranges (Table 2–2). This often exceeds the dosage schedule recommended on the product package insert; however, experience suggests that better visualization along with no apparent increase in adverse reactions justifies its continued use. One must keep in mind that serious electrolyte disturbances can result if an excessively high volume of medium is given (Standen et al., 1965). Radiologists familiar with the care of small or sick children should assume responsibility for these studies.

The ideal time sequence and desired views for urography should achieve a compromise between an adequate study and efforts to minimize radiation exposure. Four views — preliminary, three-minute, 10-minute, and a 20-minute postvoiding film—

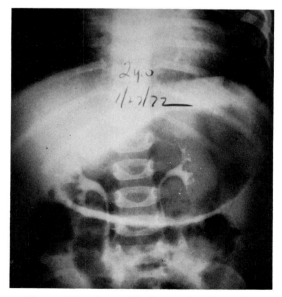

Figure 2–7. An air-filled stomach achieved with a carbonated beverage after injection of contrast medium aids in renal visualization by pushing the remainder of the intestines into the lower abdomen.

Table 2–2. Dosage of Contrast Medium for Excretory Urograms

Premature	4 ml°/kg
Newborn	3–3.5 ml°/kg
Infants and children	1–2 ml°/kg
Adolescents	0.25–0.5 ml°/kg

°300 mg iodine per ml contrast medium
(Modified from Witten, D. M., Myers, G. H., and Utz, D. C.: Emmett's Clinical Urography, Vol. 1, 4th ed. Philadelphia, W. B. Saunders Co., 1977, p. 39.)

are usually adequate. Inadequate visualization or the presence of abnormalities suggests a need for additional views, including oblique, prone, and even tomographic cuts.

Owing to reduced glomerular filtration rates, poor renal concentrating ability, and the inevitable excessive bowel gas, the usefulness of the excretory urogram is limited in the first several days of life. Martin and colleagues (1975) reviewed excretory urograms carried out in the first week of life. Twenty-eight (44 per cent) were of less than optimal quality, making interpretation difficult. We personally know of a child who had removal of a congenital hydronephrotic kidney after excretory urographic evaluation demonstrated what appeared to be a normal contralateral kidney. Unfortunately, the hydronephrotic kidney was the child's only kidney, and the contralateral "kidney" was bowel gas. Endoscopic evaluation was carried out on this child, and a "normal contralateral ureteral orifice" was thought to have been seen. If visualization of the urinary tract is indicated in the newborn, radioisotope renography offers a more reliable means. An additional advantage is the avoidance of the risk of osmotic complications, which may be associated with intravenous contrast media in that age group.

Although excretion of contrast medium indicates the presence of a functioning kidney, neither the excretory urogram nor the renogram or renal scan alone offers an accurate measure of individual renal function. Variability in the state of hydration of the patient, the amount of contrast medium injected, and overlying bowel gas and stool all influence the density of medium seen. Biochemical studies or isotope GFR determined by serum levels are the only means of reliably determining renal functional status at this time.

CYSTOGRAPHY

Perhaps the single most important radiographic diagnostic advance made in pediatric urology since the introduction of excretory urography is the cystourethrogram. The one drawback to cystography is the necessity for urethral instrumentation for adequate visualization. In some areas of the world, the contrast medium is injected percutaneously suprapubically. Although the urethra in males often can be outlined with voiding of contrast medium accumulated following an excretory urogram, dilution of the medium and poor voiding related to incomplete bladder filling often limit urethral visualization. Additionally, the inability to recognize vesicoureteral reflux limits its applicability to only the exceptional circumstance, that is, evaluation of microscopic hematuria. In almost all other indicated situations, an appropriate aphorism would be "spare the catheter, spoil the study."

It is the habit in many centers for cystography to be performed under anesthesia by the urologist at the time of cystoscopy. It is our contention that this really puts the cart before the horse. How has it been determined that cystoscopy is indicated if complete radiographic visualization of the urinary tract has not been achieved preoperatively? Cystoscopy is *not* indicated in every child who is a candidate for radiographic evaluation of the urinary tract.

Most problems related to pediatric uroradiology revolve around the personnel carrying out the studies. The radiology department that is not accustomed to carrying out complete radiographic evaluation in children should not be patronized by the pediatrician. Skill and confidence are required. The use of a small (6 to 8 F) well-lubricated feeding tube inserted gently and calmly through the urethra can be relied upon to give an excellent study without trauma or risk in virtually any patient. The reported complications of awake cystography are few (McAlister et al., 1974) and in our own personal experience relate to a single patient who had a urethral tear following inflation of a Foley catheter balloon in his urethra. The use of a straight catheter obviates that particular risk.

Radiographic visualization of the urethra for its own sake in girls is of little clinical value. There appears to be no real correlation between the configuration of the female urethra and its circumference at time of calibration (Shopfner, 1967). Little additional information is to be gained on female

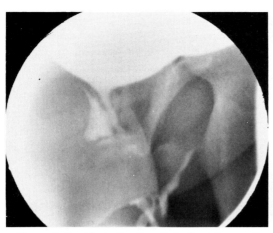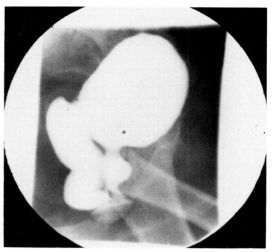

Figure 2–8. Vaginal reflux. *Left,* Partial vaginal reflux in a five-year-old girl. *Right,* Complete vaginal reflux with distention of the vagina in a four-year-old girl. (From Kelalis, P. P., King, L. R., and Belman, A. B.: Clinical Pediatric Urology, Vol. 1. Philadelphia, W. B. Saunders Co., 1976, p. 42.)

cystography beyond discovering vesicoureteral reflux and disclosing bladder outlines (Lyon, 1974). However, reflux into an ectopic ureter may be missed if a voiding film is not obtained.

One must be aware that it is common to see filling of the vagina during voiding (Fig. 2–8). This should not be viewed as a patho-

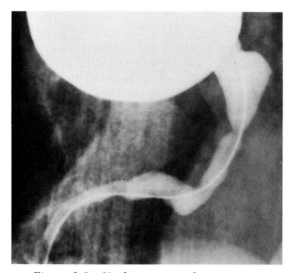

Figure 2–9. Voiding cystourethrogram in an infant with prune belly syndrome. The child is voiding around a small feeding tube, adequately filling the urethra and demonstrating absence of urethral obstruction.

logic phenomenon, although it may be helpful in understanding the underlying problem in a girl whose panties become moist immediately after standing up from the toilet (Chap. 6).

Visualization of the urethra can be achieved in almost all boys if the bladder is filled until contrast medium passes around the catheter as observed with limited fluoroscopic monitoring (Fig. 2–9). Removal of the feeding tube at this juncture will almost always assure voiding with a full stream, during which spot films may be taken. Continuous fluoroscopy during bladder filling and throughout voiding is to be condemned. Older boys will usually void on request after bladder filling is complete.

Urethrography is an essential part of the evaluation of male patients. Urethral obstruction is one of the most common findings when an identifiable cause for infection exists in boys. It is unfortunate that the age group in which urethral catheterization is most necessary (infants) is also the group in whom catheterization causes the most anxiety and is often neglected.

RETROGRADE URETHROGRAPHY

Occasionally it becomes desirable to outline the urethra by injecting contrast

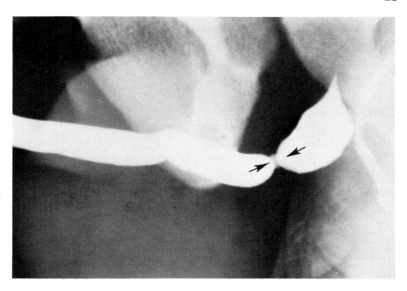

Figure 2–10. Retrograde urethrogram in an adolescent male with complaints of slow urinary stream and documented urinary tract infection. A urethral catheter could not be passed; therefore, a retrograde urethrogram was elected. Arrows demonstrate stricture just beyond the bulbous urethra. Teardrop deformity proximal to stricture (right side of picture) is the result of the normal sphincter mechanism at the urogenital diaphragm.

medium through the meatus toward the bladder neck. This procedure is useful to confirm the presence of a urethral stricture (Fig. 2–10) and may be the only means of urethral visualization if catheterization is not possible or is contraindicated, such as in the case of pelvic trauma.

RETROGRADE PYELOGRAPHY

Retrograde injection of contrast medium directly into a ureter and renal pelvis by means of cystoscopy and ureteral catheterization was one of the earliest means of radiographic visualization of the urinary tract. At present, there are few indications for its use as a primary method of outlining the collecting system. If a diagnosis cannot be made by one of the standard, less invasive studies available, the retrograde pyelogram remains a procedure of great value. Additionally, allergic reactions to iodide are virtually absent when contrast medium is injected directly into the collecting system rather than intravenously and may be the only means of complete visualization in a patient known to be allergic to iodinated compounds. Precautions should nevertheless be taken in a patient with a known iodide allergy even with retrograde pyelography.

ANTEGRADE PYELOGRAPHY AND PRESSURE FLOW STUDIES (WHITAKER TEST)

Direct puncture of the renal collecting system has become acceptable since our medical colleagues have demonstrated the benignity of renal needle biopsy. Significant hydronephrosis is a prerequisite. Indications are limited to the rare occasions when retrograde studies cannot be obtained or as a means of differentiating low pressure

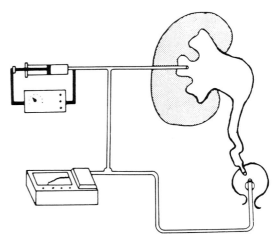

Figure 2–11. The Whitaker test—a percutaneous method of instilling fluid into the kidney at a constant flow rate with simultaneous measurement of intrapelvic pressure. (From Whitaker, R.: The Whitaker test. Urol. Clin. North Am., 6:529, 1979.)

dilatation of the urinary tract from obstruction. In conjunction with perfusion at a fixed rate, intrarenal pressure can simultaneously be measured in an effort to evaluate the flow capability of a dilated system (Fig. 2–11). This pressure-flow study is a valuable clinical tool that offers the opportunity to differentiate dilatation of the renal collecting system, which may be of no clinical consequence, from actual obstruction (Whitaker, 1973). The risk of this procedure is greater than that of retrograde studies; however, if done with caution, avoiding the area of the renal hilum and its vessels, significant complications are generally prevented. Ideally, antegrade pyelography should be done under fluoroscopic or ultrasonic control. In children, retrograde studies are best performed under anesthesia, whereas antegrade studies usually may be carried out under heavy sedation.

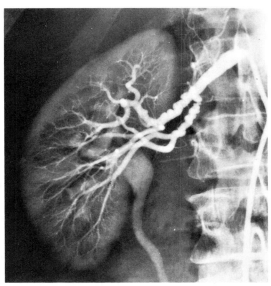

Figure 2–12. Multifocal type of fibromuscular dysplasia involving primary branches of the right renal artery and extending into the superior secondary branches. Note the characteristic "string of beads" appearance of involved portions of vessels. (From Witten, D. M., Myers, G. H., and Utz, D. C.: Emmett's Clinical Urography, Vol. 1, 4th ed. Philadelphia, W. B. Saunders Co., 1977, p. 134.)

ANGIOGRAPHY

With newer isotope scanning techniques capable of demonstrating both renal vascular flow and renal cortical function, and with the advent of computerized tomography, angiography has less application than it did several years ago. Nevertheless, situations arise in which angiography becomes essential — renal trauma and the evaluation of renal vascular hypertension are examples (Fig. 2–12). Technical skills have advanced to the state that age is not a limiting factor in these studies. Umbilical artery catheterization has been successfully employed up to 10 days of age (Emmanouilides and Rein, 1964). Femoral percutaneous access is available for angiography in older children and may, of course, be used in newborns, although an arterial cutdown may be necessary. Renal arterial thrombosis has been recently recognized as a complication of indwelling umbilical artery catheters (Merten et al., 1978).

VENOGRAPHY

Inferior vena cavography occasionally plays a role in the evaluation of the patient with a flank mass. Determination of the extent of venous spread in the presence of a Wilms' tumor and definitive diagnosis of renal vein thrombosis has proved this study invaluable. Rapid injection of the calculated dose of contrast medium over a three-second period through the femoral vein while taking both anteroposterior and lateral views will demonstrate the entire length of the inferior vena cava. The study may also be performed in small children by injecting the total calculated dose of contrast medium into a lower extremity percutaneously with the tourniquet in place. Sudden release of the tourniquet should visualize the entire vena cava. The best studies are performed by inserting a femoral or saphenous vein catheter as is done in arteriography and cardiac catheterization.

RADIONUCLIDE STUDIES

Modern diagnostic techniques available at most institutions include the capabilities for radiopharmaceutical evaluation of the urinary tract. Favorable decay characteristics (short half-life) and lower irradiation exposure to tissues makes this mode of evaluation particularly appealing in pediatrics. The ability to use minute quantities of the physiologically active molecule not only obviates the problem of allergy but, because these are injected in a bolus, also allows evaluation of the vascular as well as secretory phases of renal function.

THE RENOGRAM

The earliest tool to gain clinical acceptance that applied isotope excretion to the evaluation of renal function was the renogram (Winter, 1956). The radioactivity of I^{131}-iodohippurate sodium (Hippuran), secreted rapidly by the tubules, was picked up by radiosensitive probes placed over the renal areas. Often the inaccuracy of approximation of renal position by probe placement interfered with the quality of the study as it was done then. Modern scintiscan techniques are now being applied to renography, eliminating most of these technical problems.

Radioactive emissions picked up over the kidneys are transferred to a graph, and, in the normal situation, a typical curve results that can be broken down into three phases. The first of these, the vascular phase, is impaired in arterial vascular disease, a problem rarely seen in children. Prolongation of this segment is indicative but not diagnostic of pathologic renal arterial function. The renogram remains a useful screening test for major obstructive arterial disease. The second, or secretory, phase is representative of active renal function. Prolongation of this phase suggests impairment of tubular handling of the iodohippurate, which may be found in acute or chronic parenchymal disease. In renal transplantation, for example, prolongation of the second stage of the renogram when compared to an earlier study may be one of the first signs of kidney rejection (zumWinkel, et al., 1975). The third, or excretory, phase is of great urologic significance (Fig. 2–13). Since the renogram offers a continuous recording, it provides an objective estimate of excretion of the isotope by the collecting system (phase 3) vs. secretion of the isotope by the tubules (phase 2). Once a baseline rate is established, repeat studies may be used to evaluate whether obstruction is progressive.

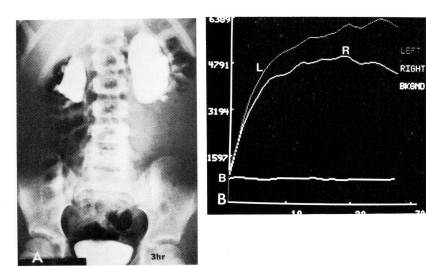

Figure 2–13. *A,* Excretory urogram three hours after injection shows bilateral delayed excretion and bilateral pyelectasis. *B,* Renographic curves show equal uptake of ^{131}I-orthoiodohippurate and bilateral delay in time of maximum activity and excretion in the kidneys. (From Bueschen, A. J., and Witten, D. M.: Radionuclide evaluation of renal function. Urol. Clin. North Am., 6:307, 1979.)

THE RENAL SCAN

Improved gamma scintillation detectors have added a new dimension to isotope imaging. Although visual detail is not comparable to standard radiographic techniques, its reduced radiation exposure makes it a viable alternative (Fig. 2–14). The large bolus effect of standard excretory urography requires excretion by glomerular filtration, whereas the radioisotope (usually ^{99m}Tc DTPA) is handled by tubular secretion, making it a more sensitive indicator of renal function. Overlying bowel gas and stool do not interfere with the image produced; therefore, bowel preparation is not required. In newborns particularly, in whom the combination of immature renal concentrating ability and excessive bowel gas often make excretory urography un-

satisfactory (Fig. 2–15), the renal scan has great appeal. Poorly functioning or abnormally positioned kidneys are also frequently more readily located by scan than by contrast media studies (Fig. 2–16).

Although the renal scan is not one of the better studies for evaluation of renal masses, it may be helpful in differentiating functioning from nonfunctioning renal tissue. This is relevant in the so-called renal pseudotumors (hypertrophied columns of Bertin). Renal cortical scanning agents, such as ^{99m}Tc DMSA, are taken up by the tubules with little excretion (Handmaker and Lowenstein, 1975). This advantage, that is, slow excretion, also becomes a disadvantage since tissue radiation exposure is higher than with more rapidly cleared substances. Improved visual resolution of the more commonly used ^{99m}Tc DTPA scan

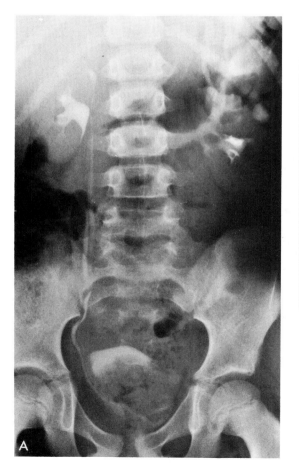

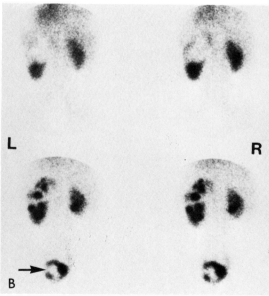

Figure 2–14. A, Excretory urogram demonstrating duplication of the right collecting system and poor visualization of the left midrenal and upper renal segments. B, Renal scan (posterior view) reveals excellent perfusion and concentration of marker in the left lower pole with a hydronephrotic picture in the early phase (top). Delayed scan demonstrates caliectasis and a filling defect in the bladder (arrow). Diagnosis: Duplication of left collecting system with obstruction of upper segment secondary to a ureterocele (filling defect in bladder).

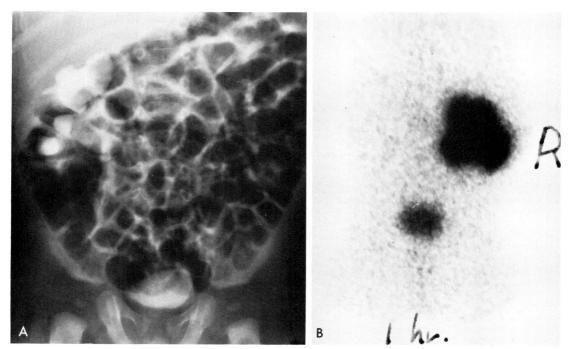

Figure 2–15.   A, Excretory urogram in newborn with right flank mass. Hydronephrotic system is visible on the right. Excessive bowel gas obscured adequate interpretation on the left. B, Delayed renal scan in the same patient (posterior view). Hydronephrosis secondary to ureteropelvic junction obstruction is evident. No isotope is present on the left to indicate renal presence or function on that side. Imagine the consequences if one had thought that a collecting system was present on the left and removal of the right hydronephrotic kidney had been elected.

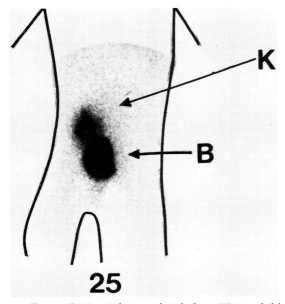

Figure 2–16.   Solitary pelvic kidney (K) in a child evaluated for urinary tract infection. Note close relationship to bladder (B) and absence of isotope in flank areas.

offers a temporary compromise in this area until more satisfactory radiopharmaceuticals are developed (Conway, 1976).

The Lasix-Stimulated Renal Scan

Very recently, the renal scan, when supplemented with Lasix, has been used as a means of differentiating nonobstructed upper tract dilatation from true obstruction (O'Reilly et al., 1978). The goal is the same as that of the pressure-flow study of Whitaker (p. 25). Although the method has not as yet been standardized, an acute diuresis stimulated by the intravenous injection of Lasix has the capability of washing isotope that has accumulated in the dilated collecting system completely out of the collecting system. One can judge the effectiveness of drainage on the basis of time (Fig. 2–17) or a plotted curve (Fig. 2–18). This relatively noninvasive study may well replace the percutaneous pressure-flow study previously described.

Radioisotopes for Renal Functional Evaluation

Even as this is being written, spectacular advances are being made that allow evaluation of individual renal function and even segmental renal function. Computer assisted appreciation of the emissions over isolated renal areas combined with simultaneous analysis of plasma disappearance offers an opportunity to determine the degree of renal function. Objective rather than subjective determinations may then be

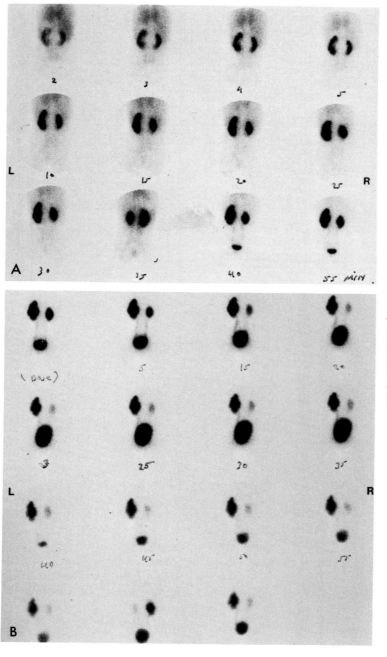

Figure 2–17. A, Isotope renal scan with delayed images demonstrating delayed drainage bilaterally. B, Continuation of scan shown in A with addition of Lasix. The right side drains rapidly by 20 minutes; however, the left side fails to drain by 55 minutes. A definite obstructive pattern secondary to ureteropelvic junction obstruction is present. (Courtesy of Dr. Massound Majd.)

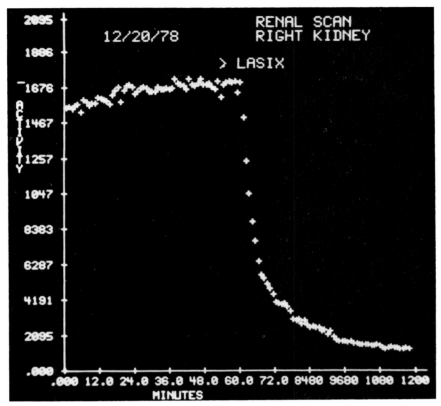

Figure 2–18. Isotope renal scan with Lasix in a child with a dilated right renal collecting system. An obstructive pattern is evident for one hour until Lasix is injected. Rapid washout ensues with prompt excretion of contrast medium. (Courtesy of Dr. Massoud Majd.)

made to aid in determining the best solution to specific problems (Kawamura et al., 1978; Piepsz et al., 1977).

Radionuclide Cystography

The nuclear cystogram is a relatively recent addition to the isotope armamentarium that has proved its worth in the detection of vesicoureteral reflux, making it singularly applicable to pediatric urology (Conway et al., 1972). Urethral catheterization is still required, after which the bladder is filled with sterile saline or water to which an isotope marker is added. Continuous oscilloscopic monitoring is begun. Since the amount in the bladder is known at any particular time (as determined by filling), the volume at which reflux occurs can be appreciated (Fig. 2–19). The continuous monitoring, which is available at no addi-

tional radiation exposure to the child, allows recognition and recording of even transient reflux. This is in sharp contrast to the radiation exposure if the same end is achieved fluoroscopically.

We have found the most practical use of isotope cystography to be the follow-up and monitoring of the patient with vesicoureteral reflux who does not appear to require immediate surgical correction. The total radiation dosage for the complete isotope cystogram has been estimated to be from 1/10th to 1/100th of that for standard radiographic cystography (Conway et al., 1974). Taking into view the possibility of repeated radiographic procedures over several years, the radiation exposure saved may be quite significant to the patient.

The only practical limitation of this study versus routine radiographic cystography is its failure to visualize the urinary

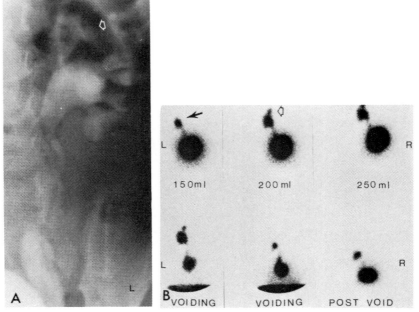

Figure 2–19. *A,* A standard radiographic cystogram demonstrates reflux into this completely duplicated left collecting system. *B,* Reflux into the lower segment of the duplicated system at 150 ml (solid arrow) and then into the upper segment at 250 ml (open arrow). Drainage is also noted to be more rapid from the upper system. (From Majd, M., and Belman, A. B.: Nuclear cystography in infants and children. Urol. Clin. North Am., 6:395, 1979.)

tract in detail and thus accurately grade the severity of the reflux. Although probably of no clinical significance, minor wisps of reflux into the distal ureter (grade 1) may be missed. Finally, isotope cystography has no capability for visualizing the urethra.

SCROTAL SCANNING

Intravenous injection of ^{99m}Tc pertechnetate, concentrating first on the internal iliac blood flow followed by pinhole collimation, isolating the area of interest to the scrotum, allows for evaluation of blood flow and perfusion of the testes. Increased perfusion is indicative of an inflammatory process (Fig. 2–20), while a "cold" area strongly suggests torsion, hematoma, or abscess (Fig. 2–21) (Holder et al., 1977). Scrotal scanning does not have the capability of locating an otherwise normal undescended testis.

ULTRASONOGRAPHY

One of the newest diagnostic modalities is the ultrasonic B-mode scan. Its non-

invasiveness along with its independence of function make it unique in the evaluation of the urinary tract. High frequency sound waves applied to the abdomen by means of a probe reflect off tissue surfaces. The return waves are then received by a transduc-

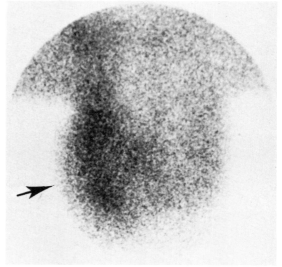

Figure 2–20. Testicular scan demonstrating increased perfusion (arrow) indicative of epididymitis. (Courtesy of Dr. Massoud Majd.)

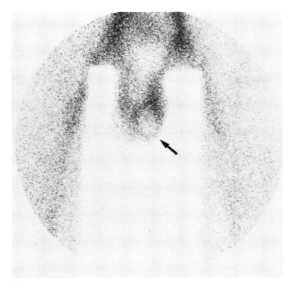

Figure 2–21. Testicular scan with cold region (arrow) indicative of testicular torsion. (Courtesy of Dr. Massoud Majd.)

er and are converted to images on an oscilloscope, which can be recorded on film and preserved for later evaluation. Experience has demonstrated characteristic patterns for normal tissue planes. In this manner, the cystic dysplastic (multicystic) kidney in a newborn (Fig. 2–22A) can be tentatively differentiated from a congenital ureteropelvic junction obstruction (Fig. 2–22B) or solid tumor (Fig. 2–22C) by noninvasive means. Additional uses for renal ultrasonography include the ability to monitor renal size, noninvasive screening for familial polycystic disease, and needle direction for either renal biopsy, cyst puncture, or antegrade pyelography (Shkolnik, 1977).

One of the major attractions of this modality in addition to its noninvasiveness is also the apparent absence of complications. Once convinced of its painlessness, small children will be totally cooperative during ultrasonography, particularly if they are allowed to observe the various oscilloscopic patterns. Technical advances suggest that we can anticipate the addition of computerized imagery gained from ultrasonic waves. It is hoped that this marriage of technical skills will provide the imagery currently offered by computerized axial tomography with no radiation exposure to the patient.

COMPUTERIZED AXIAL TOMOGRAPHY

The applicability of this newest diagnostic modality to pediatric urology has not yet been clearly demonstrated, although its effectiveness in visualizing abdominal masses is apparent (Leonidas et al., 1978). Technical problems relating to movement of both patient and bowel gas as well as absence of significant retroperitoneal fat in children to assist in the demarcation of the various structures has limited its usefulness. Additionally, the infrequency of diagnostic genitourinary dilemmas that cannot be resolved by the other various studies available has limited any extensive investigation of its use. There is no question, however, of its ability to beautifully demonstrate anatomy (Fig. 2–23).

ENDOSCOPY

Cystourethroscopy remains the ultimate diagnostic tool for the urologist. Recent advances in urologic instrumentation make it possible to perform endoscopy on even the youngest and smallest of children. By endoscopic means, completion of evaluation prior to definitive correction or as part of planning the therapeutic regimen continues as an important component of the urologic armamentarium. Retrograde pyelography (p. 25) by means of *ureteral* catheterization is still an indicated and informative study in selected situations.

INDICATIONS

With maturation of the field of pediatric urology, indications for cystoscopy in children have changed over recent years (Walther and Kaplan, 1979). Whereas not too long ago, all children with urinary infections had routine cystoscopy as part of their evaluation, there now is greater preoperative selectivity. Little justification exists for routine cystoscopy in all girls with documented urinary tract infection if the radiographic studies are completely normal.

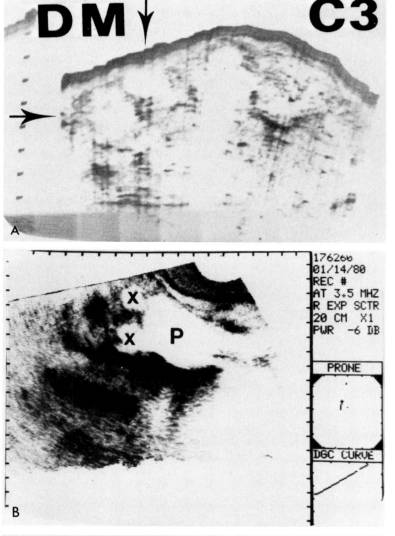

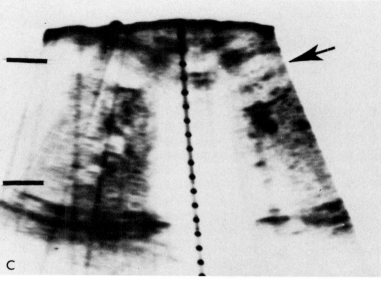

Figure 2–22. A, Transverse renal ultrasound study demonstrating multiple echo-free areas (arrows). This picture is typical of a multicystic kidney (cystic dysplasia). *B,* Longitudinal renal ultrasound study revealing a large dilated renal pelvis (P) and dilated calices (X). This could be confused with cystic dysplasia; however, function is evident on the renal scan, and this was hydronephrosis secondary to ureteropelvic junction obstruction. *C,* Transverse renal ultrasound study demonstrates normal right kidney (arrow) and a large mass on the left that has multiple internal echoes (between markers). This child had a large Wilms' tumor. (Courtesy of Dr. Barry Potter.)

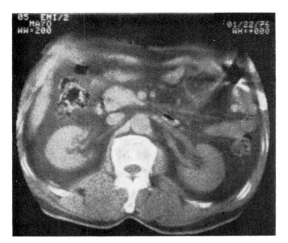

Figure 2–23. CT scan through midsection of both kidneys. Aorta, inferior vena cava, and segments of renovascular pedicle are well visualized. Length and position of the left renal vein can be seen as the vein exits from the renal hilum and courses anterior to the aorta toward the inferior vena cava. (From Witten, D. M., Myers, G. H., and Utz, D. C.: Emmett's Clinical Urography, Vol. 1, 4th ed. Philadelphia, W. B. Saunders Co., 1977, p. 351.)

Rarely, in the patient with persistent infection or an unusual clinical situation, one may justify visual evaluation of the lower genitourinary tract. If cystoscopy is performed, vaginoscopy becomes a part of that evaluation.

We still recommend cystoscopy in boys who have recurrent urinary infection even though the radiographs may appear normal. The rationale lies in the relative rarity of unexplained recurrent infections in boys and the likelihood of finding an underlying cause. However, when excellent radiographic studies fail to demonstrate a pathologic condition in the boy with a single infection, there appears to be little additional to learn at cystoscopy. Failure to respond to standard antibacterial therapy is another indication for further evaluation in either sex.

When infection remains unexplained and there is reason on a clinical or radiographic basis to suspect a renal origin, collection of urine from each kidney is a means of localization. Ureteral catheterization with culture of urine collected from the individual kidney pelvis requires cystoscopy and

anesthesia and is reserved for those patients with unusual clinical situations.

Indications for cystoscopy when urinary radiographs are otherwise normal include the evaluation of otherwise unexplained gross hematuria (p. 17) and selected instances of urinary incontinence. Both visual inspection of the ureteral orifices in children demonstrating vesicoureteral reflux and cystoscopy prior to forming a therapeutic plan when an abnormality is demonstrated on excretory urography may be desirable. Often endoscopy may be carried out under the same anesthetic preceding a definitive surgical procedure.

PROCEDURE

Endoscopy in the anesthetized child is usually quite simple and in most centers is carried out on an outpatient basis or in a short stay unit in which an overnight admission is unnecessary. Visualization of the entire urethra as well as the bladder in males is ideal. Trigonal development, ureteral orifice configuration, and, in girls, vaginoscopy, complete the study. Endoscopy also has the capability for bladder biopsy and removal of urethral or intravesical foreign bodies, when the circumstance arises.

REFERENCES

Alfrey, A. C.: The renal response to vascular injury. *In* Brenner, B. M., and Rector, F. C., Jr. (Eds.): The Kidney. Philadelphia, W. B. Saunders Co., 1976.

Chapman, Z. A., Reeder, P. S., Friedman, I. A., and Baker, L. A.: Gross hematuria in sickle cell trait and sickle cell hemoglobin C disease. Am. J. Med., 19:773, 1955.

Conway, J. J., Belman, A. B., and King, L. R.: Direct and indirect radionuclide cystography. *In* Freeman, L. M., and Beaufox, M. D. (Eds.): Radionuclide Studies of the Genitourinary System. New York, Grune and Stratton, 1974.

Conway, J. J., King, L. R., Belman, A. B., et al.: Detection of vesicoureteral reflux with radionuclide cystography: A comparison study with roentgenographic cystography. Am. J. Roentgen Radium Ther. Nucl. Med., 115:720, 1972.

Conway, J. J.: Radionuclides. *In* Kelalis, P. P., King, L. R., and Belman, A. B. (Eds.): Clinical Pediatric Urology. Philadelphia, W. B. Saunders Co., 1976.

Craig, W. A., Kunin, C. M., and DeGroot, J.: Evaluation

of new urinary tract infection screening devices. Appl. Microbiol., *26*:196, 1973.

Dolan, T. F., and Meyers, A.: A survey of office management of urinary tract infection in childhood. Pediatrics, *52*:21, 1973.

Emmanouilides, G. C., and Rein, B. I.: Abdominal aortography via the umbilical artery in a newborn infant. Radiology, *82*:447, 1964.

Gillenwater, J. Y., Gleason, C. H., Lohr, J. A., and Marion, D.: Home urine cultures by the dipstrip method: Results in 289 cultures. Pediatrics. *58*:508, 1976.

Handmaker, H., and Lowenstein, J. M.: Nuclear Medicine in Clinical Pediatrics. Chicago, Year Book Med. Publ, 1975.

Holder, L. E., Martire, J. R., Holmes, E. R., and Wagner, H. N., Jr.: Testicular radionuclide angiography and static imaging: Anatomy, scintigraphic interpretation, and clinical indications. Radiology, *125*:739, 1977.

Ingelfinger, J. R., Davis, A. E., and Grupe, W. E.: Frequency and etiology of gross hematuria in a general pediatric setting. Pediatrics; *59*:557, 1977.

Kaplan, G. W., and Brock, W. A.: Deep urethral inflammatory disease. Presented before the Section of Urology, 50th annual meeting of the American Academy of Pediatrics, Detroit, Oct. 25, 1980.

Kass, E. H.: Asymptomatic infections of the urinary tract. Trans. Assoc. Am. Phys., *69*:56, 1956.

Kawamura, J., Hosokawa, S., Yoshida, O., et al.: Validity of ^{99m}Tc dimercaptosuccinic acid renal uptake for assessment of individual kidney function. J. Urol., *119*:305, 1978.

Kunin, C. M., and DeGroot, J. E.: Sensitivity of a nitrite indicator strip method in detecting bacteriuria in preschool girls. Pediatrics, *60*:244, 1977.

Leonidas, J. C., Carter, B. L., Leepe, L. L., et al.: Computerized tomography in diagnosis of abdominal masses in infancy and childhood. Comparison with excretory urography. Arch. Dis. Child., *53*:120, 1978.

Lewy, P. R.: Renal failure and related disorders. *In* Kelalis, P. P., King, L. R., and Belman, A. B. (Eds.): Clinical Pediatric Urology. Philadelphia, W. B. Saunders Co., 1976.

Lyon, R. P.: Distal urethral stenosis. Reviews in Paediatric Urology. Johnston, J. H., and Goodwin, W. E. (Eds.): Excerpta Medica, Amsterdam, 1974.

Mandell, J., and Stevens, P. S.: Supravesical hematoma following suprapubic urine aspiration. J. Urol., *119*:286, 1978.

Marr, T. J., and Traisman, H. S.: Detection of bacteriuria in pediatric outpatients. Am. J. Dis. Child., *129*:940, 1975.

Martin, D. J., Gilday, D. C., and Reilly, B. J.: Evaluation of the urinary tract in the neonatal period. Radiol. Clin. North Am., *13*:359, 1975.

McAlister, W. H., Cacciarelli, A., and Shackelford, G. D.: Complications associated with cystography in children. Radiology, *111*:167, 1974.

Merten, D. F., Vogel, J. M., Adelman, R. D., et al.: Renal vascular hypertension as a complication of umbilical artery catheterization. Radiology, *126*:751, 1978.

Nelson, J. D., and Peters, P. C.: Suprapubic aspiration of urine in premature and term infants. Pediatrics, *36*:132, 1965.

O'Reilly, P. H., Testa, H. J., Lawson, R. S., et al.: Diuresis renography in equivocal urinary tract obstruction. Br. J. Urol., *50*:76, 1978.

Pass, R. F., and Waldo, F. B.: Anaerobic bacteriuria following suprapubic bladder aspiration. J. Pediatr., *94*:748, 1979.

Piepsz, A., Dobbeleir, A., and Erbsmann, F.: Measurement of separate kidney clearance by means of ^{99m}Tc-DTPA complex and a scintillation camera. Eur. J. Nucl. Med., *2*:173, 1977.

Pryles, C. V., and Eliot, C. R.: Pyuria and bacteriuria in infants and children. Am. J. Dis. Child., *110*:628, 1965.

Randolph, M. F., and Majors, F.: Office screening for bacteria in early infancy: Collection of a suitable urine specimen. J. Pediatr., *76*:934, 1970.

Rockoff, A. S.: Hemorrhage after suprapubic bladder aspiration. J. Pediatr., *89*:327, 1976.

Royer, P., Habib, R., Mathieu, H., and Broyer, M.: Pediatric Nephrology. Philadelphia, W. B. Saunders, Co., 1974.

Shkolnik, A.: Gray scale ultrasound of the pediatric abdomen and pelvis. *In* Current Problems in Diagnostic Radiology. Chicago; Year Book Medical Pub., 1977.

Shopfner, C. E.: Roentgen evaluation of distal urethral obstruction. Radiology, *88*(2):222, 1967.

Standen, J. R., Nogrady, M. B., Dunbar, J. S., et al.: Osmotic effects of methylglucamine diatrizoate (Renographin 60) in intravenous urography in infants. Am. J. Roentgen., *93*:473, 1965.

Walker, D.: Indications for cystoscopy in children with hematuria. Presented before the Section of Urology, 46th annual meeting of the American Academy of Pediatrics; New York, Nov. 6, 1977.

Walther, P. C., and Kaplan, G. W.: Cystoscopy in children: Indications for its use in common urologic problems. J. Urol. *122*:717, 1979.

Whitaker, R. H.: Methods of assessing obstruction in dilated ureters. Br. J. Urol., *45*:15, 1973.

Winter, C. C.: A clinical study of a new renal function test: The radioactive diodrast renogram. J. Urol., *76*:182, 1956.

Winter, C. C.: Rapid miniaturized tests for bacteriuria: Microstix and Bacturcult urine tests. J. Urol., *114*:755, 1975.

zumWinkel, K., Harbst, H., Das, K. B., and Newiger, T.: Applications of radionuclides in renal transplantation. *In* Freeman, L. M., and Blaufox, M. D. (Eds.): Radionuclide Studies of the Genitourinary System. New York, Grune and Stratton, 1974.

Chapter Three

URINARY TRACT INFECTION

General Aspects of Urinary Tract Infection

"The bladder urine is normally sterile, and the presence of any bacteria in the bladder urine is an abnormal circumstance." (Stamey, 1972.) With this admonition it then becomes the obligation of the primary care physician to recognize this abnormal state, document its presence, treat it appropriately, and determine, if possible, its underlying cause. The necessary steps to fulfill this responsibility have been delineated and are relatively simple.

INCIDENCE

SCHOOL-AGE GIRLS

There are many reported studies from various geographic areas that document the incidence of bacteriuria in school-age girls to be 3 to 5 per cent (Allen, 1965; Winberg et al., 1974). The prevalence of bacteriuria was demonstrated by Kunin and colleagues (1964) in their classic epidemiologic survey to be 0.7 per cent in five- to nine-year-old girls and 0.5 per cent in those 10 to 14 years of age. This trend toward decreasing incidence of bacteriuria with advancing age is

an important one to appreciate and one that has been substantiated by others (Meadow et al., 1969; DeLuca et al., 1963). Additional data on the same population collected by Kunin (1970) reveal that the incidence of recurrent bacteriuria for white girls is about 80 per cent, whereas in black girls it is only 60 per cent. In other words, the drop-off rate following treatment of any single episode of bacteriuria is 20 per cent in white girls and 40 per cent in black girls. Fair and coworkers (1972) also found that 80 per cent of their patients had recurrences following short-term treatment of a documented urinary tract infection. In our own experience, children with chronic urinary tract infection with evidence of bladder changes of cystitis cystica (p. 49) also had an 80 per cent recurrence rate after 12 months of continuous long-term prophylaxis (Belman, 1978).

BOYS

The incidence of asymptomatic bacteriuria in boys, other than neonates, is extremely low. In the survey by Kunin and his associates, only two of 7731 boys studied were found to have asymptomatic bacteriu-

Table 3–1.   Sex Ratio of Urinary
Tract Infections

	FEMALES	MALES
Neonate	0.4	1
1–6 mos.	1.5	1
6–12 mos.	4.0	1
1–3 yrs.	10.0	1
3–11 yrs.	9.0	1
11–16 yrs.	2.0	1

(Modified from Winberg, J., Andersen, H. J., Bergstrom, L., et al.: Epidemiology of symptomatic urinary tract infection in childhood. Acta Pediatr. Scand. (Suppl.), 252:1, 1974.)

ria. The female:male sex ratio of children with urinary tract infection at varying ages has been noted by Winberg and colleagues (1974) (Table 3–1).

NEONATES

As previously stated, the sex ratio of bacteriuria in neonates is reversed. The overall incidence of neonatal urinary tract infection has been recorded as 1.4 to 5 per 1000 live births with the male:female ratio 2.8 to 5.4:1 (Bergstrom et al., 1972; Drew and Acton, 1976). The explanation for this observation of a reversed sex ratio remains unclear, although it has been reliably documented and is even more apparent in low birth weight and premature neonates (Thrupp et al., 1973; Edelmann et al., 1973).

Newborn males have a higher incidence of sepsis than newborn females (Buetow et al., 1965) in approximately the same ratio as that for bacteriuria. The source of the bacteria in urinary tract infections in this age group is thought to be primarily hematogenous and not ascending (Stamey, 1972). Although the mature kidney prevents the filtration of bacteria from blood into urine (Stamey, 1972), it would appear that in neonates, particularly in premature infants, circulating bacteria may indeed enter the urine by filtration. If this is true, it would explain both the high incidence of bacteriuria in neonates in the absence of

obstructive urinary tract disease and the increased incidence of bacteriuria in males who as a group are more susceptible to septicemia.

ETIOLOGY

ROUTE OF ENTRY

The route of bacterial entry into the urinary tract in all age groups other than the neonate is thought to be largely retrograde (urethral) in origin, and the usual pathogens are fecal flora that contaminate the perineum. Stamey (1972) demonstrated that the organisms that cause bladder infections in women can be found on perineal culture prior to bladder invasion. In contrast to adult females in whom bacteria are virtually always found on the perineum, Stamey noted that two thirds of randomly selected girls did not have a solitary gram-negative bacterium on the introitus on routine culture. Leadbetter and Salvin (1974) reported that girls with recurrent infections also tend to have colonization of the introitus with the offending organism prior to infection just as women do. The ensuing conclusion is that the majority of normal women (and girls) have a degree of introital resistance (perineal defense mechanism) to pathogenic organisms. The mechanism of this resistance has not been elucidated. The susceptible group of females tend to allow perineal colonization with pathogenic organisms presumably secondary to the loss of this defense mechanism.

Cox and colleagues (1968) documented that colonization of the female urethra is proportional to the distance from the meatus at which cultures are taken. Bacteria are present in virtually all women at the level of the meatus and in only three fourths at a depth of 4 cm. This tends to support the urethral origin theory of route of infection. Stamey's findings that there is a high incidence of colonization by pathogenic organisms in those who are susceptible was also supported by this study.

DEFENSE MECHANISMS

Efforts have also been made to understand the mechanisms of immunologic response at the bladder level. Uehling and King (1973) recorded increased urinary IgA levels in children with chronic cystitis but were unable to appreciate any degree of resistance in this group. Indeed, it would appear that they fit into a relatively recalcitrant group despite (or because of) the apparently activated immune system. Clark and associates (1971) did not note a circulating (systemic) antibody response to cystitis. Dubroff and associates (1975), however, found a positive delayed phytohemagglutinin hypersensitivity response to cystitis equal to that of other acute infections. All this would appear to attest to the normalcy of the local and systemic immune mechanisms of children who develop urinary tract infections. It is of further interest that patients with generalized immune deficiencies are no more prone to urinary tract infection than are those without such deficiencies.

Efforts have been made to correlate immune mechanism abnormalities with upper urinary tract infection (pyelonephritis). However, there is no evidence demonstrating an abnormal response or immune deficit in this group, except for infants under two months of age (Winberg et al., 1963).

There is evidence, however, that some bacterial strains have greater nephrogenic toxicity than others. Capsular polysaccharide antigens K1, K2, K12, and K13 of *Escherichia coli* are found more commonly in upper than lower urinary tract infections (Kaijser, 1973).

Local bladder mechanisms, including frequency of urination (Cox and Hinman, 1961), have always been thought important in the prevention of urinary tract infections. Infrequent voiding allows bacteria, which enter via the urethra, more time to replicate, thus lessening the likelihood of expelling all bacteria at micturition. Apparently, surface mucopolysaccharides play a role in this intrinsic bladder defense mechanism by inhibiting the binding of bacteria to the bladder wall (Parsons et al., 1977). Interference with or inadequacy of this mechanism may be a contributing factor in the establishment and maintenance of infection in some patients.

IRRITATION

No discussion of the etiology of urinary tract infections would be complete without mentioning the possible contribution of mechanical factors. Local irritation, such as that caused by detergents (including bubble bath), types of underclothing worn, bathing, swimming, toilet hygiene, constipation, and pinworm infestation have all been implicated as significant underlying causes. Unfortunately, no data to our knowledge exist that truly substantiate a relationship between any of these agents and documented infection. This is not to say that any or all of these factors may not be responsible for lower urinary tract discomfort. In our experience, dysuria, urgency, and frequency may all result from these factors. It is important to differentiate this from bona fide infection. However, it is possible but unproved that the voiding dysfunction that may be the result of any of these could, by virtue of tissue inflammation (i.e., reduced intrinsic defense mechanisms) with or without residual urine, set the stage for true urinary tract infection to supervene.

URINARY STASIS

It has always been taught that urinary stasis increases susceptibility to urinary tract infection. It is our impression that infrequent voiding appears to play such a role by allowing bacteria that enter by the urethral pathway time to replicate in the bladder in those who void infrequently. Lapides and Diokno (1970) postulate that elevation of intravesical pressure hydrodynamically interferes with blood flow to the bladder wall when the bladder is overdistended. The bladder tissue, deprived of its normal perfusion, then loses some of its defenses against bacterial infection.

The exact mechanism behind infection in girls who void infrequently is not clinically relevant. What is relevant is remembering to inquire as to the frequency of urination in girls with recurrent infection. Simple alteration of voiding frequency or fluid intake might beneficially affect recurrent urinary tract infections. An example is an eight-year-old girl referred with a history of uncontrollable urinary tract infections. She had been evaluated urologically on more than one occasion with demonstration of a radiographically normal urinary tract. Cystoscopy and multiple urethral dilatations had been performed; however, even with long-term suppressive medication,

breakthrough infections occurred. The child, when finally appropriately questioned, admitted to urinating only two or three times daily. Urodynamic evaluation (Fig. 3–1) revealed a functional capacity of 200 ml with predictable voiding to completion at that volume on repeated studies. Further questioning revealed that this child's fluid intake was minimal and that she voided infrequently as a function of slow bladder filling. Increased oral fluid intake coupled with a low-dose suppressive antibacterial regimen resolved the problem of recurrent infection.

Most children who void infrequently attain higher than normal bladder capacities and usually have large bladders on radiographic evaluation. Whether this is habitual "holding back" in response to dysuria (from

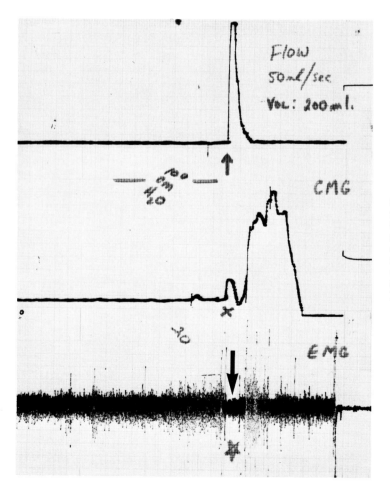

Figure 3–1. Urodynamic evaluation in an eight-year-old girl with infrequent voiding and recurrent, intractable urinary tract infections. The child was noted to void to completion repetitively at 200 ml with a normal flow rate (50 ml per sec) (upper recording) along with relaxation of her ing) as determined by sphincter EMG (arrow).

either previous infections or mechanical irritation) or the factor responsible for infection is unknown. This phenomenon is much more common in girls than boys and has been seen in association with a toilet phobia in some. Not uncommonly, constipation also exists in this group and may be part of the syndrome of acquired megacolon secondary to fissure in ano in infancy.

Another common form of urinary stasis seen in children is that which is the result of vesicoureteral reflux. During voiding a portion of the urine in the bladder is passed into the upper collecting system in this group of patients. Upon completion of micturition, with the return of intravesical pressure to normal, the refluxed urine then returns to the bladder (Fig. 3–2). This interferes with the defense mechanisms of normal bladder emptying. It is unclear as to whether the presence of reflux truly increases the risk of urinary tract infections. Govan and coworkers (1975) noted little or no change in recurrence rate of infection after cessation of reflux, although this was not the observation reported by Williams (1971). Our own feeling is that reflux does seem to increase the child's susceptibility to urinary tract infection. The salient point is that those with reflux and infection are at risk for pyelonephritis, whereas most others are at risk only for lower tract infection. Hence, the presence of reflux should be recognized at an early age, and recurrent infections prevented by medical prophylaxis.

URETHRAL NARROWING (FEMALES)

The single factor most frequently indicted by many as the underlying cause for urinary infection in girls is urethral obstruction. A variety of procedures have been offered as the best means of widening the urethra or changing its caliber to prevent turbulence and to limit the incidence of infection. There is no evidence, however, that a difference in urethral caliber exists between those patients susceptible to infection and those not susceptible to infection (Graham et al., 1967). Simple urethral dilatation is the procedure most commonly performed to enlarge urethral caliber and, to its credit, carries little or no morbidity. In a prospective study carried out by Govan and colleagues (1975), 29 patients followed for three years before and three years after urethral dilatation had no change in the incidence of recurrence. The predilation incidence was 2.08 infections per year vs. 2.19 infections per year after dilatation.

Internal urethrotomy is a procedure designed to longitudinally incise the internal urethra, disrupting the so-called "distal urethral ring" described by Lyon (1974). It is not as benign as dilatation, and there is potential for both bleeding and vesicovaginal fistula (we have seen both). Reports suggest that this procedure decreases the incidence of recurrence of infection

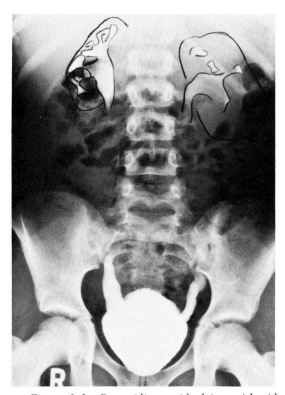

Figure 3–2. Postvoiding residual in a girl with marked vesicoureteral reflux. Note also severe bilateral renal scarring. Remaining functional renal tissue was confined primarily to the lower pole of the left kidney.

(Halverstadt and Leadbetter, 1968; Immergut and Gilbert, 1973), although in our own experience (Kaplan et al., 1973) and that of others (Walker and Richard, 1973) this has not been substantiated.

It has been suggested that an additional beneficial aspect of the various procedures to enlarge the urethral caliber in girls is to reduce lower urinary tract symptoms by diminishing urethral resistance. The subjective nature of the complaints and the multiple causative factors that might be responsible for these complaints limit one's ability to objectively judge the efficacy of these procedures. In our viewpoint, however, it would seem that none of the procedures designed to change the caliber of the female urethra predictably influences the incidence of recurrent infections or lower urinary tract symptoms. We therefore cannot support these who recommend procedures designed solely to achieve this end in view of the information presently available.

URETHRAL NARROWING (MALES)

The question of urethral meatal stenosis in males must be briefly addressed. Although urinary obstruction is generally feared when a small meatus is noted on examination, there does not seem to be a relationship between urethral meatal caliber and urinary tract infections in males (Committee from the Urology Section, American Academy of Pediatrics, 1978). Additionally, the observed size of the urethral meatus does not appear to correlate with the calibrated size (Morton, 1963) nor does the observed size of the urinary stream necessarily correlate with the "stenotic" appearance of the meatus. Therefore, what appears to be meatal stenosis on physical examination may in reality be normal (Chap. 5).

BLADDER NECK OBSTRUCTION

At this point, the question of obstruction at the bladder neck in otherwise normal children is of historical interest only. Thought to have been a major contributing factor not only to urinary infection but also to vesicoureteral reflux two or three decades ago (Lich and Maurer, 1950), surgical revision of the bladder neck is now rarely performed. In the absence of neurogenic disease, one should be extremely skeptical of the diagnosis of bladder neck obstruction or contracture in children (Chap. 5).

GENETICS

Genetic aspects may play a role in a girl's susceptibility to infection. Kunin (1970) noted a lesser incidence of asymptomatic bacteriuria and a lower recurrence rate of infection in black girls than in their white counterparts, and in the experience of one of us practicing in a predominantly black urban setting (ABB), the incidence of symptomatic urinary tract infections in black girls is extremely low. An interesting study by Fennell and colleagues (1977) suggests that recurrent bacteriuria has a familial tendency, and the follow-up study of the large group of girls with bacteriuria originally done by Kunin and associates (1964) reveals that the daughters of this group have a higher incidence of bacteriuria than normally would be anticipated (Gillenwater et al., 1979).

CLINICAL PRESENTATION

SYMPTOMS

The classical symptoms heralding the presence of urinary tract infection are known to all. One must keep in mind, however, that urgency, frequency, and urinary incontinence are nonspecific symptoms of bladder irritability and that dysuria and voluntary holding back of urine may also occur in response to introital irritation.

In infants the symptoms are less classic, and one should suspect urinary tract infection when a baby feeds poorly, has unexplained jaundice, is irritable (colic), fails to gain weight, or has diarrhea or an unexplained fever. Because of symptom nonspecificity, there is often an unfortunate delay in the recognition of urinary tract infection in the youngest and most susceptible group. Toddlers generally are unable to verbalize lower urinary tract complaints. It is not until investigations are carried out for failure to achieve urinary control at a later age that infection, which may have been of long duration, is recognized. Often the parents will then recall vague symptoms which, if appreciated in the past, might have led to earlier investigation.

In the younger age groups, urinary tract infection as a cause of fever is often missed for the same reason. Nonspecificity or absence of localizing symptoms prevents etiologic recognition. Evaluation of the child with fever of undetermined cause should always include collection of urine for culture (Chap. 2).

In older children, other than those with long-standing asymptomatic bacteriuria, the symptoms are less vague. Even in the "asymptomatic" group, however, a history of enuresis or abdominal pain can frequently be elicited if appropriate questions are asked. In the small group of patients with chronic lower urinary tract infection, symptoms often include squatting, with the child sitting on the heel of her foot in an attempt to prevent voiding. This is a response to urgent bladder contractions and is frequently associated with simultaneous crampy lower abdominal pain.

The classic triad of lower urinary tract symptoms, fever, and flank pain is highly suggestive of pyelonephritis. In younger children, flank pain is often replaced by abdominal discomfort. Cystitis alone is rarely associated with significant fever. The differentiation between isolated bladder infection and acute renal infection is clinically based on the presence of fever and systemic symptoms. The role that vesicoureteral reflux plays between renal involvement and cystitis was made clear in a study referred to by Woodard (1976) in which 90 per cent of those with vesicoureteral reflux had a past history of febrile urinary tract infections, whereas reflux was found in only 9 per cent of those with a history of nonfebrile urinary tract infec-

tions. Govan and Palmer (1969) reported similar findings. Conversely, vesicoureteral reflux was seen in 55 per cent of children with fever, leukocytosis, and culture proven urinary tract infection. In those patients presenting with a confirmed febrile urinary tract infection or a history thereof and in whom reflux is not demonstrated, transient reflux present only at the time of the acute infection is probably the underlying cause.

HEMATURIA

Infection as the underlying cause was noted in only 26 per cent of patients presenting to an outpatient clinic with gross hematuria (Ingelfinger et al., 1977). Nevertheless, one of the only circumstances in which one can feel confident making the diagnosis of urinary infection without awaiting the report of a urine culture is in the patient with the acute onset of lower urinary tract symptoms and gross hematuria. This does not ensure an underlying bacterial cause, as symptoms of lower urinary tract irritability and gross hematuria may also be a response to viral cystitis. In patients with hematuria of viral origin as well as those with bleeding due to nephritis, stone disease, lower urinary tract sarcoma, chemical cystitis (cyclophosphamide), or unexplained eosinophilic cystitis, the routine urine culture will be negative. If it is not possible to clinically determine that the cause is viral, radiographic evaluation and perhaps endoscopy are warranted.

DIAGNOSIS

There is abundant evidence that routine urinalysis alone is a poor means of making the diagnosis of urinary tract infection (Margileth and Filipescu, 1974; Pryles and Eliot, 1965). Microscopy of stained sediment is somewhat more accurate (Kass, 1956), as is examination under the phase contrast microscope (Brody et al., 1968). The immediate application of freshly collected urine or urine that has been refrigerated shortly after collection to culture media is the only reliable means of making the diagnosis of bacterial urinary tract infection. The various means of urine collection, office culture techniques, and significance of colony counts are discussed in detail in Chapter 2. The importance of documenting urinary tract infection by culture prior to treatment or evaluation cannot be overstressed.

BACTERIOLOGY

Gram-negative enteric bacteria can be anticipated as the infecting organism in most children with a bacterial urinary tract infection. The source of the bacteria is the child's own intestinal tract, and the route of infection presumably is via the perineum and urethra. E. coli is found in 80 to 90 per cent of first infections and is also the most common organism cultured on reinfection. Since most recurrences are reinfections rather than exacerbations and incompletely treated infections, E. coli serotypes would be expected to differ with subsequent episodes. This is indeed the case. Proteus mirabilis, Klebsiella, Enterobacter, Streptococcus fecalis and other enterococci, Pseudomonas, and Staphylococcus aureus are also pathogenic. In our experience, the latter two are usually found in patients who have been previously treated with antibiotics.

Occasionally, a patient is seen who has definite pyuria but in whom bacterial cultures are repeatedly negative (sterile pyuria). First it should be established that the child is not taking antibiotics and that cultures are not falsely negative. Then, before further evaluation, one should determine that the pus is not vaginal or preputial in origin by either personally supervising the urine collection or collecting the urine by catheterization or suprapubic aspiration. Once it is established that the pyuria is real, one must then consider organisms that do not readily grow on the usual culture media. Hermansson and colleagues (1974) found gram-negative staphylococci (micrococcus

3) as the invading organism in 41 per cent of sexually active adolescents with urinary tract infection. Hemophilus influenzae type b, another organism that does not readily grow on routine culture plates, has recently been seen to cause urinary tract infections (Granoff and Roskes, 1974), including epididymitis (Chesney et al., 1977) in children. Anaerobic bacteria occasionally may also be responsible for urinary tract infections (Segura et al., 1972). Other considerations include tuberculous urinary tract infections, fungi, calculi, and parasitic infestations, all rare in children. The child with sterile pyuria deserves complete urologic evaluation.

Nonpathogenic contaminating organisms can usually be recognized by the relatively small numbers of colonies grown on culture, assuming rapid plating or refrigeration of the specimen has taken place. Diphtheroids, Streptococcus fecalis, Staphylococcus albus, or Staphylococcus epidermidis are the most common. Current information suggests that those children in whom urinary pathogens can persist on the perineum or in the urethra may actually be the group at risk for or susceptible to urinary tract infections (p. 38). It is probably advisable to reculture the urine of children who are reported to have fewer than 100,000 colonies/ml of a pathogen on a fresh, appropriately handled specimen. This information reinforces the concept that it is not as important how the urine is collected for culture but how the urine is handled once collected, i.e., immediate refrigeration or medium inoculation.

TUBERCULOSIS

Tuberculous urinary tract infection in all age groups has become very uncommon in the United States and is rarely seen in children. The classic presentation of sterile pyuria in a child known to have had close contact with an infected individual suggests its possibility. Definitive diagnosis by culture must be obtained before institution of the multidrug, long-term treatment for what is basically urinary disease secondary to hematogenous spread of the primary pulmonary infection. Urographic changes of calyceal scarring and infundibular stenosis are late findings, and, because of their rarity, may fail to be recognized as secondary to tuberculosis by the inexperienced observer.

GONORRHEA

No age group is immune from genital gonorrhea. It should be suspected in males of any age with a urethral discharge or purulent balanitis or posthitis. The presence of gram-negative intracellular diplococci on gram stain of the discharge is highly suggestive, but specific culture is definitive. We have seen toddler-age males with urethral discharge of gonococcal origin apparently transmitted in the course of routine home diaper care (Meek et al., 1979). Burry (1971) reported gonococcal vulvovaginitis and possible peritonitis in prepubertal girls. Cervicitis is uncommon in the prepubertal group. Unfortunately, sexual abuse must always be considered as an underlying factor in both males and females of all societal groups.

NONBACTERIAL URINARY TRACT INFECTIONS

VIRAL INFECTION

Viral urinary tract infections, usually associated with gross hematuria and symptoms of lower urinary tract irritation lasting three to seven days, have been noted to be caused primarily by adenovirus 11 but also, more rarely, by adenovirus 21 (Mufson et al., 1973). Verification of a viral etiology is made by specific viral culture within 24 hours of onset. Unfortunately, because it takes 24 to 48 hours to obtain the results of a routine bacterial culture, it is usually too late to isolate the agent by the time a viral etiology is suspected. Determination of neutralizing antibody elevation comparing the acute levels to those at three weeks after infection was indicative of a viral etiology in

70 per cent of the suspected patients and in 100 per cent of those with culture-proven infection in the experience of Numazaki and coworkers (1973). Nonbacterial hemmorhagic cystitis has also been thought to be caused by papovirus-like particles (Hashida et al., 1976).

FUNGAL INFECTION

Fungal urinary tract infection usually results as an overgrowth following broad-spectrum antibiotic therapy in a child with an underlying pathourologic condition. The presence of foreign bodies (drainage tubes, catheters) in the postoperative period may serve as the infecting pathway. Fortunately, discontinuation of antibiotics after confirmation that urinary tract obstruction has been alleviated resolves the problem in most as treatable bacterial infection replaces the fungus. Local irrigation with an antifungal drug (amphotericin B) is rarely necessary.

Renal parenchymal fungal infection is often indicative of underlying immunologic deficiency and is not an uncommon event in the immunodepressed state (such as patients with malignant disease, neonates, diabetics, and transplant recipients.) In otherwise normal patients, the presence of fungal urinary tract infection suggests an underlying abnormality, probably obstructive in nature requiring drainage. *Candida* sp. is the yeast form that most commonly involves the urinary tract.

PROTOZOAL INFECTION

Protozoal infestation is rarely seen in the United States, although recognition of the urinary pathologic conditions caused by *Schistosoma haematobium* is important. Severe bladder fibrosis from chronic inflammation leading to a contracted bladder and ultimate development of bladder malignancy in adult years is a significant risk. Fully 90 per cent of the population in some areas of the Middle East is infested.

Trichomonas vaginalis, both as a cause

of vaginal discharge in sexually active girls and urethral complaints in sexually active boys, should be kept in mind. Wet preparation of vaginal or prostatic secretions identifying the motile flagellate confirms the diagnosis.

EVALUATION

UROGRAPHY

Confirmation of bacterial urinary tract infection in children strongly suggests the need for radiographic studies. The fact that children with both asymptomatic and symptomatic culture-proven urinary tract infection have an 80 per cent incidence of recurrence suggests that there is no statistical justification in waiting for a "second" infection prior to evaluation (Kunin, 1970; Fair et al., 1972). In addition, a retrospective review of a carefully controlled population of children seen with their "first" episode of bacteriuria demonstrated a previous infection at an earlier age in many (Winberg et al., 1974). Excretory urography and cystography (with visualization of the urethra in males) is required in all patients for adequate evaluation. The importance of cystography relates to the finding that about one third of children with documented urinary tract infections have been found to have vesicoureteral reflux (Govan and Palmer, 1969; Smellie et al., 1964). Once complete radiographic evaluation has been carried out and the urinary tract has been found normal, little would appear to be gained by repeat radiographic studies even if recurrent cystitis is a problem. In a review of 70 girls with recurrent lower urinary tract infection (cystitis) who had repeated excretory urography, no change in renal configuration was noted over a course of several years (ABB). On the other hand, those with an abnormal urinary tract may require further studies. A discussion of the radiographic evaluation of the urinary tract is presented in Chapter 2.

ENDOSCOPY

Cystoscopy in all children with proven urinary tract infection would not appear to be justified. If one accepts the premise that female urethral configuration does not play a role in the genesis of urinary tract infection (Walker and Richard, 1973) (p. 41) and if one also accepts the fact that cystography can be carried out with the child awake with no risk to life and with no lasting emotional trauma, then there is little indication for cystoscopy in the patient with an uncomplicated urinary tract infection who has normal radiographic findings. Rarely the need for further radiographic evaluation or documentation of chronic bladder changes demands completion of evaluation by endoscopy.

LOCALIZATION OF INFECTION

Occasionally the question arises as to whether infection is bladder or renal in origin or both. This need not be a concern in the child with normal radiographs but can be of importance in children with chronic infection and significant dilatation of the collecting system (Fig. 3–3). Cystoscopy, bladder urine culture, culture of the bladder wash after thorough irrigation, and split renal pelvic urine cultures obtained by differential catheterization (Table 3–2) localize the site of infection. The washout test described by Fairley and colleagues (1967) has been suggested for the same purpose, but if such information is necessary, this method seems less reliable in our opinion. If bacteria are localized to the upper urinary tract and if obstruction or significant stasis can be corrected by surgical means, reconstruction of the urinary tract is in order. In the absence of obstruction or if stasis cannot be altered, aggressive long-term antibacterial therapy should be pursued.

Differentiation between renal and bladder infection has recently been attempted by determination of the presence of antibody-coated bacteria in the urinary sediment on the assumption that such coat-

Measurement of acute serum C-reactive protein levels appears to correlate well with the clinical impression of acute pyelonephritis based on the presence or absence of fever (Wientzen et al., 1979). The overall impression one gains is that the physician can differentiate acute pyelonephritis from acute cystitis on clinical grounds. Of course, a positive urine culture is an absolute requirement in either case.

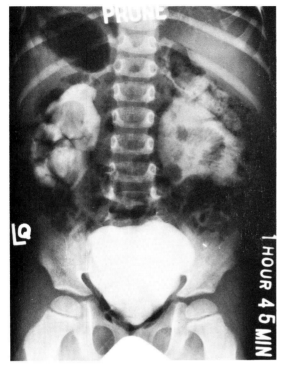

Figure 3–3. Eight-year-old boy with prune belly syndrome and repeated urinary tract infections. Marked stasis in both upper and lower urinary tracts is present.

SIGNIFICANCE OF URINARY TRACT INFECTION

KIDNEY

The potential for renal damage from urinary tract infection appears to correlate inversely with the age of the patient. There is abundant evidence that the greatest renal threat exists in neonates and infants, whereas later in childhood the likelihood of permanent damage resulting from bacterial pyelonephritis is less (Hodson and Wilson,

ing occurs as a result of renal infection. However, coating may occur with urethral and vaginal contamination (Montplaisir et al., 1977), and the specificity of the study is questionable (Hellerstein et al., 1978). In addition, the absence of radiographic evidence of either renal scarring or significant anatomic abnormality (reflux or obstruction) casts doubt on the clinical significance of the suggestion that all antibody-coated bacteria come from the kidneys.

Table 3–2.   Split Cultures

CULTURE SITE	COLONY COUNT
Bladder	100,000 *Enterococcus*, group D
Bladder wash	15,000 *Enterococcus*, group D
Left renal pelvis	25,000 *Enterococcus*, group D
Right renal pelvis	80,000 *Enterococcus*, group D

Example of split cultures that localize urinary tract infection in both kidneys as well as the bladder, thus proving the presence of upper tract infection.

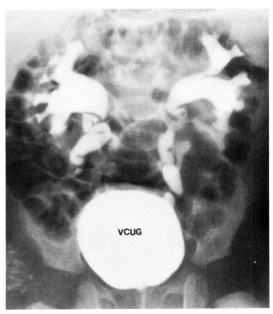

Figure 3–4. Cystogram in a six-month-old boy with a single episode of febrile urinary tract infection. The kidneys appear to be of equal size.

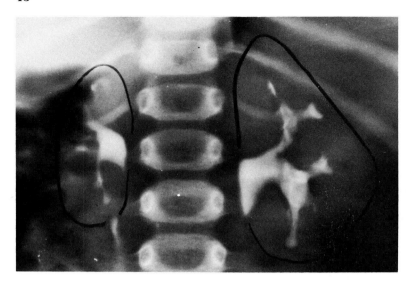

Figure 3–5. Excretory urogram in the patient discussed in Figure 3–4 two years later demonstrates a small right kidney. This picture is typical of the possible effects of bacterial pyelonephritis in infancy.

1965; Bergstrom et al., 1972). The unfortunate fact that scarring is already present at the time of initial evaluation in about half of the patients found to have vesicoureteral reflux (Govan et al., 1975) suggests that earlier episodes of infection have been missed (Figs. 3–4 and 3–5). The role that "chronic pyelonephritis" plays in childhood is unclear. The authors are unsure that this entity truly exists in the nonobstructed state.

BLADDER

In addition to the potential for renal damage associated with vesicoureteral reflux, unrecognized bladder infection in the toddler may also play an important role in disrupting toilet training. It is not uncommon in our practices to see children who present with urinary tract infection recognized only after the child was seen in consultation for day or night enuresis persisting beyond the age of four or five years. It would appear that a period exists when children learn to understand the significance of bladder stimuli, and toilet training becomes successful when central inhibitory mechanisms take control. Overstimulation or increased sensory input, such as from inflammatory bladder changes, reduces inhibitory capabilities and interferes with the ability to gain full control (Yeates, 1973). This

theory, which we hold as highly tenable, strongly suggests the need for routine periodic urine culture in the general pediatric practice. Our own experience with

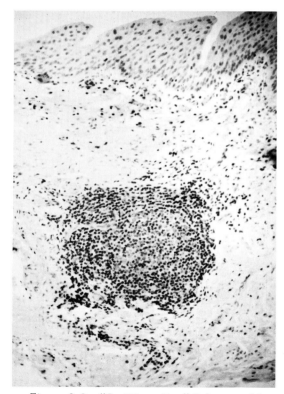

Figure 3–6. "Cystitis cystica." Submucosal lymphoid follicle (cystitis follicularis) is typical of the histologic changes seen in children with long-standing cystitis.

patients with chronic lower urinary tract infections supports the high incidence of enuresis in this group (Belman, 1978).

A group of girls exists who tend to have frequent recurrences or unremitting urinary tract infections. Endoscopic evaluation may reveal cystic mucosal changes, referred to because of their endoscopic appearance as "cystitis cystica," the results of subepithelial lymphoid proliferation (histologically cystitis follicularis) (Fig. 3–6). These changes may be an effort at an immunologic response to chronic infection (Uehling and King, 1973).

The incidence of cystitis follicularis in children has been reported to range from 2.4 per cent (Kaplan and King, 1970) to 8 per cent (Vlatkovic et al., 1977) of the total of those with urinary tract infections. Its occurrence in boys is extremely rare and in that sex suggests a significant underlying anatomic pathologic condition.

RECURRENCE RATE

As determined by Kunin, (1970), the recurrence rate of uncomplicated urinary tract infection in girls is apparently related more to "statistical likelihood" than the anatomic configuration of the urinary tract. After each infection, another infection within a two-year period is found in about 80 per cent of white girls regardless of whether the infection was the first one or a recurrence. The recurrence rate in black girls is 60 per cent. After two years without infection, recurrences tend to be infrequent, although the population in question has a higher incidence of infection when becoming sexually active than statistically anticipated. This is probably an important point for the primary physician to keep in mind. Those girls who had urinary tract infections in childhood should be checked for asymptomatic bacteriuria when sexually active and when pregnant.

Socioeconomic status and the presence of vesicoureteral reflux did not affect infection recurrence rate in Kunin's series, although one must assume that the reflux in question in those patients was mild or surgical correction would have been carried out. Race and age, however, did play a role; older children and black girls tended to have fewer recurrences.

OTHER SITES OF URINARY TRACT INFECTION

PROSTATE

In our experience, actual infection of the prostate has not been recognized in the patient population in question. Even in young pubertal males this would be a most uncommon diagnosis, possibly related to the frequent emptying of prostatic ducts with sexual activity. Prostatic abscesses secondary to bacterial sepsis have been reported (Mann, 1960), but the event is extremely uncommon.

URETHRA

Chronic or recurrent urethritis in women is frequently offered as the etiology for otherwise unexplainable lower urinary tract symptoms. Documentation of this diagnosis is difficult and often subjective. Fortunately, it is seldom offered as a cause for lower urinary tract symptoms in girls. Irritation of the delicate periurethral mucosa by detergents or by abrasion may be responsible for symptoms of frequency, urgency, and dysuria.

In prepubertal boys, unexplained dysuria is a not infrequent complaint. Actual confirmation of urethritis by noting a purulent discharge is the exception in this group, and an explanation for the symptoms is lacking. Some of these boys have terminal hematuria or blood staining on their underwear, suggesting either inflammatory or traumatic origins. A forceful urinary stream causing acute distension of the urethra is a cause speculated by one of us (ABB), and unexplained mild inflammation of the posterior urethra is offered by the other (GWK). Endoscopy has demonstrated erythema in the area of the prostatomembranous urethra in some of those with terminal hematuria (GWK). In those with hematuria, supportive and symptomatic treatment (reassurance, liberal fluid intake, and sitz baths) is recommended after confirming by voiding cystourethrography that no significant underlying pathologic condition exists.

It is unlikely that normal masturbatory activity is responsible for either dysuria or terminal hematuria, although in one of our rather disturbed patients, repeated self-instrumentation with a pencil was the cause of a bloody urethral discharge, dysuria, and urethral injury leading to urinary retention.

Bacterial urethritis in the form of gonorrhea is a common presenting complaint in the adolescent male population. Forms of sexually transmitted nonbacterial urethritis, referred to as nonspecific urethritis, are also seen. Chlamydia and T-strain mycoplasma have been found on culture in patients with urethral discharge (Segura et al., 1972). Other recognized causes include *Candida albicans, Trichomonas vaginalis,* and herpes simplex virus.

A little-known problem in pediatrics that can occur in adolescents is a self-induced urethritis in an individual who is overly concerned about the possibility of gonorrhea. The following is the usual scenario: A young man has sexual intercourse, feels guilty, and starts looking for a urethral discharge. He strips his penis repeatedly and finally notes a clear discharge, which persists until the cycle is interrupted. Treatment is simply one of reassurance after confirming that no actual infection is present.

EPIDIDYMIS

Epididymitis in the prepubertal male is uncommon and suggests underlying urinary infection and a pathologic anatomic condition. The child presenting with an acutely swollen hemiscrotum must initially be considered to have torsion of the spermatic cord. Isotope scrotal scan, if available, may be helpful in the differentiation between torsion and other diagnostic possibilities (Chaps. 2 and 9). If clinical differentiation between epididymitis and torsion is not possible, emergency surgical exploration becomes mandatory. The clinical distinction between torsion and epididymitis may, at times, be extremely difficult. Delay in diagnosis leads to testicular death in the child with torsion, whereas exploration entails no additional risk to life beyond that of anesthesia in the child with epididymitis.

Children with proven epididymitis should have a urine culture, excretory urography, and cystourethrography. Deviant development of the terminal wolffian duct with an ectopic ureter into the seminal vesicle or ejaculatory duct may be responsible for the development of epididymitis. Additionally, urethral obstruction causing increased intraurethral pressure in association with bacterial infection can occasionally cause retrograde filling of the ejaculatory duct and vas deferens leading to epididymitis.

ORCHITIS

In our experience, orchitis independent of other scrotal pathologic conditions is extremely rare in the prepubertal population. The association of orchitis with mumps virus in adults is recognized. In younger children, other more significant causes, such as torsion, should first be considered when confronted with a child who has scrotal swelling.

REFERENCES

Allen, T. D.: Pathogenesis of urinary tract infections in children. N. Engl. J. Med., *273*:1421, 1965.

Belman, A. B.: Clinical significance of cystitis cystica in girls: Results of a prospective study. J. Urol., *119*:661, 1978.

Bergstrom, T., Larson, H., Lincoln, K., and Winberg, J.: Studies of urinary tract infection in infancy and childhood. III. Eighty consecutive patients with neonatal infection. J. Pediatr., *80*:858, 1972.

Brody, T., Webster, M. C., and Kark, R. M.: Identification of elements of urinary sediment with phase contrast microscopy. J.A.M.A., *206*:1777, 1968.

Buetow, K. C., Klein, S. W., and Lane, R. B.: Septicemia in premature infants. Am. J. Dis. Child., *110*:29, 1965.

Burry, V. F.: Gonococcal vulvovaginitis and possible peritonitis in prepubertal girls. Am. J. Dis. Child., *121*:536, 1971.

Chesney, P. J., Saari, T. N., and Mueller, G.: Acute epididymo-orchitis due to Hemophilus influenzae type b. J. Pediatr., *91*:368, 1977.

Clark, H., Ronald, A. R., and Turck, M.: Serum antibody response in renal versus bladder bacteriuria. J. Infect. Dis., *123*:539, 1971.

Committee from the Urology Section of the American Academy of Pediatrics: Urethral meatal stenosis in males. Pediatrics *61*:778, 1978.

Cox, C. E., and Hinman, F. J.: Experiments with induced bacteriuria, vesical emptying and bacterial growth in the mechanism of bladder defense to infection. J. Urol., *86*:739, 1961.

Cox, C. E., Lacy, S. S., and Hinman, F., Jr.: The urethra and its relationship to urinary infection. II. The urethral flora of the female with recurrent urinary infection. J. Urol., *99*:632, 1968.

DeLuca, F. G., Fisher, J. H., and Swenson, O.: Review of recurrent urinary tract infections in infancy and early childhood. N. Engl. J. Med., *268*:75, 1963.

Drew, J. H., and Acton, C. M.: Radiologic findings in newborn infants with urinary infection. Arch. Dis. Child., *51*:628, 1976.

Dubroff, L. M., Duckett, J. W., and Corriere, J. N., Jr.: Phyto-hemagglutinin lymphocyte stimulation in children with recurrent urinary tract infections. Urology, 5:744, 1975.

Edelmann, C. M., Ogwo, J. E., Fine, B. P., and Martinez, A. B.: The prevalence of bacteriuria in full-term and premature newborn infants. J. Pediatr., 82:125, 1973.

Fair, W. R., Govan, D. E., Friedland, G. W., and Filly, R. A.: Urinary tract infections in children. West. J. Med., *121*:366, 1972.

Fairley, K. F., Bond, A. G., Brown, R. B., et al.: Simple test to determine the site of urinary tract infection. Lancet, 2:427, 1967.

Fang, L. S. T., Tolkoff-Rubin, N. E., and Rubin, R. H.: Efficiency of single-dose and conventional amoxicillin therapy in patients with urinary tract infection localized by the antibody-coated bacteria technique. N. Engl. J. Med., *298*:413, 1978.

Fennell, R. S., Wilson, S. G., Garin, E. H. et al.: Bacteriuria in families of girls with recurrent bacteriuria. Clin. Pediatr., *16*:1132, 1977.

Gillenwater, J. Y., Harrison, R. B., and Kunin, C. M.: Natural history of bacteriuria in school girls. A long-term case control study. N. Engl. J. Med., *301*:396, 1979.

Govan, D. E., Fair, W. R., Friedland, G. W., and Filly, R. A.: Management of children with urinary tract infection. Urology, 6:273, 1975.

Govan, D. E., and Palmer, J. M.: Urinary tract infection in children. The influence of successful antireflux operations in morbidity from infection. Pediatrics, *44*:677, 1969.

Graham, J. B., King, L. R., Kropp, K. A., et al.: The significance of distal urethral narrowing in young girls. J. Urol., 97:1045, 1967.

Granoff, D. M., and Roskes, S.: Urinary infection due to Hemophilus influenzae, type b. J. Pediatr., *81*:414, 1974.

Halverstadt, D. B., and Leadbetter, G. W., Jr.: Internal urethrotomy and recurrent urinary tract infection in female children. I. Results in the management of infection. J. Urol., *100*:297, 1968.

Hashida, Y., Gaffney, P. C., and Yunis, E. J.: Acute hemorrhagic cystitis and papovirus-like particles. J. Pediatr., 89:85, 1976.

Hellerstein, S., Kennedy, E., Nussbaum, L., and Rice, K.: Localization of the site of urinary tract infections by means of antibody-coated bacteria in the urinary sediments. J. Pediatr., 92:188, 1978.

Hermansson, B., Bollgren, I., Bergstrom, T., and Winberg, J.: Coagulase negative staphylococci as cause of symptomatic urinary infections in children. J. Pediatr., 84:807, 1974.

Hodson, C. J., and Wilson, S.: Natural history of pyelonephritic scarring. Br. Med. J., 2:191, 1965.

Immergut, M. A., and Gilbert, E. C.: Internal urethrotomy in recurring urinary infections in girls. J. Urol., *190*:126, 1973.

Ingelfinger, J. R., Davis, A. E., and Grupe, W. E.: Frequency and etiology of gross hematuria in a general pediatric setting. Pediatrics, 59:557, 1977.

Kaijser, B.: Immunology of E. coli: K antigen and its relation to urinary tract infection. J. Infect. Dis., *127*:670, 1973.

Kaplan, G. W., and King, L. R.: Cystitis cystica in childhood. J. Urol., *103*:657, 1970.

Kaplan, G. W., Sammons, T. A., and King, L. R.: A blind comparison of dilatation, urethrotomy and medication alone in the treatment of urinary infections in girls. J. Urol., *109*:917, 1973.

Kass, E. H.: Asymptomatic infections of the urinary tract. Trans. Assoc. Am. Phys., 69:56, 1956.

Kunin, C. M.: The natural history of recurrent bacteriuria in school girls. N. Engl. J. Med., 28:1443, 1970.

Kunin, C. M., Deutscher, R., and Paquin, A., Jr.: Urinary tract infection in school children: An epidemiologic, clinical and laboratory study. Medicine, *43*:91, 1964.

Lapides, J., and Diokno, A. C.: Persistence of the infant bladder as a cause for urinary infection in girls. J. Urol., *103*:243, 1970.

Leadbetter G. W., Jr., and Slavin, S.: Pediatric urinary tract infection. Significance of vaginal bacteria. Urology, 3:581, 1974.

Lich, R., and Maurer, J. E.: The surgical relief of vesical neck obstruction in children. South Surg., *16*:127, 1950.

Lyon, R. P.: Distal urethral stenosis. *In* Johnston, J. H., and Goodwin, W. E. (Eds.): Reviews in Pediatric Urology. Amsterdam, Excerpta Medica, 1974.

Mackie, G. G., and Stephens, F. D.: Duplex kidneys. A correlation of renal dysplasia with position of the ureteral orifice. J. Urol., *114*:274, 1975.

Mann, S.: Prostatic abscess in the newborn. Arch. Dis. Child., 35:396, 1960.

Margileth, A. M., and Filipescu, N.: Initial urinary tract bacterial infection. An overview of clinical features, management and outcome in 64 children. Clin. Proc. Child. Hosp. Nat. Med. Ctr., 30:175, 1974.

Meadow, S. R., White, R. H. R., and Johnston, N. M.: Prevalence of symptomless urinary tract disease in Birmingham school children. I. Pyuria and bacteriuria. Br. Med. J., 3:31, 1969.

Meek, J. M., Askari, A., and Belman, A. B.: Prepubertal gonorrhea. J. Urol., *122*:532, 1979.

Montplaisir, S., Corteau, C., and Roche, A. J.: Antibody-coated bacteria on contaminated urine specimen. N. Engl. J. Med., 296:758, 1977.

Morton, H. G.: Meatus size in 1000 circumcised children from two weeks to sixteen years of age. J. Fla. Med. Assoc., *50*:137, 1963.

Mufson, M. A., Belshe, R. B., Horrigan, T. J., and Dollar, L. M.: Cause of acute hemorrhagic cystitis in children. Am. J. Dis. Child., *126*:605, 1973.

Numazaki, Y., Kumaska, T., Yano, N., et al.: Further study on acute hemorrhagic cystitis due to adenovirus II. N. Engl. J. Med., *280*:344, 1973.

Parsons, C. L., Greenspan, C., Moore, S. W., and Mulholland, S. G.: Role of surface mucin in primary antibacterial defense of bladder. Urology, *9*:48, 1977.

Pryles, C. V., and Eliot, C. R.: Pyuria and bacteriuria in infants and children. The value of pyuria as a diagnostic criterion of urinary tract infections. Am. J. Dis. Child., *110*:628, 1965.

Salvatierra, O., Jr., and Tanagho, E. A.: Reflux as a cause of end stage kidney disease: Report of 32 cases. J. Urol., *117*:441, 1971.

Segura, J. W., Kelalis, P. P., Martin, W. J., and Smith, L. H.: Anaerobic bacteria in the urinary tract. Mayo Clin. Proc., *47*:30, 1972.

Segura, J. W., Smith, T. F., Weed, L. A., and Pettersen, G. R.: Chlamydia and nonspecific urethritis. J. Urol., *117*:720, 1977.

Smellie, J. M.: Medical aspects of urinary infection in children. J. R. Coll. Phys., *1*:189, 1967.

Smellie, J. M., Hodson, C. J., Edwards, D., and Normand, I. C. S.: Clinical and radiological features of urinary infection in childhood. Br. Med. J., *2*:1222, 1964.

Stamey, T. A.: Urinary Infections. Baltimore, Williams and Wilkins, 1972.

Thrupp, L. D., Hodgman, J. E., Karelitz, M., and Coblentz, D.: Transurethral reflux during cleansing procedure for clean-voided urine specimens in low-birth weight infants. J. Pediatr., *82*:1057, 1973.

Uehling, D., and King, L. R.: Secretion immunoglobulin A excretion in cystitis cystica. Urology *1*:305, 1973.

Vlatkovic, G., Bradic, I., Gabric, V., and Batinic, D.: Cystitis cystica: Characteristics of the disease in children. Br. J. Urol., *49*:57, 1977.

Walker, D., and Richard, G. A.: A critical evaluation of urethral obstruction in female children. Pediatrics *51*:272, 1973.

Wientzen, R. L., McCrackey, G. H., Petruska, M. L., et al.: Localization and therapy of urinary tract infections of childhood. Pediatrcs, *63*:467, 1979.

Williams, D. I.: The natural history of reflux—a review. Urol. Int., *26*:350, 1971.

Winberg, J., Andersen, H. J., Bergstrom, T., et al.: Epidemiology of symptomatic urinary tract infection in childhood. Acta Paediatr. Scand. (Suppl.), *252*:1, 1974.

Winberg, J., Andersen, H. J., Hanson, L. A., and Lincoln, K.: Studies of urinary infection in infancy and childhood. Br. Med. J., *2*:524, 1963.

Woodard, J. R.: Genitourinary infections. *In* Kelalis, P. P., King, L. R., and Belman, A. B. (Eds.): Clinical Pediatric Urology. Philadelphia, W. B. Saunders Co., 1976.

Yeates, W. K.: Bladder function in normal micturition. *In* Kolvin, I., MacKeith, R. C., and Meadow, S. R. (Eds.): Bladder control and Enuresis. Clinics in Developmental Medicine, 48/49, 1973.

Treatment of Urinary Tract Infection

With the first section of this chapter as background, it is now appropriate to consider, in general terms, the treatment of urinary tract infections. It constantly must be kept in mind that we are treating patients, not laboratory results or radiographs. The goals of treatment are to restore the patient to a state of well-being, alleviate symptoms, render the urine sterile, minimize renal damage, and, it is hoped, minimize cost, both monetary and emotional. To treat a patient with urinary infection intelligently, one must proceed through a decision-making process of several steps. One should first attempt to determine the site of infection. This is usually accomplished by an estimation of the severity of the illness when the patient initially presents. Cystitis is a minor illness and usually produces lower urinary tract symptoms only. Children with urinary tract infections who present with high fever,

prostration, and gastrointestinal symptoms usually have renal involvement. Because upper urinary tract infection potentially may lead to renal damage, a more aggressive mode of therapy must be chosen for those judged to have upper as opposed to lower tract infection.

In this same context, it must be decided whether the child can be treated as an outpatient or if hospitalization is indicated. Most neonates, even if asymptomatic, are best treated in the hospital because of their decreased immune competence and the intensity of antibiotic therapy required (Winberg, 1972). The decision for hospitalization of older infants and children is made largely on clinical grounds. Parents are often alarmed by high fevers, but if the parent can cope with the situation, fever in and of itself is not an indication for hospitalization. However, it is imperative that the child receive adequate doses of medication and adequate fluids. Consequently, those children, regardless of age, whose clinical picture includes vomiting or dehydration may require hospitalization so that parenteral routes of fluid and antibiotic administration can be afforded them.

One much neglected aspect of treatment is the decision as to whether or not some form of urinary or surgical drainage of the infection is required. In some children, particularly those with vesicoureteral reflux, who have marked dysuria and are voiding poorly, the insertion of an indwelling catheter either per urethra or suprapubically may be of dramatic benefit in resolving the acute stages of the infection. Additionally, it must be remembered that renal cortical and perinephric abscesses do still occur and that such problems often require surgical drainage for their resolution.

The next decision is whether or not high tissue levels of antibiotics are required or whether a high concentration in the urine will be sufficient to produce the desired result. Most of the antibiotics that are used for urinary tract infection produce very high urinary levels but only some of these agents will produce high tissue levels (Stamey et al., 1965). The agents that produce high tissue levels usually do so when administered by a parenteral route, and, again, hospital treatment may be required to achieve this. Obviously, tissue levels are not required for the treatment of cystitis but may be required for the treatment of pyelonephritis in an attempt to minimize renal scarring. Occasionally, bacterial resistance to commonly employed agents in children with cystitis alone requires the use of agents administered parenterally.

One must also decide the purpose of treatment. Ideally one would like to permanently eradicate all bacteria from the urinary tract with a single course of medication. However, as has been stated in the previous sections, this is not always possible. Certainly bacteria can be eradicated on a temporary basis, but unless the clinical situation dictates treatment, it is futile to treat a child with a complex problem in which there is no hope of permanently sterilizing the urinary tract only to have

recurrence with a resistant organism. Perhaps the best example of this dilemma is the patient who requires an indwelling catheter for prolonged periods of time (e.g., in traumatic paraplegia). In this instance, if one treats the bacteriuria that is uncovered on urine culture, it will be possible to sterilize the urine temporarily, but within a short period of time there will be further bacteriuria with an organism that is now resistant to the antibiotic previously used. If this patient was asymptomatic at the time of initial treatment and if for some reason in the course of the illness this individual developed a clinical pyelonephritis, there might then be no medication with which to treat the patient effectively. The point of this example is that there are clinical situations in which it is best to ignore bacteriuria and to treat the patient only at indicated intervals.

The last decision to be made is the length of treatment. It is common practice to treat septic neonates and infants with 10 days to two weeks of intensive antibiosis (Lincoln et al., 1970). Similarly, most physicians would employ a similar regimen in any child with acute pyelonephritis. There is some evidence that one to five days of therapy may be sufficient to completely eradicate bacteria from the lower urinary tract in uncomplicated cases without recurrence of infection (Fang et al., 1978). Ten days of treatment remains the more popular course of treatment for "simple cystitis," but there are still some who recommend six weeks or even three months of treatment for a single episode of uncomplicated cystitis.

Situations exist where it is preferable to utilize suppressive courses of medication. A classic example of this is the child with cystitis follicularis (cystitis cystica). It has been shown that low-dose, long-term medication (such as nitrofurantoin 25 mg once or twice daily or sulfisoxazole 250 mg to 500 mg two or three times daily for 6 to 12 months) can protect the child from multiple recurrences of infection while on medication (Belman, 1978). Similar courses of medication are effectively utilized for children who are known to have vesicoureteral reflux.

Because the majority of urinary tract

infections are caused by *E. coli* and because most are exquisitely sensitive to agents such as sulfonamides (Kunin, 1972), there is a tendency to blindly administer such agents to patients suspected of having urinary tract infections without documentation. Urine culture is essential to diagnosis, and it is far wiser in the long run to obtain sensitivity testing upon which to base therapy of any given infection. This is not to be interpreted as a mandate for awaiting the results of sensitivity tests to initiate therapy. To reiterate, we are treating patients, and one of our goals is symptomatic relief. Once fresh urine has been collected and refrigerated or submitted for culture and sensitivity, it is perfectly appropriate to commence therapy in a child strongly suspected of having urinary tract infection. Should the culture prove sterile, therapy should be discontinued. Additionally, if the patient is not responding to the agent that was initially blindly selected, the results of the bacterial sensitivity study offer a guide to better therapy.

If therapy is efficacious, it is anticipated that the patient will become asymptomatic within 24 to 48 hours and the urine will be rendered sterile (Stamey et al., 1965). If this is not the case, one must reevaluate therapy and must be prepared to change to a more appropriate agent. Additionally, in the patient who is quite ill, failure to respond to therapy within 48 hours suggests the need for obtaining an excretory urogram at that time; this study will demonstrate whether an anatomic lesion is present that is preventing a response to medical management.

BACTERIAL SENSITIVITY TESTS

When discussing sensitivity tests, one must remember that the terms sensitive and resistant refer to bacterial growth in the presence of specific concentrations of antimicrobial agents. For effective treatment of urinary tract infections, we are more often concerned with urine rather than serum levels. Most sensitivity tests are reported in terms of antibiotic concentration achievable in serum. With most antibiotics, the urinary concentration far exceeds that achieved in serum or tissue. Hence, bacteria will often be killed by drugs to which they are "resistant" in vitro because testing occurred at a lower concentration than that achieved in urine.

The most widely used method for sensitivity testing is the disc method, in which the radius of an antibiotic inhibition zone in an agar medium surrounding an antibiotic-impregnated disc indicates the sensitivity of that particular bacterium to the antibiotic in question. This method of testing has the merits of being simple and relatively inexpensive. Some agents, particularly sulfas, do not diffuse well from the antibiotic disc into the agar, and, consequently, organisms may be reported as resistant when they are quite sensitive. Other methods of testing include the tube dilution method and agar dilution method. These methods, which are time-consuming and consequently expensive, come into play when dealing with organisms that are resistant to the usual agents. These methods are utilized in the minimum-inhibitory concentration test, which has of late come into vogue. However, as was previously pointed out, urine levels rather than tissue levels seem to be of most clinical significance, and studies of this type are rarely necessary in the management of the usual urinary tract infection.

ANTIBACTERIAL AGENTS

SULFONAMIDES

Sulfonamides have long been utilized in the treatment of urinary tract infection. They have their greatest utility in the treatment of simple cystitis, are the least expensive agents available, have few side effects, and are well tolerated by children. They act by competitively blocking the conversion of para-aminobenzoic acid to folic acid (Feingold, 1963). About 75 per cent of the oral dose is absorbed. Free sulfonamide is excreted by the kidney by filtration and tubular secretion. Although high tissue levels are not achieved, excellent urine levels result. Sulfonamides are most effective against *E. coli* but also may be effective against other gram-negative and gram-positive organisms. Sensitivity testing for sulfonamides is not particularly useful when the disc method is employed.

Sulfonamides do affect the gastrointestinal flora slightly when used for long-term therapy, but in spite of this, they are effective agents for both short-term acute therapy of uncomplicated infections as well as low-dosage, long-term prophylaxis. These agents displace protein-bound bilirubin; hence, in the neonate they may interfere with bilirubin excretion and cause kernicterus. Once the infant has passed through the period of "physiologic jaundice," these agents can be utilized if so desired. Toxicity is low. Admittedly, some patients are allergic to sulfas, but fortunately most reactions are of a minor cutaneous nature, such as urticaria. There have been some problems with major hypersensitivity reaction, such as Stevens-Johnson syndrome, to long-acting sulfas, and for this reason this form is not widely utilized at present (Salvaggio and Gonzalez, 1959). The most widely used agent is sulfisoxazole, employed in a dose of 150 mg per kg body weight per day given in four to six divided doses orally (Vaughan and McKay, 1975).

NITROFURANTOIN

Nitrofurantoin is quite useful in the treatment of simple cystitis and is also a very useful agent for long-term, low-dose suppressive therapy. Its precise mode of action is unknown, but it is thought to interfere with early stages of the bacterial Krebs cycle (AMA, 1971). It is well absorbed from the gastrointestinal tract and has minimal effect on bowel flora. Tissue levels are low; because it is excreted almost entirely in the urine by glomerular filtration, urinary levels are quite high. Urinary alkalinization increases urine levels while acidification increases tissue levels. It works well against most *E. coli* organisms and enterococci, although it is not particularly effective against *Klebsiella*, *Proteus*, or *Pseudomonas*.

One of its major disadvantages is that it may produce nausea or vomiting in some children. This can be minimized by administering the agent immediately following a meal. The nausea that is produced by the suspension and the tablet form can be further minimized by utilizing the macrocrystals of nitrofurantoin, supplied in capsule form. For the small child who is unable to swallow a capsule, the contents of the capsule can be emptied and administered in dry form on a piece of bread, in peanut butter, or in mashed potatoes. If the crystals are dissolved in a liquid, the macrocrystal effect is lost. In neonates, the drug can produce a hemolytic anemia due to glutathione instability; consequently, it should not be used in this age group. Additionally, the drug is ineffective in patients with significant renal impairment. Adverse effects are rare but do include peripheral neuropathy and pulmonary infiltrates. The usual dose for nitrofurantoin is 6 mg per kg per day given orally in four divided doses (Vaughan and McKay, 1975).

TRIMETHOPRIM-SULFAMETHOXAZOLE

The trimethoprim-sulfa combination is a newer agent that appears to be quite useful in the management of simple cystitis as well as long-term antibacterial suppression. The trimethoprim-sulfa combination does have a slight effect on bowel flora, but because it is a lipid-soluble agent it has the advantage of entering prostatic secretions in the adult male and vaginal secretions in the female (Stamey and Condy, 1975). This latter characteristic appears to be of particular utility in its effectiveness as a prophylactic agent. The trimethoprim moiety interferes with dihydrofolic acid reductase while the sulfa moiety blocks the conversion of para-aminobenzoic acid to dihydrofolic acid. The combination is effective against many gram-positive and gram-negative organisms. It is well absorbed from the gastrointestinal tract and gives high serum and urine levels. Because trimethoprim is related to 6-mercaptopurine, hematologic difficulties might be anticipated. Only rarely have such problems been observed with its use. The drug is available as a suspension containing 40 mg trimethoprim and 200 mg of sulfamethoxazole per 5 ml. The dose employed is 10 mg per kg trimethoprim and 50 mg per kg sulfamethoxazole per day in two to three divided doses (Howard and Howard, 1978).

NALIDIXIC ACID

Nalidixic acid is an antibacterial agent that produces good urinary levels and is effective against many gram-negative organisms. It is especially effective against *Proteus*. It was thought that bacterial resistance was a particular problem with this agent, but it has recently been shown that this is more a problem of insufficient dosage rather than an inherent property of the agent (Stamey and Bragonzi, 1976). Its mode of action is unknown, but it is thought to interfere with DNA synthesis. Nalidixic acid is well absorbed from the gastrointestinal tract. The drug is rapidly inactivated by the liver so that much of it is excreted in an inactive form. One unique pediatric side effect has been the development of pseudotumor cerebri in some children administered this agent (Anderson et al., 1971). The recommended dose is 50 mg per kg per day administered orally in two to four divided doses (Vaughan and McKay, 1975).

METHENAMINE MANDELATE AND METHENAMINE HIPPURATE

These agents are readily absorbed from the gastrointestinal tract and remain inactive until they are excreted by the kidney and concentrated in the urine. Methenamine in an acid urine is converted to the bactericidal agent formaldehyde. Mandelic acid and hippuric acid are urinary acidifiers and have some inherent but weak antibacterial action. Both agents are of utility for suppressive therapy but are not particularly effective for therapy of acute infections. Their efficacy can be enhanced by supplementary urinary acidification, such as with ascorbic acid. Both agents can cause dysuria when administered in high doses, and methenamine mandelate has on rare occasion produced hemorrhagic cystitis in and of itself (Ross and Conway, 1970). The recommended dose for these agents is 40 to 50 mg per kg per day given orally in two to three divided doses (Vaughan and McKay, 1975).

PENICILLINS

The penicillins as a class are probably the most widely used of the antibiotics. They all share a basic nucleus. Modifications of the side chains have marked effects on absorption, resistance to acid destruction, resistance to penicillinase, and spectrum of activity (Goodman and Gilman, 1970). All penicillins act by blocking mucopeptide synthesis in the cell wall so that the bacterium is unprotected from its high internal osmotic pressure, causing cell lysis (Goodman and Gilman, 1970). This effect occurs only in growing cells. Because grampositive bacteria have relatively more mucopeptide in their cell walls and higher internal osmotic pressure than gram-negative bacteria, they are as a group more susceptible to the penicillins.

Penicillin G. Most gram-negative organisms are not susceptible to penicillin G as measured by standard disc assay. However, because penicillin G is rapidly excreted in urine by glomerular filtration and tubular secretion, extremely high urine levels can be achieved in patients with normal renal function, and the drug is very effective against *E. coli* and *Proteus* sp. (Stamey et al., 1965). Its major toxicity is allergy manifested by rashes or anaphylaxis; the mortality of the latter when it occurs is approximately 10 per cent.

Ampicillin. Ampicillin is the most widely used of the penicillins in treatment of urinary tract infection. Its gram-negative spectrum is excellent, probably because of better organism penetrance and resistance to gram-negative β-lactamase. It is an excellent agent for treatment of both cystitis and pyelonephritis. It is not well absorbed from the gastrointestinal tract, so that high fecal levels do occur and may produce diarrhea. This can prove a management problem, especially in infants. Because only 20 per cent is protein-bound, a high proportion of the absorbed dose is excreted in the urine by both filtration and secretion (Goodman and Gilman, 1970). Both serum and urine concentrations are achieved. There is cross reactivity between ampicillin and penicillin; consequently, this agent should not be administered to patients with a history of penicillin allergy. Another problem that is encountered in 25 per cent of women (and presumably girls) receiving ampicillin is the development of a secondary vulvovaginitis which may result in recrudescence of lower tract symptoms. The usual dose of ampicillin is 50 to 200 mg per kg per day given in divided doses every six to eight hours. This agent can be administered either orally or intravenously (Vaughan and McKay, 1975).

Amoxicillin. Amoxicillin is a derivative of ampicillin that has the advantage of producing less diarrhea because its gastrointestinal absorption is superior to that of ampicillin. It is slightly more expensive than ampicillin. This drug is administered orally in a dose of 20 mg per kg per day in divided doses (Vaughan and McKay, 1975).

Carbenicillin. Carbenicillin is an agent that is especially useful in the treatment of *Pseudomonas* and indole positive *Proteus* species. It is available as tablets or as a parenteral solution. When used parenterally for urinary tract infections in children, the usual dose is 50 to 200 mg per kg per 24 hrs given every four to six hours IM or IV (Vaughan and McKay, 1975). Unfortunately, it is somewhat expensive and, in our experience, has not been predictably effective as an oral agent.

CEPHALOSPORINS

Cephalosporins are agents that have proved highly effective in the management of urinary tract infections in children. Their mode of action is thought to be similar to that of the penicillins. Gastrointestinal absorption of most of the cephalosporins is poor, necessitating parenteral administration for many of the agents in this class. However, when appropriately administered, high tissue levels as well as high urine levels are achieved. Excretion is by both glomerular filtration and tubular secretion. These agents are usually effective against most of the gram-negative and gram-positive pathogens. Although there can be some cross reactivity in patients who are allergic to penicillin, in general, these agents can be cautiously administered to patients with a penicillin allergy. In other regards, they are relatively nontoxic. Those agents of greatest utility are cefazolin, cephalothin, cephaprin, and cephalexin. Cefazolin is administered parenterally in a dose of 25 to 50 mg per kg per day either IM or IV. Cephalothin is administered in a dose of 80 to 160 mg per kg per day either IM or IV. Cephaprin is used in a dose of 40 to 80 mg per kg per day in four divided doses IV or IM. Cephalexin is well absorbed from the gastrointestinal tract. Hence, it can be administered orally in a dose of 25 to 100 mg per kg per day in four divided doses and is an excellent choice for treatment of the febrile child with presumed pyelonephritis produced by an ampicillin-resistant organism (Vaughan and McKay, 1975).

AMINOGLYCOSIDES

The aminoglycosides are agents that are well tolerated by children and are of special utility in the treatment of difficult urinary tract infections. They interfere with protein synthesis by binding proteins of the bacterial ribosomes. The bacterial cells misread the messenger-RNA codons and rapidly die. The aminoglycoside spectrum is largely gram-negative.

Table 3-3. Antimicrobial Agents — Use in Renal Failure

| | Maintenance Dose Intervals | | | | Significant Dialysis of Drug‡ | EHL, hr‡ | Toxic Effects °Remarks |
| | | Renal Failure† | | | | | |
Drug	Normal	Mild	Moderate	Severe			
Amphotericin B°	Q24h	Q24h	Q24h	Q24-36h (×1.5)	No (H)	Nonrenal 18-24	Nephrotoxic, renal tubular-acidosis, hypokalemia °Blood level essential for optimal therapy
Cephalosporins Cephalexin	Q6h	Q6h	Q6-12h (×2)	Q18-24h° (×3-4)	Yes (HP)	Renal (extra-renal) 0.6-1	°May be ineffective for urinary tract infections
Cephaloglycin	Q6h	U	U	U°	No (P)	Renal Hepatic	°May be ineffective for urinary tract infections
Cephaloridine	Q6h°	Q6h	Q12h (×2)	Q24-36h (×4-6)	Yes (HP)	Renal 1.5	Nephrotoxic °Dose should be limited to less than 4 gm/day
Clindamycin	Q6h	Q6h	Q6h	Q6h	No (HP)	Hepatic (Renal) 2	—
Chloroquine°	Q24h	U	U	U°°	?	Nonrenal 48	°Refers only to dose for uncomplicated *Plasmodium vivax* °°For prolonged treatment, cut dose
Colistimethate	Q12h	Q24h (×2)	Q36-60h (×3-5)	Q60-90h (×5-8)	Yes (P) No (H)	Renal 1.5-2	Nephrotoxic, peripheral neuropathy, respiratory paralysis; toxicity probably unrelated to dosage
Ethambutol	Q24h	Q24h	Q24-36h (×1.5)	Q48h (×2)	?	Renal 6-8	Decreased visual acuity
Gentamicin	Q8h	Q8-12h (×1.5)	Q12-24h (×1.5-3)	Q48h° (×6)	Yes (H) No (P)	Renal 2	Ototoxic, nephrotoxic, respiratory paralysis; incidence less than with colistin or kanamycin °Specific formula available
Nalidixic acid	Q8h	U	U	U	?	Renal° 1.5-2	°Inactive nontoxic metabolites accumulate

Drug					Dialysis	Excretion (EHL)	Toxicity / Comments
Neomycin	Q6h	Q6h	Q12h (×2)	Q18–24h* (×3–4)	Yes (H) No (P)	Renal 2	Nephrotoxic, ototoxic, respiratory paralysis; *May be absorbed better in cirrhotic patients
Nitrofurantoin	Q8h	Q8h	Q8h	Avoid*	Yes (H)	Renal 0.3	Peripheral neuritis, pulmonary fibrosis; *Ineffective
Pentamidine	Q24h	Q24h	Q24h	Q48h (×2)	?	Renal*	*Fixed in renal tissue, may cause direct toxicity
Penicillins*	–	–	–	–	–	–	*All agents in this group may cause allergic interstitial nephritis; convulsion may occur with very high blood levels
Carbenicillin	Q4h	Q4h	Q6–12h (×1.5–3)	Q12–16h (×3–4)	Yes (HP)**	Renal Hepatic 1.5	*Group toxicity; **May add to peritoneal dialysate at desired serum level (eg, 100 µg/ml); Coagulopathy, acidosis at high blood levels
Cloxacillin	Q6h	U	U	U	No (H)	Hepatic Renal 0.5	*Group toxicity
Dicloxacillin	Q6h	U	U	U	No (H)	Renal Hepatic 0.5	*Group toxicity
Nafcillin	Q6h	U	U	U	No (H)	Hepatic 0.5	*Group toxicity
Rifampin	Q24h	U	U	U	?	Hepatic 1.5	–
Tetracyclines Doxycycline	Q12–24h	U	U*	U*	No (HP)	Renal Hepatic 8	Group drug of choice for extrarenal infections in patients with renal disease; *Not useful in urinary tract infections
Minocycline	Q12h	U*	Q8–24h** (×1.5–2)	Q24–36h** (×2–3)	?	Hepatic 8	*Not useful in urinary tract infections; **Antianabolic; increases BUN; potentiates acidosis

†U indicates unchanged.

‡H indicates hemodialysis; P, peritoneal hemodialysis. EHL indicates excretion or inactivation normal half-life in hours.

(From Bennett, W. N., Singer, I., and Collins, C. H.: Guide to drug usage in adult patients with impaired renal function. J.A.M.A., 223:991, 1973.)

Gentamicin. Gentamicin is probably the most widely used of these agents in children. It has a wide gram-negative spectrum and is especially useful against *Pseudomonas*. The usual dose is 3 to 6 mg per kg per day IM or IV in two to three divided doses (Vaughan and McKay, 1975). As is true of all the aminoglycosides, it is cleared by glomerular filtration. It is widely distributed in body tissues. It can be ototoxic, particularly to the vestibular cells, especially with high serum levels. Ototoxicity is noted in about two per cent of patients. Nephrotoxicity occurs in three to six per cent of patients and is manifested by proteinuria and elevated serum creatinine. Nephrotoxicity is especially frequent when combinations of gentamicin and cephalosporins are employed (Bennett). Both ototoxicity and nephrotoxicity are usually transient but unfortunately occasionally may be permanent.

Kanamycin. Kanamycin has the same spectrum as gentamicin but is less effective against *Pseudomonas*. Although it can be given intravenously, such use often results in thrombophlebitis. Additionally, compatibility with intravenous fluids is often a problem. Hence, it is usually given intramuscularly in a dose of 6 to 15 mg per kg per day in two doses. Although available as a capsule, it is not absorbed from the gastrointestinal tract. When used in high doses or for prolonged periods, it may also be ototoxic and can cause deafness. Additionally, it can cause neuromuscular blockade in anesthetized patients. Nephrotoxicity may also occur with this agent.

Tobramycin. A newer aminoglycoside, tobramycin, has the advantage of particular efficacy against *Pseudomonas*. Its dosage and toxicity are the same as those of gentamicin, but it is said to be less nephrotoxic than gentamicin.

TETRACYCLINES

Tetracyclines should be avoided in children under eight years whenever possible because they stain the permanent teeth. The need for their use is extremely unusual in modern-day practice because so many other agents are available. However, in the unusual situation in which their use is indicated, they can be administered in a dose of 25 to 50 mg per kg per day divided into four doses (Vaughan and McKay, 1975). They act by inhibiting the enzyme aminoacyl transferase and RNA from binding to ribosomal receptor sites, thereby inhibiting protein synthesis (Goodman and Gilman, 1970).

CHLORAMPHENICOL

Chloramphenicol is an agent that has the advantage of being excreted completely by the liver; consequently, it can be used in full dosage in urinary tract infection and renal failure. However, its major side effect is aplastic anemia, and for that reason it should be used only in very specific situations and then only when dictated by sensitivity tests. When necessary, it is used in a dose of 25 to 50 mg per kg per 24 hr in four divided doses.

TREATMENT IN RENAL FAILURE

The dynamics of antibiotic detoxification and excretion are usually deranged in the child with renal failure. Hence, antibiotic doses need to be adjusted in such patients to avoid adverse reactions. Certain drugs, those that depend on renal function for their efficacy, are useless in these patients. With those drugs that are effective in renal impairment, the frequency of administration rather than the amount administered is the factor most often in need of modification. Table 3–3 provides a guide to drug therapy in renal failure.

ANTIBIOTIC COST

Another factor in drug selection is cost. Table 3–4 provides a cost comparison of antibiotics, but because drug costs vary widely and geographically, this is intended

Table 3–4. Outpatient Antibiotic Cost Comparison

DRUG	AVERAGE ORAL DOSE*	DAILY COST (TABLETS OR CAPSULES)**
Ampicillin	250 mg q 6 h (1 gm/day)	$ .55
Amoxicillin	250 mg q 8 h (750 mg/day)	1.20
Sulfisoxazole	500 mg q 6 h (2 gm/day)	.12
Trimeth/Sulfa	2 tabs q 12 h (4 tabs/day)	.68
Cephalexin	250 mg q 6 h (1 gm/day)	4.00
Tetracycline	500 mg q 6 h (2 gm/day)	.24
Carbenicillin	382 mg q 6 h (1528 mg/day)	5.20
Nitrofurantoin	50 mg q 6 h (200 mg/day)	1.60
Penicillin VK	250 mg q 6 h (2 gm/day)	.24
Dicloxacillin	250 mg q 6 h (1 gm/day)	.60
Erythromycin	250 mg q 6 h (1 gm/day)	.72
Clindamycin	150 mg q 6 h (600 mg/day)	2.35

*For fully grown teenager. The dosages listed are given primarily for comparative purposes. These doses are not offered as a guide to therapy, which should be individualized for each patient.

**Suspension may be more than twice as expensive, depending on the drug.

Modified from Children's Hospital Medical Center (Boston) Bacteriology-Epidemiology Newsletter 5:6, 1978.

only as a guide to relative, not absolute, cost.

PREVENTION

The only reliable means of preventing urinary tract infection in the susceptible individual is with continuous antibacterial prophylaxis. Nevertheless, in some patients a few simple steps can be carried out to help reduce the incidence of recurrences.

HYGIENE

As indicated previously, much has been made in the past of perineal hygiene. It would seem that this is an inconsequential problem. However, it must be emphsized that some mothers are unduly compulsive, and it is suspected strongly that vulvitis is produced in some children by overzealous attempts at perineal cleansing. It is our practice to suggest to such mothers that the area be left completely alone. If there is evidence of vulvar irritation, soothing sitz baths in bicarbonate or colloidal oatmeal solutions are occasionally of benefit. Another adjunct is the use of bland ointments, sometimes with steroids added, to protect the irritated perineum.

CONSTIPATION

There does seem to be some relationship between constipation and genesis and perpetuation of urinary tract infection; for this reason, an attempt is made in those children in whom this history is elicited to improve their defecatory habits with the use of high-fiber diets. These diets are at variance to that of most American children, and many simply will not tolerate them. However, many new cereals high in fiber are available and are quite palatable. In instances in which a change in bowel habits is felt to be of importance and dietary manipulation fails, mineral oil in large doses is utilized. If mineral oil is used, the children need a supplement of B vitamins to assure that they do not become depleted of these substances. Enemas and suppositories may be necessary during the early phases of emptying an overdistended bowel. However, their long-term use is to be avoided as these may further irritate the perineum and consequently may lead to further voiding dysfunction.

PINWORMS

Pinworm infestation, by producing perineal irritation, is occasionally incriminated in the genesis of urinary tract infection.

Where this is indeed the case, such infestations are appropriately treated. Rarely the worms themselves may be identified. However, usually one must actually seek out eggs using the Scotch Tape test (Vaughan and McKay, 1975).

Clothing

Some authors have recommended the avoidance of nylon panties and tight-fitting clothing. We would put this in the same category as changes in perineal hygiene and cannot really see the rationale for this recommendation. It is true that occasionally a child will present with sham syndrome (p. 64) secondary to contact dermatitis to some new article of clothing, but this situation is usually quite evident.

Urinary Analgesics

We do not generally recommend phenazopyridine (Pyridium) for children with dysuria for two reasons. Firstly, the azo dye stains clothing and sheets. Secondly, they are potentially toxic compounds as the tablets are not dividable and overdosage may result in methemoglobinemia. For those children who hold back voiding because of dysuria, sitz baths are often beneficial in promoting urination. The use of catheterization to empty the bladder in this situation is unnecessary and may provoke further dysuria and fear; it only compounds the problem. If the bladder must be emptied, suprapubic aspiration or an indwelling catheter for several days is preferable.

Hydration

It is often suggested that fluid intake be increased in children with urinary tract infection to dilute the bacterial concentration and to increase urinary frequency. If the child is cooperative, so much the better, but often the child will not cooperate with attempts to increase fluid intake. In those children with acute pyelonephritis who are quite ill, hydration and diuresis can be maintained intravenously.

Frequent voiding may be beneficial in reducing bladder bacterial concentration if the bladder is completely emptied. Once again, one has to be somewhat practical. This is an adjunct that can be utilized well in the older cooperative child, but the younger child often simply will not cooperate with this regimen, and for that reason it is best avoided.

Urinary Acidification

Urinary acidification is of adjunctive value because bacterial growth is inhibited by an acid urine. Acidification is best achieved with ascorbic acid tablets 250 mg several times a day, cranberry juice several times daily, or methenamine several times daily. However, acidification alone is not successful as treatment.

SPECIFIC THERAPY

Our approach to the treatment of these children is pragmatic. In the asymptomatic child, we await the result of the urine culture prior to initiation of treatment. If the culture was carried out by office techniques or if the colony count is below 10^5 organisms, a repeat culture should be done before medication is prescribed.

In the child with isolated lower urinary tract symptoms and a positive urinalysis, treatment is begun after collection of a fresh specimen, which is then appropriately handled. Our preference is to employ sulfa, sulfa-trimethoprim, or nitrofurantoin rather than one of the synthetic penicillins for initial therapy. The length of treatment does not appear to be very significant; more than one week of therapy in those children with cystitis alone is probably not necessary. Reculture after 48 to 72 hours of treatment establishes an appropriate response to treatment. Radiographic evaluation is then recommended as previously indicated.

Those children who present with a febrile urinary tract infection (≥100°F P.O.) but who are otherwise relatively well, able to take oral fluids, and not dehydrated are started on ampicillin, amoxicillin, or cephalexin until the results of the culture return. These offer the multiple advantages of an oral bactericidal drug. Cephalexin is used in the child who has had previous treatment for urinary tract infection and in whom penicillin resistance is anticipated. Follow-up culture is performed to ensure response. After 10 days of treatment, therapy is changed to one of the urinary antiseptics recommended for cystitis alone. These are administered as low-dose prophylaxis until radiographic studies of the urinary tract are performed four to six weeks later. The likelihood that an abnormality will be found in this group approaches 50 per cent; therefore, recurrences should be prevented until evaluation is completed, if possible.

Those children with febrile urinary tract infections who are obviously septic, dehydrated, or vomiting should be hospitalized. Our first choice of drugs is an intravenous aminoglycoside. It is possible that renal damage may be minimized if aminoglycoside therapy is started immediately (Ransley). Blood and urine cultures as well as any other appropriate bacteriologic studies should be obtained prior to starting therapy. Urine for culture is collected by catheterization or suprapubic aspiration, if necessary.

Treatment with appropriate bactericidal medication should be maintained for 10 days. Complete uroradiographic evaluation in this group is essential. Prior to hospital discharge, an excretory urogram or renal scan should be obtained to rule out obstruction. If negative, cystography can be delayed for several weeks as long as the child is maintained on suppressive medication.

In children with frequently occurring lower urinary tract infections, cystitis follicularis, or vesicoureteral reflux, long-term antibacterial suppressive medication is indicated. A low dose of the least expensive, least toxic, and best tolerated medication is recommended. Sulfisoxazole 500 mg twice a day, nitrofurantoin 25 mg twice a day or at bedtime, or trimethoprim 50 mg and sulfamethoxazole 400 mg at bedtime may suffice. Urine culture is advisable every three to four months while the child is maintained on such medication.

CLINICAL EXAMPLES

To best illustrate the application of the foregoing material, let us utilize some specific clinical examples:

Acute Pyelonephritis. A three-month-old infant presents with a temperature of 104° and no other symptoms. Examination in the office reveals no localizing findings. Urine obtained from a clean, bagged specimen contains 15 to 20 WBC/HPF and 4+ bacteriuria. A catheterized specimen is obtained and is immediately cultured. Because clinical judgment suggests that this child can be treated as an outpatient, amoxicillin is administered orally in a dose of 20 mg per kg per day in four divided doses. The mother is given a supply sufficient for 10 days. The child is next seen 48 hours later. If the child is then well, another urine specimen is obtained for repeat culture to prove that therapy has been effective. The patient is again seen 14 days after the onset of illness for reexamination and urine culture to prove that therapy was successful. Sulfisoxazole three times a day is then started as prophylaxis, and urinary radiographs, which demonstrate bilateral vesicoureteral reflux, are taken four weeks later.

To vary this example somewhat let us say this child was initially seen at 10 A.M. That evening the mother calls back, stating that the child is now vomiting and is unable to retain the medication. At that time, arrangements are made for admission to the hospital, and an aminoglycoside is administered intravenously. The repeat culture is obtained at 48 hours, and if the child is afebrile, tolerates feedings well, and the urine is now sterile, therapy is converted to appropriate bactericidal oral medication, and the child is discharged 48 hours later. Follow-up care continues as described before.

Acute Cystitis. A four-year-old girl presents with a two-day history of dysuria, day wetting, secondary enuresis, and a tinge of blood on the toilet tissue after voiding. Her temperature is 99° and she outwardly appears quite well. Previous urologic evaluation has been negative. Examination reveals a small postvoiding residual as determined by palpation and percussion. Rectal examination reveals a large mass of hard stool in her rectal ampulla. A clean-catch midstream urine specimen contains 30 to 40 WBC/HPF, 5 to 8 RBC/HPF and 4+ bacteriuria. This urine is submitted for culture and sensitivity, and the child is given sulfisoxazole in a dose of 150 mg per kg per 24 hrs in three divided doses. The mother is instructed to have the child sit in a tub of warm water with 4 to 5 T of baking soda in the water for 10 minutes four times a day. She is asked to attempt to increase the child's fluid intake without this becoming an odious task. Phenazopyridine is not utilized. The mother is instructed that the child should become asymptomatic within 24 to 48 hours. She should continue the medication for 10 days, and a repeat culture should be obtained in approximately two weeks. If the child is not asymptomatic promptly, the child is reevaluated, and the urine is recultured at 48 hours.

Sham Syndrome. The previously described patient is improved at 48 hours, but the culture has proved to be sterile. Medication is discontinued, although the adjunctive measures are continued, and the child is kept under observation.

Chronic Cystitis. A seven-year-old girl is seen with a history of multiple episodes of urinary tract infection, all manifested by lower tract symptoms. Evaluation has included cystoscopy, which has demonstrated cystitis follicularis (cystitis cystica). At the time of cystoscopy, it was seen that the trigone was grossly elevated by a large mass of stool in the rectal ampulla. The child is placed on six to 12 months therapy with nitrofurantoin 25 mg twice a day and is given 1 T of mineral oil every morning with instructions to have a bowel movement every evening. A B-complex vitamin is ad-

ministered in the evening. The child's urine is surveyed at six-week to three-month intervals while on medication to ascertain that her urine is indeed remaining sterile. If her urine has remained sterile for six to 12 months, medication is withdrawn and the urine is recultured. If the child promptly becomes reinfected, suppressive therapy is once again instituted for another 12 months. Once the child has achieved regular, soft stools at predictable intervals, the mineral oil is withdrawn.

URINARY TRACT TUBERCULOSIS

Urinary tract tuberculosis, although uncommon in the United States, is still seen with sufficient frequency to warrant discussion. Modern therapy is largely chemotherapeutic, but surgical intervention occasionally may be required. The agents of greatest utility include isoniazid, para-aminosalicylic acid (PAS), ethambutol, streptomycin, and rifampin (Medical Letter, 1977). Isoniazid 10 to 20 mg per kg per day (maximum dose per day 500 mg) is usually included in treatment regimens but can be neurotoxic. Pyridoxine is usually given concomitantly to prevent isoniazid-induced pyridoxine deficiencies.

PAS can cause gastrointestinal upsets, and patients may need up to 24 tablets daily. Consequently, it has been largely replaced by ethambutol 15 to 25 mg per kg per day. This drug can cause optic neuritis, which may be detected by repeated examination of visual and color acuity. The other mainstays of antituberculosis therapy are streptomycin and rifampin. Streptomycin must be given by injection and can cause vestibular damage. Hence, rifampin in a dose of 10 to 20 mg per kg per day, 600 mg per day maximum, is usually substituted for streptomycin. Other drugs of benefit but with significant toxicity include pyrazinamide, ethionamide, cycloserine, viomycin, kanamycin, and capreomycin. It has been suggested that steroids be administered early in the course of the treatment of urogenital tuberculosis to prevent the formation of ureteral strictures (Claridge, 1970), but there is little experience with this modality. In all likelihood, it would not be harmful and might indeed be of some benefit.

GONORRHEA

Confirmation of the diagnosis of genital gonorrhea is made by immediate culture on Thayer-Martin medium. If immediate inoculation is not possible, transport in an anaerobic medium is recommended. We have had success using a standard Culturette,* however.

Treatment of genitourinary gonorrhea in children has not been standardized. The recommendations of the Center for Disease Control published in 1975 are noted in Table 3–5.

NONBACTERIAL INFECTIONS

VIRAL INFECTION

Although viruses (for example, rubella virus) can be cultured from neonatal kidneys at autopsy, there is no evidence to suggest that there are any clinical situations in which there are viral upper urinary tract infections. Consequently, the use of antiviral agents (for example, ARA-G) are not of clinical importance. Viral infections of the lower urinary tract do occur but are self-limited and require no specific therapy.

FUNGAL INFECTIONS

Candidal infections of the urinary tract are becoming more common, especially in neonates who have been treated for respira-

*Scientific Products, American Hospital Supply Corp.

Table 3–5. Recommended Treatment Schedule for Gonococcal Infection in Pediatric Patients

Uncomplicated vulvovaginitis and urethritis:
  75,000 to 100,000 units/kg. aqueous procaine penicillin G intramuscularly, 25 mg./kg. probenecid orally
  Patients allergic to penicillin < 6 yrs. old — 40 mg./kg./day erythromycin in 4 doses for 7 days; >6 yrs. old — 25 mg./kg. tetracycline initially then 40 to 60 mg./kg./day in 7 doses for 7 days
Complicated infections:
  75,000 to 100,000 units/kg./day aqueous crystalline penicillin G intravenously in 4 doses for 7 days or
  75,000 to 100,000 units/kg./day procaine penicillin G intramuscularly in 2 doses for 7 days
  Pts. allergic to penicillin <6 yrs. old — 60 to 80 mg./kg./day cephalothin in 4 doses for 7 days; >6 yrs. old — 60 to 80 mg./kg./day cephalothin or 15 to 20 mg./kg./day tetracycline in 4 doses for 7 days

(From J. Ped., 86:794, 1975.)

tory distress in neonatal intensive care units. These are usually blood-borne and manifest themselves as a candidal septicemia. Unrecognized, these can result in the formation of fungous balls in the upper urinary tract. Therapy for these children is directed toward their underlying disease, but the finding of *Candida* in the urine of an infant is not something to be taken lightly. Since most such infections are indeed systemic, they are best treated with amphotericin B intravenously in a dose of 0.25 mg per kg per day, increasing the dose level to 1 to 1.5 mg per kg per day. As an alternative, a newer agent, 5-fluorocytosine, can be administered orally in a dose of 250 mg per kg. Yet a newer (but as yet unavailable) agent is chlortrimazole. This, too, is administered orally in a dose of 100 mg per kg per day in four divided doses.

Adjuncts to the therapy of fungal infections of the urinary tract occasionally include direct instillation of antifungal agents into the urinary tract. Bladder irrigation with amphotericin solution may suffice for candidal cystitis. When fungous balls are present, it may be necessary to irrigate the upper urinary tract. Although it is often possible to do this through an indwelling catheter in the adult, in the child if this is to be accomplished, it usually necessitates placement of a nephrostomy tube (Keller et al., 1977).

Schistosomiasis

The major parasite that affects the urinary tract is *Schistosoma haematobium.* Fortunately, this is not seen in this country; it is endemic in Egypt. Antimony compounds, such as stibophen (antimony sodium dimercaptosuccinate) in a dose of 8 mg per kg IM once or twice a week for five doses, are somewhat effective and are the only agents readily available in this country for the treatment of this disorder. The drug of choice is niridazole in a dose of 25 mg per kg per day orally for five to seven days. This drug is available from the Center for Disease Control (Medical Letter, 1978).

Trichomoniasis

Treatment of trichomonal vaginitis, urethritis, cystitis, and prostatovesiculitis has been revolutionized with metronidazole (Flagyl). However, there has been some recent concern in reference to the carcinogenic and mutagenic side effects of this drug (Medical Letter, 1975).

Nonspecific Urethritis

All forms of urethritis not proved to be gonococcal in origin are referred to as nonspecific urethritis. *Chlamydia trachomatis* and T mycoplasma are suspected as being causative agents. Treatment with tetracycline hydrochloride 500 mg four times daily for seven days is effective in most cases. Nonresponders should be evaluated for *Trichomonas vaginalis.*

REFERENCES

AMA Drug Evaluations. Chicago, 1971, p. 423.

Anderson, E. E., Anderson, B., Jr., and Nashold, B. S.: Childhood complication of nalidixic acid. J.A.M.A., *216*:1023, 1971.

Belman, A. B.: The clinical significance of cystitis cystica in girls. Results of a prospective study. J. Urol., *118*:661, 1978.

Bennett, W. M.: Personal communication.

Claridge, M.: Ureteric obstruction in tuberculosis. Br. J. Urol., *42*:688, 1970.

Drugs for parasitic infection. The Medical Letter, *20*:17, 1978.

Drugs for treatment of tuberculosis. The Medical Letter, *19*:97, 1977.

Fang, L. S. T., Tolkoff-Rubin, N. E., and Rubin, R. H.: Efficacy of single-dose and conventional amoxicillin therapy in urinary tract infection localized by the antibody-coated bacteria technique. N. Engl. J. Med., *298*:413, 1978.

Feingold, D. S.: Antimicrobial chemotherapeutic agents: The nature of their action and selective toxicity. N. Engl. J. Med., *269*:900, 1963.

Goodman, L. S., and Gilman, A.: The Pharmacological Basis of Therapeutics, 4th ed., New York, MacMillan Co., 1970.

Howard, J. B., and Howard, J. E.: Trimethoprim-sulfamethoxazole vs. sulfamethoxazole for acute urinary tract infections in children. Am. J. Dis. Child., *132*:1085, 1978.

Is Flagyl dangerous? The Medical Letter, *20*:13, 1975.

Keller, M. A., Sellers, B. B. Jr., Melish, M. E., Kaplan, G. W., Miller, K. E., and Mendoza, S. A.: Systemic candidiasis. Am. J. Dis. Child., *131*:1260, 1977.

Kunin, C. M.: Detection, Prevention and Management of Urinary Tract Infection. Philadelphia, Lea and Febiger, 1972, pp. 56, 153.

Lincoln, K., Lidin-Janson, G., and Winberg, J.: Treatment trials in urinary tract infection with special reference to the effect of antibiotics on the faecal flora. *In* Kincaid-Smith, P., and Fairly, K. F.: Renal Infection and Renal Scarring. Melbourne, Mercedes Publishing Services, 1970.

Ransley, P.: Personal communication.

Ross, R. R., Jr., and Conway, G. F.: Hemorrhage cystitis following accidental overdose of methenamine mandelate. Am. J. Dis. Child., *119*:86, 1970.

Salvaggio, J., and Gonzalez, F.: Severe toxic reactions associated with sulfamethoxypyridazine (Kynex). Ann. Intern. Med., *51*:60, 1959.

Stamey, T. A., and Bragonzi, J.: Resistance to nalidixic acid. A misconception due to underdosage. J.A.M.A., *236*:1857, 1976.

Stamey, T. A., and Condy, M.: The diffusion and concentration of trimethoprim in human vaginal fluid. J. Infect. Dis., *131*:261–266, 1975.

Stamey, T. A., Govan, D. E., and Palmer, J. M.: The localization and treatment of urinary tract infections: The role of bactericidal urine levels as opposed to serum levels. Medicine, *44*:1, 1965.

Vaughan, V. C., III, and McKay, R. J.: Nelson's Textbook of Pediatrics, 10th ed. Philadelphia, W. B. Saunders Co., 1975.

Winberg, J., quoted by Stamey, T. A.: Urinary Infections. Baltimore, Williams & Wilkins Co., 1972, pp. 124–125.

Chapter Four

VESICOURETERAL
REFLUX

HISTORY

Protecting the kidneys from the potential ravages of bacterial infections is the raison d'etre for the intact antireflux ureterovesical junction. Recognition of the importance of the anatomic relationship between the ureter and bladder dates back in published literature at least to Paré (1575), although Bell (1912) is often credited, and then, more recently, to the early part of this century with studies by Sampson (quoted by Stephens and Lenaghan, 1962). In 1924 Bumpus performed cystography in more than 1000 patients, identifying an incidence of reflux in 8.6 per cent of the general urologic population. At about the same time, Gruber (1929) carried out experimental studies in various laboratory animals, discovering that reflux was not an uncommon finding and in some rodents appeared to be normal. Although a correlation was noted between the degree of anatomic development of the trigone and the predictability of reflux, the clinical importance of the prevention of retrograde flow of urine from the bladder to the ureters and collecting system in humans was not appreciated.

Meredith F. Campbell, the father of pediatric urology, appreciated the simplicity of retrograde cystography as a diagnostic tool as early as 1930 and advocated its use on a regular clinical basis in children. He was also keenly aware of the risk of performing cystograms in children with active urinary tract infections and the likelihood of provoking secondary sepsis by forcing bacteria into the kidneys. The choice between gaining information of poorly understood disease outlined radiographically (reflux) and the risk of making the child sicker by virtue of the investigation put the clinician of that generation into very difficult straits. Antireflux surgery had not been developed, antibiotic therapy was in its infancy, and there was little appreciation of the danger of infected bladder urine continuously seeding the renal collecting system.

A quiescent period followed, and it was not until the early 1950s that reflux again achieved appreciable recognition. J. A. Hutch recorded reflux in adults with acquired neurogenic pathologic conditions (1952). Distortion of the ureterovesical junction by an adjacent diverticular outpouching in this group of patients was thought to be a significant causal factor (Fig. 4–1). In addition, renal deterioration secondary to infection and reflux reawakened an interest in vesicoureteral reflux in children. In 1955 Hutch and colleagues reported the first series of antireflux surgery in children.

Unfortunately, the discovery of reflux in patients with neurogenic disease added a perspective to the problem that then took years to resolve. The acquired paraureteral

67

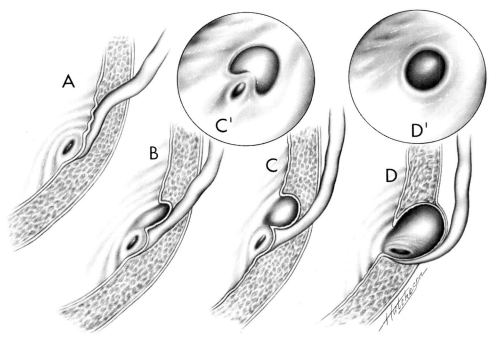

Figure 4–1. Development of paraureteral saccule or diverticulum leading to displacement of submucosal and intramural ureter with subsequent loss of the muscular support and resultant incompetence of the ureterovesical angle. The ureteral orifice can be displaced within the diverticulum and lost to cystoscopic view. (From Kelalis, P. P., King, L. R., and Belman, A. B.: Clinical Pediatric Urology, Vol. 1. Philadelphia, W. B. Saunders Co., 1976, p. 283.)

diverticulum reported by Hutch (1952) that distorted the ureterovesical junction was the consequence of secondary bladder outlet obstruction in those with neurogenic disease. Similar diverticula adjacent to the intravesical ureter also occur on a congenital basis and contribute to reflux in some children. However, bladder outlet obstruction is not present in this group. Unfortunately, whether it was the coexistence of paraureteral diverticula and reflux in the segment of the pediatric population first studied or the persistent desire of urologists to explain most urinary problems on the basis of obstruction, an era was ushered in that lasted, in some regions, for two decades. During that period the demonstration of vesicoureteral reflux was taken as prima facie evidence of bladder outlet obstruction (Stewart, 1961). The natural outcome was that surgical correction of the problem revolved around revision of the bladder neck by transurethral resection or, more commonly, by Y-V plasty (Fig. 4–2). This was done either as a first-stage procedure in the correction of reflux or as a combined ap-

proach. Although others attempted to suggest that reflux was not always associated with obstruction, most believed it was a major contributing cause (Garrett et al., 1962).

Bladder neck obstruction became an epidemic disease, its existence "objective-

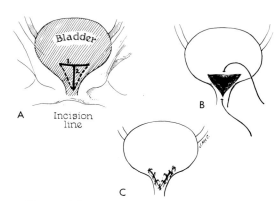

Figure 4–2. Operative technique of Y-V vesicourethroplasty: normal bladder is interspersed between disrupted "obstructive ring." (From Kaplan, G. W., and King, L. R.: An evaluation of Y-V vesicourethroplasty in children. Surg. Gynecol. Obstet., *130*:1059–1066, 1970. Reproduced by permission of Surgery, Gynecology, and Obstetrics.)

ly" verified by the presence of bladder trabeculation noted endoscopically and relative narrowing of the bladder outlet seen on voiding urethrography in girls. Unfortunately, unrecognized at the time was the ubiquity of fine to mild bladder trabeculation on endoscopic evaluation in children when compared to adults and the poor correlation between urethral appearance on voiding urethrography in girls and the actual measured urethral size. Also absent at the time was an understanding of the idiopathic nature of childhood lower urinary tract infections. Therefore, many children with vesicoureteral reflux and urinary tract infection had bladder neck revision in association with ureteral reimplantation on an empiric basis in an effort to control both infection and reflux. Each was thought to be secondary to a degree of outlet obstruction and, to that degree, interdependent.

Fortunately, pediatric urology has matured over the last 20 years, and concerted efforts have been made to better understand the natural history of the various pathologic processes involved. This is probably most true in the case of vesicoureteral reflux. Whereas the relatively high incidence of reflux in children and its relative rarity in adults could be interpreted as evidence of the seriousness of the problem — that children with reflux do not survive until adulthood — the high degree of spontaneous resolution of vesicoureteral reflux began to be appreciated in the mid-1960s (Baker et al, 1966). The purpose of this chapter is to acquaint the primary physician with the concepts underlying the treatment of the patient with vesicoureteral reflux.

THE URETEROVESICAL JUNCTION

The prevention of vesicoureteral reflux is dependent upon the configuration of the ureterovesical junction. Multiple factors come into play. The extravesical ureter extending from the ureteropelvic junction to the ureteral hiatus at the bladder is comprised of musculature that pursues an intertwining course. As the ureter passes through the hiatus at the bladder wall (Wal-

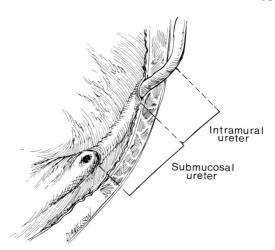

Figure 4-3. Normal ureterovesical junction. (From Harrison, J. H., Gittes, R. F., Perlmutter, A. D., et al.: Campbell's Urology, Vol. 2, 4th ed. Philadelphia, W. B. Saunders Co., 1979, p. 1597.)

deyer's space), it becomes the intravesical ureter. At this junction, the direction of the ureteral muscle becomes more longitudinal with an increased concentration of fibers on the floor of the intravesical ureter. These longitudinal muscles continue beyond the ureteral orifice to become part of the superficial trigone and then into the bladder neck. The result is fixation of the distal ureter at the base of the bladder. From its entrance at the muscular hiatus to its orifice, the ureter pursues a submucosal course, commonly called the submucosal tunnel. It is this segment of ureter, measuring only about 1 cm in length, that seems to be most influential in the prevention of reflux (Fig. 4-3).

THE ANTIREFLUX MECHANISM

The earliest understanding of the antireflux mechanism was based on the appreciation of a simple principle. The submucosal ureter, with its sparse muscular roof, is compressed against the bladder muscle, which supports its floor during increased intravesical pressure (voiding), effectively closing it — like stepping on a straw. This flap valve mechanism is most certainly responsible for the absence of demonstrable reflux in cadavers and, in all likelihood, plays a role in life too. The ratio of distal ureteral diameter to submucosal tunnel length is quite significant in the prevention of vesicoureteral reflux. In the normal urinary tract, this ratio of width to length is 1:5, whereas in a group with reflux it was found by Paquin (1960) to be only 1:1.4. Assuming that the point of entrance of the ureter at the muscular hiatus is fairly constant in humans, the more lateral the orifice position, the shorter will be the submucosal tunnel and the more likely will be reflux (Fig. 4–4).

Fixation of the ureter at the trigone by the incorporation of its extended longitudinal fibers makes the intravesical portion relatively immobile during voiding. This may be of greatest importance in preventing reflux when intravesical pressure is exceptionally high. Finally, Stephens and Lenaghan (1962) noted that the degree of devel-

opment (maturation?) of the longitudinal muscles of the most distal ureter contributes to its competency. Contraction of these muscles conveys the bolus of urine, flattens the ureter, and closes its lumen behind that bolus. The decreasing incidence of reflux with age supports the concept of some maturational or growth process being involved.

EMBRYOLOGY*

The budding of the ureter from the wolffian duct near its cloacal junction is an extremely significant step in the development of the urinary tract (Fig. 4–5). Formation of the kidney is dependent upon this bud stimulating the nephrogenic elements. Division of the cloaca by the urorectal septum, budding of the ureter, and development of the lower spine all occur during the fifth to sixth gestational week.

With further growth, the distal wolffian duct is absorbed into the base of the bladder, playing an important role in the formation of the internal male genitalia, forming the ipsilateral prostate, seminal vesicle, and ejaculatory duct. The remnants of the wolffian duct in females, which is completely resorbed at about the tenth week, is called Gartner's canal (or duct).

The distal ureter becomes incorporated into the base of the bladder as part of the absorption of the wolffian duct, accounting for the intravesical location of the ureteral orifices (Fig. 4–6). Failure of complete incorporation of the ureteral bud into the bladder base results in a juxtavesical or extravesical location of the ureteral orifice. Predictable extravesical ectopic locations include the bladder neck or urethra in either sex, prostate or seminal vesicle in males, and along the course of Gartner's duct in females (Fig. 4–7).

In duplication of the collecting system,

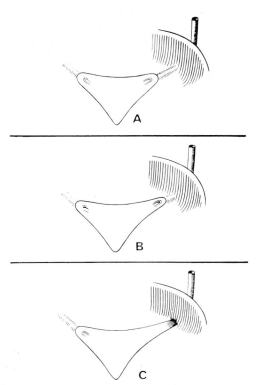

Figure 4–4. Drawings of trigone and ureter to demonstate *A*, the normal length of the submucosal segment of the ureter; *B*, congenital shortening; *C*, absence of this segment. (From Stephens, F. D.: Congenital Malformations of the Rectum, Anus, and Genitourinary Tracts. Edinburgh, E. & S. Livingstone, Ltd., 1963.)

*Adapted from Gray, S. W., and Skandalakis, J. E.: Embryology for Surgeons. Philadelphia, W. B. Saunders Co., 1972, and Arey, L. B.: Developmental Anatomy, 7th ed. Philadelphia, W. B. Saunders Co., 1974.

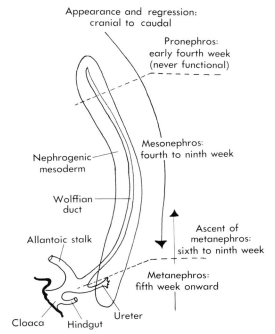

Figure 4–5. Diagram of the development of mesonephric structures of the human embryo. Development, maturation, and regression proceed caudad. Only the most caudal portion of the nephrogenic mesoderm persists to become the adult kidney. This organ then moves cranial to reach its normal position in the abdomen. (From Gray, S. W., and Skandalakis, J. E.: Embryology for Surgeons. Philadelphia, W. B. Saunders Co., 1972, p. 444.)

two embryonic ureteral buds instead of one meet the nephrogenic mass (Fig. 4–8A). These ureters then cross one another as they migrate into the bladder to conform to the constant relationship of the upper renal segment ureteral orifice being situated lower in the bladder than the lower renal segment ureteral orifice (Weigert-Meyer law).

Recent theories have been proposed that help explain the development of the abnormal ureterovesical junction (Mackie et al., 1975). As previously mentioned, one of the initial steps in the development of the urinary tract is the absorption into the base of the bladder of the distal portion of the wolffian duct, including the ureteral bud. If the fetal ureteral bud originates too close to the bladder base, its orifice will be more lateral than normal when the absorptive process is complete. The resultant intravesical portion of that ureter will be shorter than normal, thus serving as a less efficient valve

mechanism. Reflux then becomes more likely.

Corroboration of this embryologic explanation would appear to exist when anatomic abnormalities are discovered in association with duplication of the collecting system. In virtually all patients with a duplicated system in whom vesicoureteral reflux is discovered, that reflux is noted to extend into the lower segment of the duplicated system. Embryologically, the ureteral bud to the lower pole renal segment originates closer to the bladder than the bud to the upper renal pole. Upon absorption of these duplicated buds into the bladder, the bud closer to the bladder, the one that will become the lower pole ureter, ends up with its orifice more laterally placed in the trigone (Fig. 4–8C). Therefore, it stands a higher risk of having a shorter submucosal tunnel and is more likely to be involved in reflux. The theory goes on to state that the more abnormally originating ureteral bud may strike a less central portion of the nephrogenic mass, increasing the possibility of abnormal renal development (Fig. 4–9).

This total concept is appealing in that it offers an embryologic explanation for vesicoureteral reflux. In addition, the genesis of the dilated, poorly functioning kidney associated with severe reflux but in which an underlying history of urinary tract infection is absent also becomes understandable. So-

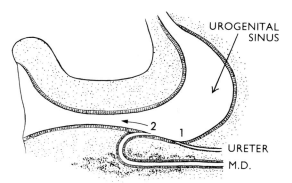

Figure 4–6. Diagrammatic parasagittal section showing the entrance of the ureter into the bladder at the site of Chwalle's membrane (1), and the loop of the mesonephric duct (M. D.), which will straighten out as the lower orifice (2) is carried downward to the site of the müllerian tubercle in the urethra. (From Williams, D. I.: The development of the trigone of the bladder. Br. J. Urol., 23:123–128, 1951.)

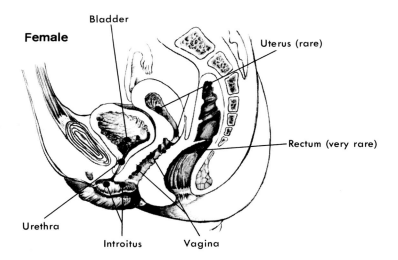

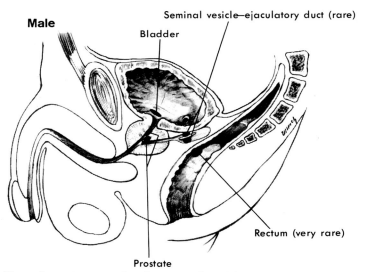

Figure 4–7. Sites of ectopic ureteral orifices in girls and boys. (From Harrison, J. H., Gittes, R. F., and Perlmutter, A. D., et al.: Campbell's Urology, Vol. 2, 4th ed. Philadelphia, W. B. Saunders Co., 1979, p. 1757.)

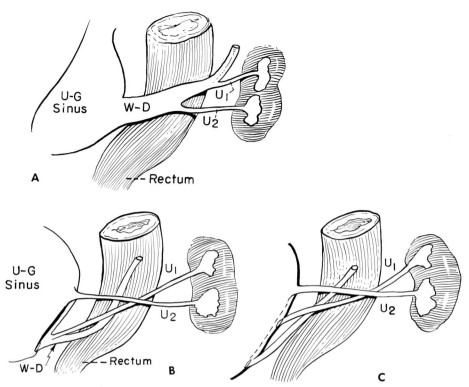

Figure 4–8. Development of duplicated collecting system. U-G, urogenital: W-D, wolffian duct; U, ureter. (From Kelalis, P. P., King, L. R., and Belman, A. B.: Clinical Pediatric Urology, Vol. 1. Philadelphia, W. B. Saunders Co., 1976, p. 510.)

called reflux nephropathy, which has been attributed by some to the back pressure of reflux alone in those children with severe reflux and in whom no history of urinary

tract infection can be elicited (Salvatierra and Tanagho, 1977) is then explained as a developmental abnormality. In most patients with reflux nephropathy, however,

Figure 4–9. Relationship of orifice zones in bladder and urethra and points of origin from wolffian duct is shown, as well as relationship of bud position on wolffian duct and nephrogenic blastema. Point A corresponds with the site of origin of the normal ureteral bud. It meets the midportion, or most "healthy" part of the nephrogenic mass. Point D corresponds with a bud that might be "outside" the bladder, associated with a paraureteral diverticulum. The corresponding renal substance might be significantly abnormal with a resultant dysgenetic unit, including massive reflux and a nonfunctioning or poorly functioning kidney. Point H would also be associated with a poorly formed kidney; however, the ureteral orifice would be more caudal, that is, ectopically located in the vaginal vestibule (Gartner's duct) or in the seminal vesicle. (From Mackie, G. G., and Stephens, F. D.: Duplex kidneys: A correlation of renal dysplasia with position of the ureteral orifice. J. Urol., *114*:274, 1975.)

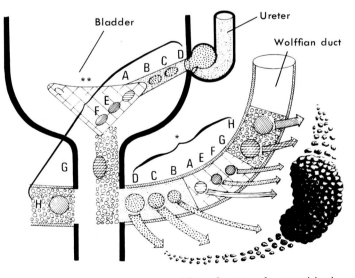

*Site of origin of ureteral bud
**Ultimate orifice position

the changes are more likely the product of unrecognized pyelonephritis in early infancy resulting in severe renal damage such as that shown in Figure 4–15.

FACTORS INFLUENCING REFLUX

PARAURETERAL DIVERTICULUM

Anatomic distortion of the ureterovesical junction may promote reflux. As Hutch (1952) had noted in his investigation of the group of patients with neurogenic disease and reflux, many had a diverticulum adjacent to the refluxing ureteral orifice. Paraureteral diverticula may also occur in otherwise normal children as congenital defects and potentially may contribute to reflux by weakening the supporting wall behind the

ureter as the bladder fills and the diverticulum distends (Fig. 4–1). The presence of a paraureteral diverticulum considerably reduces the chances of reflux resolving without a surgical procedure; however, it does not preclude it.

DUPLICATION OF THE COLLECTING SYSTEM

As mentioned in the section on embryology, reflux into the lower segment of a duplicated system is a likely finding (Fig. 4–10). Duplication of the collecting system is noted to occur in about 1 of 500 in the general population. However, Ambrose and Nicholson (1962), in a review of 75 children with known reflux, reported the incidence of duplication in that group as 1 in 4.5. Our own experience suggests that the

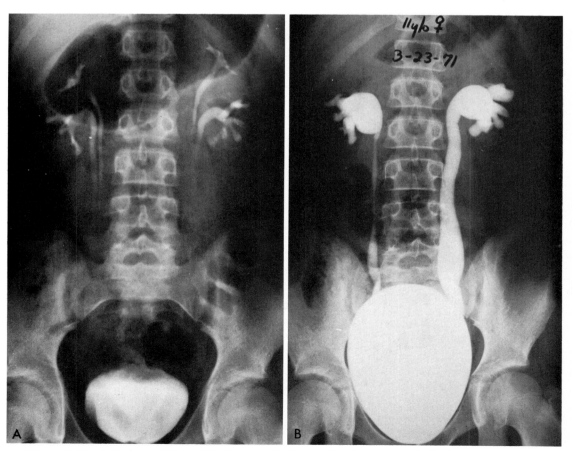

Figure 4–10. A, Complete bilateral duplication of urinary collecting systems. B, Grade 2B (III/V) vesicoureteral reflux into lower systems of duplication.

incidence is 1 in 6, adding corroboration of the frequency of a refluxing ureterovesical junction in this group.

OBSTRUCTION

Reflux is noted to occur in about 50 per cent of patients with congenital posterior urethral valves. In about 25 per cent of these, the reflux will disappear with time after relief of the obstruction (Williams et al., 1973). In adults with acquired non-neurogenic outlet obstruction such as prostatic hypertrophy, on the other hand, vesicoureteral reflux is not a common finding. It would appear that the intact ureterovesical junction is capable of withstanding increased intravesical pressure and that a degree of intrinsic developmental abnormality must be present for reflux to coexist with obstruction.

CYSTITIS

Edema at the ureterovesical junction secondary to cystitis may distort a partially incompetent valve, resulting in transient vesicoureteral reflux. The relationship between infection and reflux has been recognized since 1924 (Bumpus), and attempts to demonstrate it in laboratory animals by injection of saline in the region of the ureteral orifice have been successful (Auer and Seager, 1937). Unfortunately, this point was at one time overemphasized. Shopfner (1970) suggested that specific antibacterial medication resulted in early cessation of reflux in 85 per cent of patients. Although this figure may be moderately close to the true incidence of the spontaneous resolution of reflux, it is more likely that time, maturation, and growth are more responsible than short-term treatment of infection. Nevertheless, to avoid categorizing that group of patients with transient reflux as "refluxers," it is advisable to allow acute bladder changes to resolve by waiting four to six weeks following urinary tract infection before carrying out a cystogram.

In the clinical situation in which a child has a febrile urinary tract infection suggesting an episode of pyelonephritis but reflux is not demonstrated when radiographs are carried out four to six weeks after definitive treatment, one may conclude, nevertheless, that reflux had occurred during that acute episode.

GENETICS

There is strong evidence that the tendency toward reflux is genetically dictated, possibly through the degree of development of the submucosal tunnel (intravesical ureter) (Burger and Smith, 1971). In an evaluation of siblings of children with documented reflux, Dwoskin (1976) found that 26.5 per cent of asymptomatic siblings also have vesicoureteral reflux. Because reflux resolves spontaneously in many without its presence being recognized, the exact familial incidence is difficult to evaluate. Absence of reflux in any particular family member of the proband does not guarantee that the individual did not have reflux in the past. With two affected family members, Burger and Burger (1974) found that the chances of a third member having reflux is 13.6 per cent. More recent data (Noe) suggest this figure is much higher.

This is supported also by the knowledge that reflux is uncommon in blacks. In the experience of one of us practicing in an area in which a large segment of the population is black, the ratio of vesicoureteral reflux in black girls to white girls with urinary tract infection is 1:3.4 (Askari and Belman, unpublished data). Our conclusion is that radiographic evaluation should be reserved in black girls for those with febrile urinary tract infection or in those in whom infection cannot be readily controlled.

We do not recommend radiographic evaluation in asymptomatic siblings of a child with known vesicoureteral reflux but would suggest that these children have extra attention paid to their urinary tracts and that urine cultures should be carried out in each on a regular basis (every four months for the first year, every six months until four years of age, then annually until age seven). A urine culture should be done with each febrile illness, and aggressive antibiotic therapy should be initiated at the first sign of pyelonephritis. Radiographic evaluation is then pursued upon documentation of infection. However, if more than one child in a family is known to have reflux, radiographic evaluation of the remainder of the siblings should be strongly considered.

INCIDENCE

The actual incidence of vesicoureteral reflux in the general population is unknown. This is understandable since it is not a finding that can be determined at autopsy but one that requires special studies. For many years it has been recognized that reflux occurs more often in children than adults (Baker et al, 1966). Our general impression is that it is present in 1 in 200 white girls.

In reports throughout the Western world, 30 per cent of girls presenting with urinary tract infection are found to have reflux (Smellie, 1972). Govan and colleagues (1975) reported a somewhat higher figure of 50 per cent, whereas Kunin and associates (1960), in their initial survey of children with asymptomatic bacteriuria, noted an incidence of 19 per cent.

Scott (1977) in a review of 262 British children with vesicoureteral reflux, found that a lag of two years existed between the onset of symptoms (urinary tract infection) and the recognition of reflux. The peak incidence of urinary tract infection was two to three years, with 70 per cent occurring before age five years. The peak age of reflux was four to six years. This should not be interpreted to mean that reflux is the result of infection since reflux is a congenital problem in virtually every circumstance. Instead, it points out the delay in evaluation in children with urinary tract infection.

Children with renal scarring found on excretory urography have a much higher incidence, with two thirds or more having reflux (Bourne et al, 1976; Scott and Stansfield, 1968). In a review by Vermillion and Heale (1973) of adults with classical pyelo-nephritic scarring, slightly more than half were found to have reflux on cystograms, and on endoscopic evaluation an additional 35 per cent had abnormally placed ureteral orifices and would have been expected to reflux in the past.

Vesicoureteral reflux is the rule in some laboratory animals (Gruber, 1929) and has recently been demonstrated to occur in 80 per cent of infant rhesus monkeys (Roberts and Riopelle, 1977). This would appear not to be the case in humans, as Peters and coworkers (1967) did not observe reflux in 66 premature babies. However, 85 per cent of the children studied were black. Lich and associates (1964) also found no reflux in 26 newborns studied within the first two days of life. (The race of these children is not noted). Booth and colleagues (1975) reported a fetus found to have vesicoureteral reflux at 25 weeks of gestation as noted accidentally at the time of intrauterine transfusion. This reflux persisted at one year of life. In a review of 28 additional fetal cystograms, reflux was not noted in any. On the other hand, Drew and Acton (1976) found reflux in almost half of a group of newborns with documented bacteriuria. The clinical significance of the last observation is not completely appreciated at this time.

It is not known if the preponderance of recognized reflux in females is due to an actual sex predisposition or a skewing of the figures based on the higher incidence of urinary tract infections and, therefore, greater numbers of radiographic studies in females. It is of interest that in neonates with bacteriuria, a group statistically dominated by males, reflux is quite common. Our impression is that reflux occurs equally in males and females.

THE DIAGNOSIS OF REFLUX

The diagnosis of reflux is made radiographically and requires urethral catheterization. Although many continue to perform cystography under anesthesia, the risk to life is hard to justify. Additionally, dynamic studies with the patient awake appear to be more reliable in demonstrating reflux than sleep cystograms (Vlahakis et al., 1971). One must also take into consideration that the radiation dosage from overzealous fluoroscopy to identify minimal transient reflux is not clinically indicated. An alternative, the isotope cystogram, offers continuous monitoring during all phases of bladder filling and voiding, with minimal radiation exposure (Chap. 2). Additionally, it is a more sensitive study for determining reflux than the standard cystogram (Fig. 4–11).

Occasionally, changes on an IVP alone are suggestive of vesicoureteral reflux. Calyceal abnormalities, renal scarring, decreased renal size, ureterectasis, ureteral tortuosity, and linear streaks indenting the collecting system, the result of redundant, overstretched mucosa, may all be indicative

of vesicoureteral reflux (Fig. 4–12). Since the incidence of reflux is so high in children and can exist and be significant in the presence of a normal excretory urogram, it is strongly recommended that all children evaluated for urinary tract infection have a separate, catheterized cystogram as part of their initial study.

GRADING REFLUX

Dwoskin and Perlmutter (1973) brought a degree of standardization to the nomenclature of reflux by grading its extent. Grade I involves only the lower ureter and is often called a "whisp" of reflux. Because of its slight degree, Grade I reflux may be

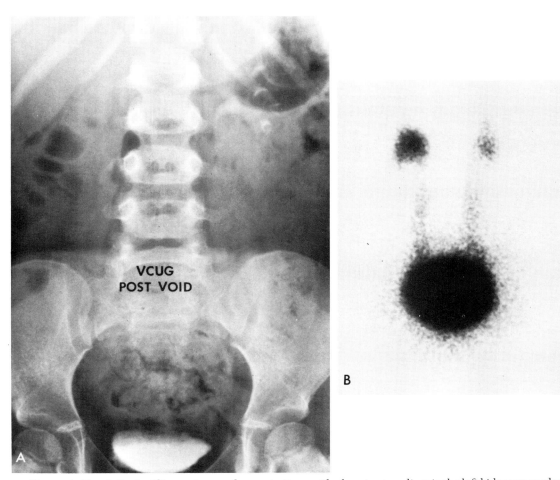

Figure 4–11. *A,* Postvoiding cystogram demonstrating residual contrast medium in the left kidney secondary to reflux. *B,* Isotope cystogram in the same patient reveals significant bilateral reflux.

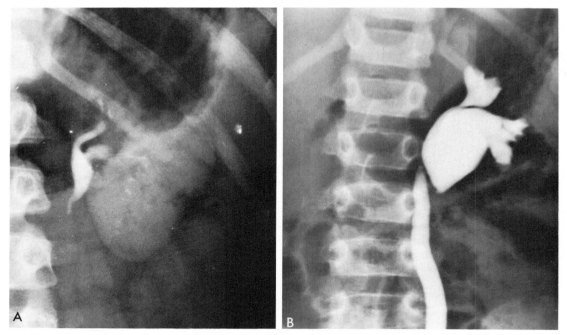

Figure 4–12. A, Excretory urogram demonstrating linear mucosal stria of the renal pelvis. B, Cystogram in the same child revealing marked vesicoureteral reflux with distension of the collecting system.

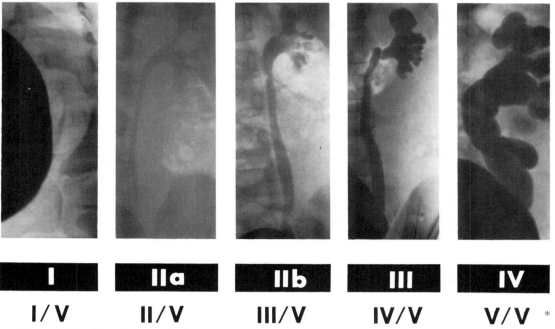

Figure 4–13. Classification of reflux according to the volume of urine seen to reflux on the cystogram. Grade I: Lower ureteral filling only. Grade IIa: Ureteral and pelviocalyceal filling without dilatation. Grade IIb: Ureteral and pelviocalyceal filling with mild calyceal blunting but without clubbing and without dilatation of the pelvis or tortuosity of the ureter. Grade III: Ureteral and pelviocalyceal filling, calyceal clubbing, and minor to moderate pelvic dilatation without tortuosity of the ureter. Grade IV: Massive ureteral dilatation and tortuosity. (From Dwoskin, J.Y., and Perlmutter, A. D.: Vesicoureteral reflux in children: A computerized review. J. Urol., 109:888–890, 1973.) *The international grading system as it compares to the Dwoskin-Perlmutter system.

missed unless oblique views are performed and may not be picked up by the isotope cystogram. However, since urine is not conveyed all the way to the kidney and drainage is rapid, Grade I reflux is, in almost all circumstances, of little clinical significance. The exception would be the child with uncontrollable infections and repeated pyelonephritis, as mentioned previously. Grade II involves complete reflux to the collecting system and is further subdivided into Grade IIa, in which there is no dilatation of the collecting system, and Grade IIb, in which there is fullness of the collecting system but no calyceal clubbing or ureteral tortuosity. With Grade III, there is calyceal blunting, ureteral tortuosity, and dilatation, while those with Grade IV have massive reflux and severe pyelocalyceal and ureteral changes. More recently an international classification has been introduced that breaks reflux into five grades. Grade IIa becomes II/V and IIb becomes III/V. Dwoskin and Perlmutter's Grade III becomes IV/V and Grade IV becomes V/V (Fig. 4–13).

For purposes of communication, we recognize the importance of classification; however, the significance of reflux should not be based only on radiographic findings. Although the grade of reflux correlates quite well with the degree of development of the ureterovesical junction, it is not absolute, and further evaluation should be carried out so that treatment of each patient will be individualized on the basis of history of infection, radiographic changes, and the degree of development of the ureterovesical junction as observed endoscopically.

SIGNIFICANCE OF VESICOURETERAL REFLUX

REFLUX AND URINARY TRACT INFECTION

Infection of the renal collecting system and medulla apparently emanates from bacteria traveling retrograde from the bladder. Whether this is absolute or not is conjecture. Lymphatic contamination is also likely and may be the source of infection in an obstructed unit in the absence of reflux. Males, in whom bladder sterility is protected by urethral length, may also develop bacteriuria in this way. It would appear, however, that the vast majority of individuals with classic pyelonephritic scarring have had infection in combination with reflux (Lenaghan et al., 1976).

In reviews of urinary radiographs of children and adults, the finding of renal scarring is strong evidence that vesicoureteral reflux is present or had existed in the past. In Scott and Stansfeld's series (1968), reflux was found in 85 per cent of children with renal scarring. Hutch and colleagues (1969) and Filly and associates (1974) found a similar high correlation between scarring and reflux. Vermillion and Heale (1973) in a review of adults with radiographic evidence of renal scarring, found that reflux could still be demonstrated in half and that the endoscopically assessed configuration of the ureterovesical junction was abnormal and had probably been incompetent in the past in virtually all of the remainder. In the absence of reflux, renal scarring is very rare and has been noted to be present in from less than one per cent (Govan et al., 1975) to 10 per cent (Dwoskin and Perlmutter, 1973) of children with urinary tract infection.

The effectiveness of the normal flap-valve mechanism at the ureterovesical junction is virtually complete. Radioactive labeled sulfur colloid placed in the bladders of dogs with an intact ureterovesical junction does not migrate into the ureters (Corriere et al., 1967). On the other hand, in the presence of reflux as demonstrated in rats, carbon particles placed in the bladder were found to enter the kidney and outline the course of the intrarenal lymphatic system. A wedge-shaped configuration from the renal fornices is demonstrated that corresponds to the pattern seen in pyelonephritic scarring (Corriere and Murphy, 1967).

It would appear that the primary factor that determines if scarring will occur is the configuration of the renal papillae. Those that are cone-shaped prevent intrarenal reflux, whereas those that are concave tend to allow urine (and bacteria in children with urinary tract infection) to enter the collecting tubules. Upper and lower pole renal papillae tend toward a concave configuration. This corresponds with the finding that scarring is more common in the renal poles (Ransley and Risdon, 1978).

It is becoming increasingly clear that the origin of pyelonephritic scarring of the type described by Hodson (1967) is unique to childhood. In all the reviews mentioned previously, it must be pointed out that scarring was already present at the time of evaluation — and yet as mentioned earlier, girls with urinary tract infection do not usually present for evaluation until school age, that is, about three to five years old. If the radiographic changes seen are secondary to bacterial renal infection, then we must be missing episodes of infection, and children presenting beyond infancy with their "first" urinary tract infection have had previous episodes. This is supported by the studies of Winberg and colleagues (1974), who have longitudinally followed small children for several years and discovered that those with urinary tract infections in the school-age years were most likely to have had previous episodes at an earlier age. The conclusion reached is that unrecognized or poorly managed urinary tract infection, most certainly associated with vesicoureteral reflux and pyelonephritis, is responsible for the relatively high incidence of renal scarring seen at "initial" presentation.

Of further interest is the apparent unique susceptibility of the younger kidney to this type of damage. Hodson (1967) states that atrophic pyelonephritis is distinctly a disease of childhood and that it is not initiated in adults (or for that matter much after the age of five years). However, in some young individuals with recurrent infections or even chronic cystitis and associated reflux, renal damage is not evident. Efforts have been made to explain the susceptibility of some kidneys to scarring. Rolleston and associates (1974) suggested that intrarenal reflux (Fig. 4–14), a phenomenon not generally seen after age five, is responsible. Experimental studies in piglets, an animal with kidneys architectually similar to those of humans, would tend to substantiate this explanation (Hodson et al., 1975). In fact, Bourne and coworkers (1976) went so far as to state that intrarenal reflux is an absolute indication for antireflux surgery.

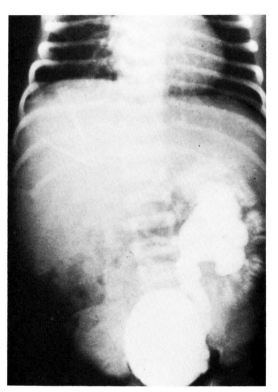

Figure 4–14. Intrarenal reflux. Note the wedge-shaped distribution corresponding to pyramids.

The experimental changes provoked in piglets by Hodson (1975) required a degree of bladder outlet obstruction in addition to alteration of the ureterovesical junction to produce significant reflux. Ransley and Risdon (1978), in an attempt to duplicate Hodson's results, found that renal scarring did not occur in piglets unless bacteriuria accompanied the vesicoureteral reflux. Additionally, scarring corresponded with the areas of intrarenal reflux. Nevertheless, they demonstrated that maintaining urine sterility alone is adequate in preventing scarring (or progression of scarring) even in those animals with pyelotubular (intrarenal) backflow. This supports our clinical experience.

The apparent sensitivity of some infants to damage from renal infection can be seen in the effect on kidney growth. Uniform failure of growth following a single episode of acute pyelonephritis in infancy (Fig. 4–15) may be responsible for what later may be called a primary hypoplastic kidney in an individual not known to have had previous urinary tract infection. In all

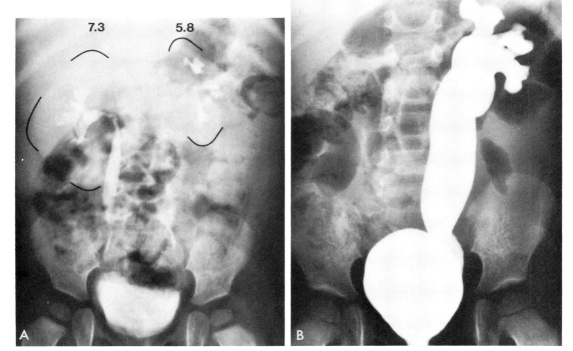

Figure 4–15. *A,* Small left kidney on an excretory urogram in a nine-month-old girl with documented U.T.I. at three weeks and 10 weeks requiring hospitalization. *B,* Cystogram demonstrating the severity of her reflux.

likelihood, this was the result of pan-pyelonephritis arrested spontaneously or by antibiotics before total destruction resulted. If both kidneys are involved, reflux nephropathy may be the end result.

STERILE REFLUX

Though all would agree that vesicoureteral reflux and urinary tract infection are a potentially serious combination, some highly respected members of the urologic community firmly believe that in special circumstances the hydrostatic effect of reflux alone can cause significant renal damage and that infection may never have been present to play an influential role (Salvatierra and Tanagho, 1977). (Salvatierra notes that this occurs only in those with severe Grade IV/V or Grade V/V reflux.)*

For this reason, the necessity for early surgical intervention in those with moderate reflux is advocated by some as a means

_____
*Personal communication

of protecting the kidneys (Mayor et al., 1975). Others (Stamey, 1972; King et al., 1974), including the present authors, feel that there is no conclusive evidence to support the concept that sterile reflux is harmful. Although reviews by Stickler and colleagues (1971) and Lloyd-Still and Cotton (1967) document progressive renal deterioration in a minority of patients with severe reflux and scarring in whom infection is absent, many were known to have had episodes of infection in childhood. Based on the common experience of children presenting in childhood with their "first" urinary tract infection in whom renal scarring is already present, the absence of a positive history does not rule out the possibility of the event.

A case in point is a family previously reported (Lewy and Belman, 1975). A father and three sons presented, all with severe reflux and renal scarring. None had a history of urinary tract infection, and the erroneous conclusion reached by the authors was that sterile reflux caused the damage. A sister, born while the remainder of the family was under urologic care, was screened at birth and also was found to have bilateral vesicoureteral reflux. Immediate continuous prophylactic antibacterial medication was instituted with urines periodically collected for culture. No episodes of urinary tract infection occurred, and evaluation over the next three years revealed no evidence of renal scarring or growth failure. Although this one case is not absolute evidence that reflux in the absence of infection does not cause renal damage, it is a single example of many such children followed carefully over several years. Other examples include children with incidental reflux in whom no history of urinary tract infection is known with normal kidneys despite moderate reflux (Fig. 4–16).

It is evident that renal damage, once established, can be progressive even when infection is controlled. In the milder situation, scarring may take up to two years after the acute episode to be evident on radiographs (Filly et al., 1974; Hodson and Wilson, 1965). Some of the patients reported by Salvatierra and Tanagho (1977) and Stickler and coworkers (1971) with Grades IV/V to V/V reflux and many with severe renin-mediated hypertension went on to dialysis and renal transplantation in spite of prevention of infection or ureteral reimplantation. Although bacterial pyelonephritis in the absence of obstruction is not generally a progressive disease, a small group with severe reflux appear to exist who are at higher risk for progressive renal failure.

The suggestion that a focus of dysplasia may predispose the kidney to a greater susceptibility for scarring (Bialestock, 1963), is supported by the theory of Mackie and colleagues (1975). They conclude that an abnormal ureteral bud stimulating a less than optimal segment of the metanephric blastema results in an abnormal refluxing renal unit from birth (p. 71). The implication is that those children with severe reflux must be recognized as early as possible, infection prevented, and the reflux corrected. It must be repeated, however, that this group represents a small minority.

EVALUATION OF THE CHILD WITH REFLUX

After reflux is recognized radiographically, further appreciation of the ureterovesical junction can be gained endoscopically. Lyon and colleagues (1969) first described

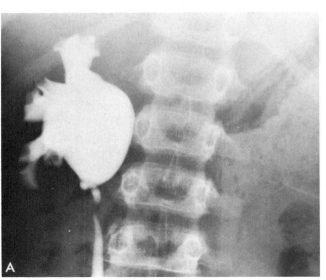 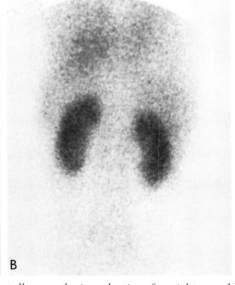

Figure 4–16.   *A,* Right vesicoureteral reflux picked up incidentally on urologic evaluation of an eight year old boy with no history of urinary infections. *B,* Renal scan (two minutes postinjection) revealing normal kidneys bilaterally.

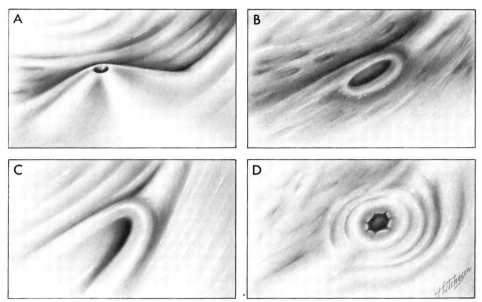

Figure 4–17.   Lyon classification of orifice morphology in primary reflux. *A*, Normal or volcano-shaped orifice as noted at cystoscopy. *B*, Stadium orifice. It is usually slightly more lateral than the normal orifice and somtimes is associated with reflux. The intravesical ureter, however, is usually well developed, and reflux associated with such orifices will usually stop with growth. *C*, Horseshoe orifice. Part or most of the intravesical ureter is represented by the longitudinal muscle in ridges above and below the orifice. The proximal submucosal ureter may be well formed but is usually short and reflux will often persist. *D*, A golf-hole orifice is most lateral in position and lacks any vestige of an intravesical ureter. Associated reflux is quite persistent and usually continues after full growth is achieved. (From Kelalis, P. P., King, L. R., and Belman, A. B.: Clinical Pediatric Urology, Vol. 1. Philadelphia, W. B. Saunders Co., 1976, p. 350.)

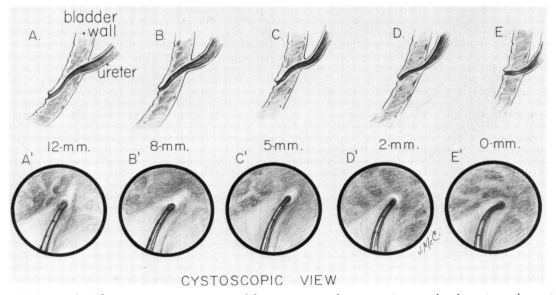

Figure 4–18.   The cystoscopic appearance of the ureterovesical junction. A ureteral catheter is used to estimate the length of the submucosal tunnel. The ureter is drawn as normal in diameter to emphasize the appearance of the flap elevated by the catheter. (From Kelalis, P. P., King, L. R., and Belman, A. B.: Clinical Pediatric Urology, Vol. 1. Philadelphia, W. B. Saunders Co., 1976, p. 356.)

the relationship between orifice configuration, orifice position, and the competency of the antireflux mechanism. Competent ureters generally can be anticipated to have their orifices in the normal trigonal position and have a cone-like shape. As the orifice is found more laterally positioned, it assumes a rounder appearance and is more likely to reflux. In the most severe form, the orifice is gaping and assumes a "golf hole" appearance (Fig. 4–17). By grading orifice location alphabetically with A being normal and C being moderately lateral but not quite "golf-hole," Lyon and associates (1969) noted that 40 per cent of those ureters with their orifices in the B position, 80 per cent in the C position, and virtually all those with a "golf-hole" orifice had reflux.

In an effort to lend additional objectivity to the evaluation of the ureterovesical junction, measurement of actual submucosal tunnel length can be achieved by the passage of a ureteral catheter under endoscopic control at the time of cystoscopy. The length of mucosa elevated by the catheter also correlates with orifice configuration and incidence of reflux (Fig. 4–18).

The timing of endoscopic evaluation of ureteral orifice configuration and the length of the submucosal tunnel is dependent upon the degree of reflux. Patients with mild reflux (Grades I and II) either may be evaluated immediately or may be placed on antibacterial prophylaxis for a period of six months with an isotope cystogram carried out at the end of that time. In a small but reasonably significant number, reflux will have ceased at the end of that period, and further evaluation may not be necessary. In those in whom reflux continues, endoscopic evaluation may then be carried out for purposes of prognostication.

PROGNOSIS

From the carefully documented Australian study by Lenaghan and coworkers (1976), in which a group of 102 patients were followed for up to 18 years without surgical intervention, a number of enlightening facts can be gleaned. The younger the age at presentation, the greater are the chances of ultimately "outgrowing" vesicoureteral reflux. Sixty-eight per cent of those presenting before 12 months had resolution of reflux by age 14 years. In 86 per cent of that group, the reflux had ceased by age nine, and in half it had ceased by age six. This corresponds with the animal studies of Roberts and Riopelle (1977) in which a group of rhesus monkeys demonstrated to have reflux were followed from birth and were all noted to outgrow the reflux by 36 months.

Thirty-seven per cent of children presenting to Lenaghan and colleagues (1976) between ages two and three years stopped refluxing by age 14 years, but none as early as age seven. Finally, only 26 per cent of those children presenting over age three years had cessation of reflux by age 14. Our conclusion is that those in whom reflux is likely to resolve spontaneously are naturally selected out as age increases, and a "hard-core" group remains in whom the ureterovesical abnormality is more severe. The data presented by King and coworkers (1974) suggests that in the United States, the peak incidence of recognition of reflux is between three to five years, whereas its disappearance is spread out between six and 11 years in those in whom reflux will cease spontaneously (Fig. 4–19). Smellie and associates (1975) reported that reflux can be anticipated to remit spontaneously in 85 per cent of those with mild to moderate reflux and in 41 per cent of those with more severe involvement. One must be aware, however, that many years may elapse before disappearance of reflux is complete.

The clinical questions that then arise are (1) how long can a patient be safely followed with known vesicoureteral reflux, and (2) is the presence of reflux harmful? The report by Edwards and others (1977) from Great Britain suggests that long-term prophylaxis is safe and effective in preventing scarring. It appears to be fairly evident that the combination of reflux and urinary tract infection is required before renal damage will occur in otherwise normal kidneys.

In the study of Lenaghan and colleagues (1976), renal deterioration as noted by the presence of scarring on excretory urography was seen in 21 per cent of those

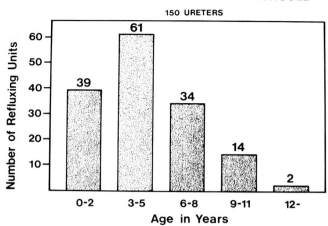

AGE AT WHICH REFLUX DIAGNOSED

150 URETERS

Figure 4–19. *Upper,* The age at which reflux was diagnosed in 150 refluxing ureters in patients in whom the reflux eventually stopped with nonoperative management. *Lower,* The age at which reflux stopped in the same patients. Cessation of reflux was related to the degree of derangement of the ureterovesical junctions at the time of diagnosis and to the degree of hydronephrosis. No special tendency for reflux to stop at puberty has been noted. (From Kelalis, P. P., King, L. R., and Belman, A. B.: Clinical Pediatric Urology, Vol. 1. Philadelphia, W. B. Saunders Co., 1976, p. 360.)

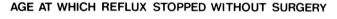

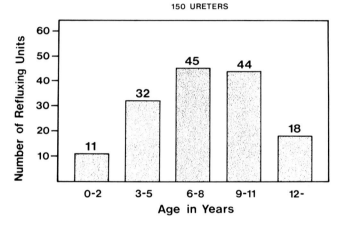

AGE AT WHICH REFLUX STOPPED WITHOUT SURGERY

150 URETERS

with initially normal radiographs, and progression of scarring was seen in 66 per cent of those presenting with an abnormal pyelogram. However, the patients in this study were not free of infection during the follow-up period, and intervening urinary tract infection was documented in virtually all those in whom new changes were noted. The authors suggest, in an addendum to the published data, that the course might have been favorably influenced by low-dose continuous prophylactic antibacterial agents in this group of patients. In the children followed by King and associates (1974) a group maintained on antibacterial prophylaxis, only seven of 163 with known reflux without surgical correction had renal growth failure or new parenchymal scarring noted. In each of these, urinary tract infection occurred during the follow-up period.

Concluding that reflux and infection are indeed a threatening combination that can cause renal damage in younger children and morbidity (fever and flank pain) in older children and adults, it would appear reasonable to try to differentiate between those who have a chance of "outgrowing" reflux from those who might benefit from early surgical correction. Ureteral orifice configuration (Fig. 4–20), length of the ureteral submucosal tunnel (Fig. 4–21), and degree of ureterectasis on the excretory urogram (Fig. 4–22) all correlate fairly well in terms of predicting the eventual outcome of reflux. Patients with patulous (golf-hole) ureteral orifices and significantly shortened submucosal tunnels (less than 3 mm) as measured by inserting a 4 F ureteral catheter under cystoscopic observation have an extremely small chance of "outgrowing"

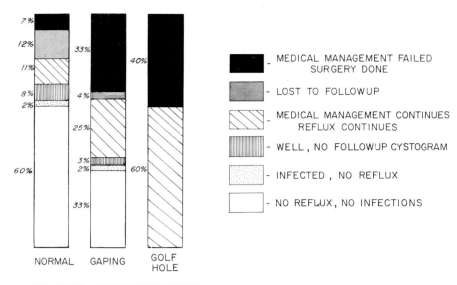

ORIFICE CONFIGURATION

Figure 4–20.   This graph depicts the relationship between the morphology of the refluxing orifice, as judged by the initial cystoscopy, and the outcome of the trial of nonoperative management in children followed for four to 10 years. The orifices initially regarded as "normal" in appearance include those of the type classified by Lyon as having a "stadium" configuration, whereas gaping orifices were primarily those of the horseshoe variety. Note that when all vestiges of an intravesical ureter are absent, resulting in a "golf-hole" orifice, reflux has not been found to correct itself with growth. (From Kelalis, P. P., King, L. R., and Belman, A. B.: Clinical Pediatric Urology, Vol. 1. Philadelphia, W. B. Saunders Co., 1976, p. 363.)

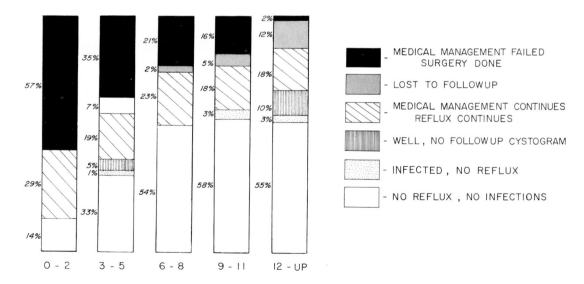

LENGTH OF INTRAMURAL URETER IN MILLIMETERS

Figure 4–21.   This graph depicts the relationships between the estimated length of the intravesical ureter at the time of diagnosis and the outcome of a trial of nonoperative management in 247 refluxing units in which the tunnel length was estimated in patients followed from four to 10 years. There is a nearly linear relationship between original tunnel length and eventual cessation of reflux, indicating the importance of this parameter. (From Kelalis, P. P., King, L. R., and Belman, A. B.: Clinical Pediatric Urology, Vol. 1. Philadelphia, W. B. Saunders Co., 1976, p. 359.)

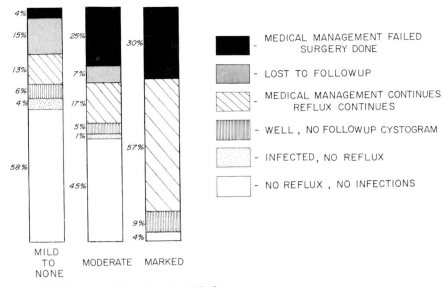

Figure 4–22. The more striking the degree of hydronephrosis, as judged by the initial intravenous pyelogram, the more likely it is that reflux will persist and that antireflux surgery will be indicated because of recurrent infection. (From Kelalis, P. P., King, L. R., and Belman, A. B.: Clinical Pediatric Urology, Vol. 1. Philadelphia, W. B. Saunders Co., 1976, p. 362.)

reflux and should be considered for early reimplantation after a period of control of urinary tract infection has been achieved.

In the majority, however, the orifice configuration and length of submucosal tunnel will suggest that the reflux will resolve with time. The interval required is unpredictable, however. The urine must be maintained sterile during that period. Low-dose sulfisoxazole, nitrofurantoin, or combination sulfamethoxazole-trimethoprim have been extremely successful in attaining long-term urine sterility. In most patients, one teaspoon of the suspension twice daily and, in some, one teaspoon at bedtime alone is adequate to prevent recurrences. It is important, however, to administer the drug continuously — it is not advisable to stop medication at any time, even to carry out a urine culture. If breakthrough infection occurs, the bacterium will be resistant to the ongoing drug and will grow on culture in spite of the presence of the ineffective antibiotic.

Rarely, a child will present in whom infection cannot be controlled or in whom the family situation precludes reliable long-term medical management. In these circumstances, early antireflux surgery is indicated

unless the clinical picture suggests that a risk for renal damage does not exist in that particular child. Some kidneys do not become scarred in spite of infection in the presence of reflux. As noted in Figure 4–19, it may take years for the reflux to resolve. It must be left to the individual clinician to decide whether it is preferable to maintain a child on continuous medication with its unknown risks or to recommend surgical correction.

REFLUX NEPHROPATHY AND THE ASK-UPMARK KIDNEY

A small percentage of otherwise healthy adolescents and young adults are discovered to have severe hypertension and moderate to severe azotemia. Most are girls, and vesicoureteral reflux can be identified in almost all. No other underlying renal disease is present. Although some give no history of previous urinary tract infection, the radiographic findings are strongly suggestive of bacterial pyelonephritis. This entity has been labeled reflux nephropathy and has a poor prognosis. Most proceed to uremia and require dialysis or transplantation (Lloyd-Still and Cotton, 1967). Correction of reflux at the time of recognition has not apparently improved the prognosis (Stickler et al., 1971).

Another process, also responsible for hypertension and associated with vesicoureteral reflux, is segmental "hypoplasia," or the Ask-Upmark kidney. Severe renal insufficiency is not a part of this clinical picture; however, total renal function is reduced in many patients.

Recent data suggest that the underlying cause of this entity also relates to reflux in conjunction with urinary tract infection (Arant et al., 1979). The hypertension associated with it is of renal etiology and is likely of origins similar to those seen with reflux nephropathy. Both problems most likely originate in infancy and reiterate the importance of recognizing and preventing urinary tract infections in that susceptible age group.

SURGICAL CORRECTION OF REFLUX (URETERONEOCYSTOSTOMY)

There are a number of approaches to the surgical correction of vesicoureteral reflux, all of which are basically designed to achieve the same end result, the creation of a new, relatively long ureteral submucosal tunnel. The earliest attempts at the correction of reflux in children date to Hutch and colleagues in 1955. However, the principles outlined in the operation introduced by Politano and Leadbetter in 1958 continue to form the framework for the majority of the methods presently in use. Basically, all intravesical procedures involve freeing the ureteral orifice, dissecting the ureter from its muscular hiatus, creating a submucosal tunnel of adequate length, and reanastomosing the distal ureter to the bladder, generally in the area of the trigone (Fig. 4–23). Artificial valves are not implanted.

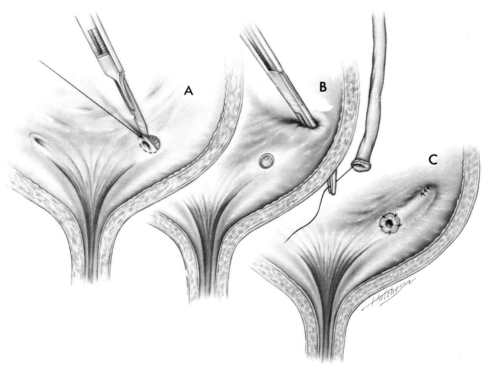

Figure 4–23.   Politano-Leadbetter technique of ureteroneocystostomy. (From Kelalis, P. P., King, L. R., and Belman, A. B.: Clinical Pediatric Urology, Vol. 1. Philadelphia, W. B. Saunders Co., 1976, p. 373.)

The success of modern ureteroneocystostomy in the uncomplicated situation in which the ureter is not greatly dilated exceeds 90 per cent. For this reason, early surgical management has been advocated by some (Wacksman et al., 1978). However, the same group in whom surgery is most likely to be successful — those with little or no ureteral dilatation as seen on excretory urography — are most likely to "outgrow"

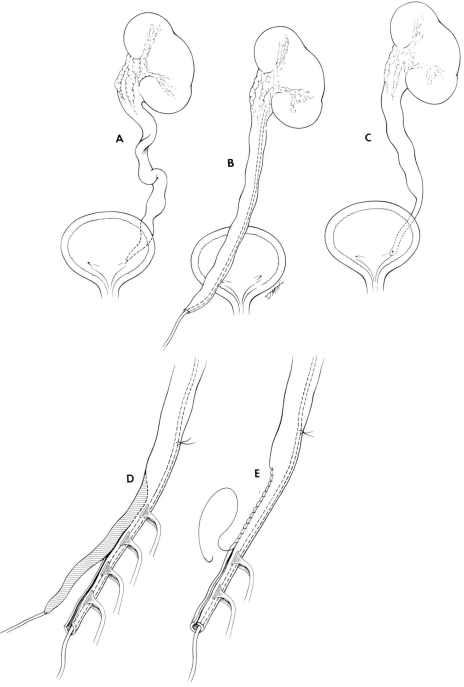

Figure 4–24.   Technique of ureteral caliber reduction. (From Kelalis, P. P., King, L. R., and Belman, A. B.: Clinical Pediatric Urology, Vol. 1. Philadelphia, W. B. Saunders Co., 1976, p. 390.)

reflux. The idea of continuous antibacterial prophylaxis, the risk (although small) of breakthrough infections, and the necessity for repeated radiographic evaluation with the possibility of surgical intervention necessary in the long run is more than some families (and physicians) can accept. It must be appreciated, however, that an occasional complication of ureteral reimplantation is ureteral stenosis and subsequent renal damage. The incidence of renal damage from complications of this type versus that from continued reflux remains one of the unanswered questions when trying to determine the correct recommendation in the care of the child with reflux.

URETERAL TAPERING AND REIMPLANTATION

In refluxing megaureters, tapering of the distal ureter may be necessary to achieve the necessary ratio of submucosal tunnel length to ureteral diameter (5:1) for a successful antireflux mechanism (Fig. 4–24). The success rate for reimplantation in this situation is significantly diminished, and surgery of this type should be performed only by individuals with a great deal of experience with this procedure. The results can be quite gratifying; however, excessive mobilization and devascularization of the ureter may end in severe distal ureteral obstruction, a problem often more complex than the original pathologic condition.

REFERENCES

Ambrose, S. S., and Nicholson, W. P., III: The cause of vesicoureteral reflux in children. J. Urol., 87:688, 1962.

Arant, B. S., Sotelo-Avila, C., and Bernstein, J.: Segmental "hypoplasia" of the kidney (Ask Upmark). J. Pediatr., 95:931, 1979.

Askari, A., and Belman, A. B.: Vesicoureteral reflux in black girls. Unpublished data.

Auer, J., and Seager, L. D.: Experimental local bladder edema causing urine reflux into the ureter and kidney. J. Exp. Med., 66:741, 1937.

Baker, R., Maxted, W., Maylath, J., and Shuman, I.: Relation of age, sex, and infection to reflux: Data indicating high spontaneous cure rate in pediatric patients. J. Urol., 95:27, 1966.

Bialestock, D.: Renal malformations and pyelonephritis: The role of vesicoureteral reflux. Aust. N. Z. J. Surg., 33:114, 1963.

Booth, E. J., Bell, T. E., McLain, C., and Evans, A. T.: Fetal vesicoureteral reflux. J. Urol., 113:258, 1975.

Bourne, H. H., Conden, V. R., Hoyt, T. S., and Nixon, G. W.: Intrarenal reflux and renal damage. J. Urol., 115:304, 1976.

Bumpus, H. C., Jr.: Urinary reflux. J. Urol., 12:341, 1924.

Burger, R. H., and Burger, S. E.: Genetic determinants of urologic disease. Urol. Clin. North Am., 1:419, 1974.

Burger, R. H., and Smith, C.: Hereditary and familial vesicoureteral reflux. J. Urol., 106:845, 1971.

Campbell, M. F.: Cystography in infants and in childhood. Am. J. Dis. Child., 39:386, 1930.

Corriere, J. N., Jr., Kuhl, D. E., and Murphy, J. J.: The use of ⁹⁹ᵐTc labeled sulfur colloid to study particle dynamics in the urinary tract. Invest. Urol., 4:570, 1967.

Corriere, J. N., and Murphy, J. J.: Vesicoureteral reflux and the intrarenal lymphatic system in the rat. Invest. Urol., 4:556, 1967.

Drew, J. H., and Acton, C. M.: Radiologic findings in newborn infants with urinary infection. Arch. Dis. Child., 51:628, 1976.

Dwoskin, J. Y.: Sibling uropathology. J. Urol., 115:726, 1976.

Dwoskin, J. Y., and Perlmutter, A. D.: Vesicoureteral reflux in children: A computerized review. J. Urol., 109:888, 1973.

Edwards, D., Normand, I. C. S., Prescod, N., and Smellie, J. M.: Disappearance of vesicoureteral reflux during long-term prophylaxis of urinary tract infection in children. Br. Med. J., 2:285, 1977.

Filly, R. A., Friedland, G. W., Govan, D. E., and Fair, W. R.: Urinary tract infections in children. Part II. Roentgenologic aspects. West. J. Med., 121:374, 1974.

Garrett, R. A., Rhamy, R. K., and Carr, J. R.: Nonobstructive vesicoureteral regurgitation. J. Urol., 87:350, 1962.

Govan, D. E., Fair, W. R., Friedland, G. W., and Filly, R. A.: Management of children with urinary tract infections. Urology, 6:273, 1975.

Gruber, C. M.: A comparative study of the intravesical ureter. J. Urol., 21:567, 1929.

Hodson, C. J.: The radiological contribution toward the diagnosis of chronic pyelonephritis. Radiology, 88:857, 1967.

Hodson, C. J., and Wilson, S.: Natural history of pyelonephritis scarring. Br. Med. J., 2:191, 1965.

Hodson, C. J., Maling, T. M. J., McManamon, P. J., and Lewis, M. G.: The pathogenesis of reflux nephropathy (chronic atrophic pyelonephritis). Br. J. Radiol. (Suppl.), No. 13, 1975.

Hutch, J. A.: Vesicoureteral reflux in the paraplegic: Cause and correction. J. Urol., 68:457, 1952.

Hutch, J. A., Bunge, R. B., and Flocks, R. H.: Vesicoureteral reflux in children. J. Urol., 74:607, 1955.

Hutch, J. A., Chisholm, E. R., and Smith, D. R.: Summary of pathogenesis of a new classification for urinary tract infection. J. Urol., 102:758, 1969.

King, L. R., Kazmi, S. O., and Belman, A. B.: The natural history of vesicoureteral reflux. Outcome of a trial of nonoperative therapy. Urol. Clin. North Am., 1:441, 1974.

Kunin, C. M., Southhall, I., and Paquin, A. J.: Epidemiology of urinary tract infections. N. Engl. J. Med., 263:817, 1960.

Lenaghan, D., Whitaker, J. G., Jensen, F., and Stephens, F. D.: The natural history of reflux and long term effects of reflux on the kidney. J. Urol., 115:728, 1976.

Lewy, P. R., and Belman, A. B.: Familial occurrence of nonobstructive, noninfectious vesicoureteral reflux with renal scarring. J. Pediatr., 86:851, 1975.

Lich, R., Jr., Howerton, L. W., Goode, L. S., et al.: The ureterovesical junction in the newborn. J. Urol., 92:436, 1964.

Lloyd-Still, J., and Cotton, D.: Severe hypertension in childhood. Arch. Dis. Child., 42:34, 1967.

Lyon, R. P., Marshall, S., and Tanagho, E. A.: The ureteral orifice. Its configuration and competency. J. Urol., 102:504, 1969.

Mackie, G. G., Awang, H., and Stephens, F. D.: The ureteric orifice: The embryologic key to radiologic status of duplex kidneys. J. Pediatr. Surg., 10:473, 1975.

Mayor, G., Genton, N., Torrado, A., and Guignard, J. P.: Renal function in obstructive nephropathy: Long term effect of reconstructive surgery. Pediatrics, 56:740, 1975.

Noz, H. N.: Personal communication.

Paquin, A. J., Jr., Marshall, V. F., and McGovern, J. H.: The megacystis syndrome. J. Urol., 83:634, 1960.

Peters, P., Johnson, E. D., and Jackson, J. H., Jr.: The incidence of vesicoureteral reflux in the premature child. J. Urol., 97:259, 1967.

Politano, V. A., and Leadbetter, W. F.: An operative technique for the correction of vesicoureteral reflux. J. Urol., 79:932, 1958.

Ransley, P. G., and Risdon, R. A.: Reflux and renal scarring. Br. J. Radiol. (Suppl.), 14, 1978.

Roberts, J. A., and Riopelle, A. J.: Vesicoureteral reflux in the primate. II. Maturation of the ureterovesical junction. Pediatrics, 59:566, 1977.

Rolleston, G. L., Maling, T. M. J., and Hodson, C. J.: Intrarenal reflux and the scarred kidney. Arch. Dis. Child., 49:531, 1974.

Salvatierra, O., Jr., and Tanagho, E. A.: Reflux as a cause of end stage kidney disease: Report of 32 cases. J. Urol., 117:441, 1977.

Scott, J. E. S.: The management of ureteric reflux in children. Br. J. Urol., 49:109, 1977.

Scott, J. E. S., and Stansfeld, J. M.: Ureteric reflux and kidney scarring in children. Arch. Dis. Child., 43:468, 1968.

Shopfner, C. E.: Vesicoureteral reflux: Five year reevaluation. Radiology, 95:637, 1970.

Smellie, J.: Do urinary infections really matter in children? Proc. R. Soc. Med., 65:513, 1972.

Smellie, J. M., Edwards, D., Hunter, N., Normand, I. C. S., and Prescod, N.: Vesicoureteral reflux and renal scarring. Kidney Int. (Suppl.), 8:65, 1975.

Stamey, T. A.: Urinary infections in infancy and childhood. In Urinary Infections. Baltimore, Williams and Wilkins, 1972.

Stephens, F. D.: The anatomic basis and dynamics of vesicoureteral reflux. In Congenital malformations of the Rectum, Anus and Genitourinary Tracts. Edinburgh, E. and S. Livingstone, Ltd., 1963.

Stephens, F. D., and Lenaghan, D.: The anatomical basis and dynamics of vesicoureteral reflux. J. Urol., 87:669, 1962.

Stewart, C. M.: Panel on ureteral reflux in children. J. Urol., 85:119, 1961.

Stickler, G. B., Kelalis, P. P., Burke, E. C., and Segar, W. E.: Primary intestitial nephritis with reflux: A cause of hypertension. Am. J. Dis. Child., 122:144, 1971.

Vermillion, C. D., and Heale, W. F.: Position and configuration of the ureteral orifice and its relationship to renal scarring in adults. J. Urol., 109:579, 1973.

Vlahakis, E., Hartman, G. W., and Kelalis, P. P.: Comparison of voiding cystourethrography and expression cystourethrography. J. Urol., 106:414, 1971.

Wacksman, J., Anderson, E. E., and Glenn, J. F.: Management of vesicoureteral reflux. J. Urol., 119:814, 1978.

Williams, D. I., Whitaker, R. H., Barratt, T. M., et al.: Urethral valves. Br. J. Urol., 45:200, 1973.

Winberg, J., Anderson, H. J., Bergstrom, T., Jacobsson, B., Lawson, H., and Lincoln, K.: Epidemiology of symptomatic urinary tract infection in childhood. Acta Paediatr. Scand. (Suppl.), 252:1, 1974.

Chapter Five

OBSTRUCTIVE
UROPATHY

After vesicoureteral reflux, obstruction is the abnormality most often sought when evaluating the urinary tract in children. There are no exact figures which tabulate the overall incidence of childhood obstructive lesions, although data are available indicating the incidence of some specific types of obstruction. There is no question that many children with obstructive lesions will be seen in any busy pediatric urologic practice.

PATHOPHYSIOLOGY OF OBSTRUCTION

Over a period of time, obstruction relentlessly damages the urinary tract; the exact mode by which this occurs is not completely known. The degree to which the kidney is damaged by any given obstruction depends upon the completeness and the duration of that obstruction. Obstruction results in some changes in renal blood flow. When the ureter is occluded acutely, renal blood flow initially increases (Selkurt, 1963). However, as the duration of obstruction increases, renal blood flow begins to decrease, and eventually reaches very low levels (Vaughan et al., 1970). In experimental animals, when the acute obstruction is relieved, renal blood flow will then increase

and once again will reach a level approximately two thirds of its preobstructed value (Kerr, 1954). Renin production may be stimulated by ureteral obstruction (Vaughan et al., 1970; Belman et al., 1968).

Increases in intraureteral pressure are transmitted to the renal pelvis and consequently to the renal tubules. Because filtration pressure (the net difference between capillary blood pressure and intraluminal pressure) is decreased in this situation, there is a resultant fall in glomerular filtration rate. Initially, this fall in glomerular filtration rate is inversely proportional to the rise in intra-ureteral pressure. However, when the ureteral pressure rises to a level equaling 40 per cent of the mean arterial pressure, glomerular filtration rate begins to fall faster than the ureteral pressure rises (Malvin et al., 1964). Nevertheless, glomerular filtration never completely ceases. Even after ureteral obstruction is complete, glomerular filtration will continue but at a much-reduced rate. The number of functional nephrons will progressively decrease with increasing time. This, too, effectively decreases the amount of glomerular filtrate (Vaughan et al., 1973).

Renal tubular function is also diminished by ureteral obstruction. If an acute obstruction is present and a water and salt diuresis is produced, urine osmolality will increase as the ureteral pressure increases, possibly because the renal tubules become more permeable to solutes (Lorentz et al., 1972). In chronic obstruction, during water and salt diuresis, urine osmolality also increases but for a different reason — an increase in urine sodium concentration occurs at the same time there is a fall in free water clearance. However, if the urine sodium concentration is corrected for glomerular filtration rate, one discovers that there really is an increased salt loss and an increased free water clearance. Obstruction diminishes glomerular filtration to a lesser degree than it diminishes renal blood flow; consequently, more filtrate reaches the distal nephron. As a result, there is decreased ability to dilute or to concentrate urine. The ability to acidify urine is also decreased (Berlyne, 1961).

In the early phases of obstruction, pressures within the proximal renal tubules rise but do not surge with a superimposed diuresis. Once tubular pressures rise to a level that equals intraureteral pressure, a superimposed diuresis will cause both tubular and ureteral pressures to rise to about 30 to 50 cm of water pressure (Weaver, 1968). In acute obstruction both ureteral pressure and diameter increase. Ureteral wall tension increases, but the ureteral peristaltic waves decrease in amplitude. As obstruction becomes chronic, the ureteral radius and volume increase. In this decompensated ureter, intraluminal pressure may be normal even though ureteral wall tension is high. Peristalsis will continue as long as infection is absent, but it is ineffective as it does not cause approximation of the ureteral walls (Ruse and Gillenwater, 1973).

If glomerular filtration actually continues despite the presence of obstruction, what happens to this increased fluid deposited within this closed space? Fluid is removed as it is produced by pyelotubular, pyelocalyceal, and pyelointerstitial backflow. The renal lymphatics seem an important part of this process (Goodwin and Kaufman, 1956). Because reabsorption is slow, it must be recognized that when an obstructive lesion has produced a steady state, any rise in intrarenal pressures because of a diuresis will potentially produce further renal damage.

INFRAVESICAL OBSTRUCTION

When there is an obstruction below the level of the bladder, in addition to the changes mentioned before, intravesical pressure initially rises. Urethral urine flow rate may fall in response to this pressure rise, but in most instances, urine flow rates are initially maintained because the detrusor muscle hypertrophies. After a further period of time, the detrusor can no longer hypertrophy; consequently, urine flow then decreases, and intravesical pressures also begin to fall (Fig. 5–1). However, at any given point in time, resistance to flow can be calculated because resistance $= \dfrac{\text{pressure}}{\text{flow}}$. With obstruction, resistance to flow is increased (O'Donnell et al., 1967).

Additionally, in the course of infravesical obstruction, the detrusor hypertrophies so that sacculation of the detrusor occurs. The areas about the ureteral orifices are specific points of weakness; consequently, periureteral sacculation is especially frequent. Such saccules may on rare occasion obstruct the ureter; in some instances, they render the ureterovesical junction incompetent so that vesicoureteral reflux may also occur (Chap. 4). Additionally, with marked detrusor hypertrophy, there can be secondary hypertrophy of the bladder neck; the bladder neck then may, in and of itself, act as an obstruction. With obstruction more distal to the bladder, that is, in the urethra, there is dilation of the urinary tract proximal to the point of obstruction as well as a decreased flow distal to the point of obstruction.

COMPLICATIONS OF OBSTRUCTION

In addition to the previously mentioned effects of obstruction, two others must be considered; both relate to the continued presence of large volumes of stagnant urine. The first of these is infection. There is no question that the emptying of the urinary tract or any portion thereof is an important facet of the normal bodily defense mechanisms against infection (Chap. 3). Consequently, when there is a large pool

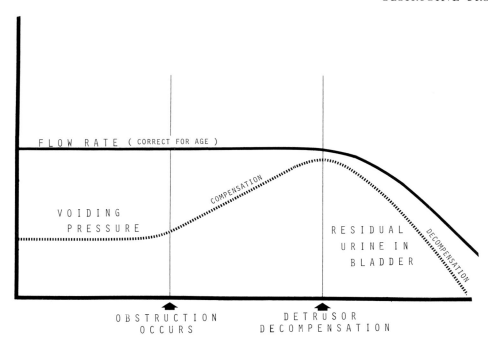

Figure 5–1. Physiologic parameters following bladder outlet obstruction. (From Kelalis, P. P., King, L. R., and Belman, A. B.: Clinical Pediatric Urology, Vol. 1. Philadelphia, W. B. Saunders Co., 1976, p. 295.)

of stagnant urine, the stage is set for the development of urinary tract infection (O'Grady and Cattell, 1966). The exact source of this infection is not always clear. In many instances, it may be ascending via the urethra but in others it may be either hematogenous or lymphogenous in origin. Once infection has occurred, it is quite difficult, in the presence of obstruction, to rid the urinary tract of bacteria for two reasons. First, there is a large pool of stagnant urine in which bacteria can grow; secondly, the delivery of antibiotics to the area by a damaged kidney is greatly reduced because of reduced renal function.

A second consequence of obstruction and urinary stasis is the propensity to form renal calculi. Fortunately, this does not occur frequently, probably because the urine produced by an obstructed kidney is too dilute for nucleation. However, should some process occur that can promote nucleation of a stone, such as infection, a stone can form rather rapidly, thereby setting the stage for further obstruction and further infection.

Obviously, the longer an obstruction has been present, the less the chance that renal function will return when the obstruction is relieved. In a Swiss study of children with obstructive uropathy, it was found that relief of obstruction prior to one year of age usually resulted in excellent return of function. Between one and two years of age, return of function was somewhat variable and often did not occur; renal function following relief of obstruction usually was stable. After two years of age, despite relief of obstruction, there often was, with time, continued loss of renal function (Mayor et al., 1975).

It must be recognized additionally that all dilation of the urinary tract is not necessarily due to obstruction. Many of the detrimental effects of obstruction are secondary to increased pressures within the system. Whitaker (1973) has shown that many dilated urinary tracts are not functionally obstructed in that even with diuresis there is no pressure rise within the system. Presumably such nonobstructive dilations are harmless if infection or stones do not supervene (Fig. 5–2). Operative intervention for such nonobstructive dilation is often fruitless. However, it is incumbent upon the responsible physician to prove that true obstruction is absent.

CLINICAL PICTURE

The mode of presentation of children with urinary tract obstruction is quite variable. In the neonatal period, children with urinary tract obstruction will often present with a palpable mass. Roughly 50 per cent of all abdominal masses are urinary in origin (Melicow, 1959). In infancy, two thirds of the renal masses are produced by hydronephrosis (Wedge et al., 1971). Another common mode of presentation is urinary tract infection, presumably because the obstructed urinary tract is more susceptible to infection than is the normal tract. Ten per cent of infants without masses presenting

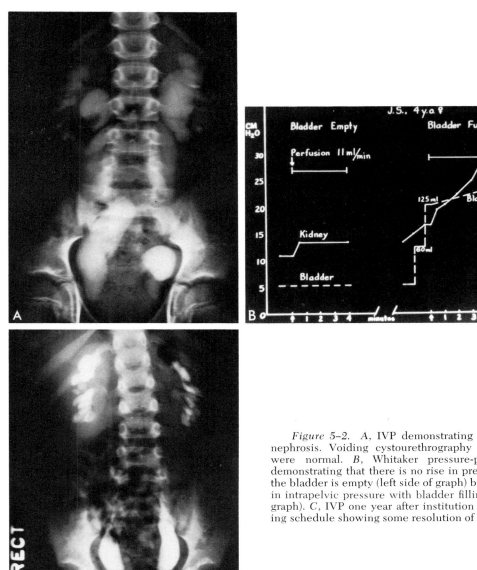

Figure 5–2. A, IVP demonstrating bilateral hydronephrosis. Voiding cystourethrography and cystoscopy were normal. *B*, Whitaker pressure-perfusion study demonstrating that there is no rise in pressure so long as the bladder is empty (left side of graph) but a definite rise in intrapelvic pressure with bladder filling (right side of graph). *C*, IVP one year after institution of a timed voiding schedule showing some resolution of hydronephrosis.

with urinary tract infection in one review were found to have hydronephrosis (Drew and Acton, 1976).

Another mode of presentation, especially in children, is abdominal pain. Why chronically distended kidneys should suddenly be painful is not clear. However, it is presumed that there is a diuresis, further distending the already distended urinary tract, resulting in pain. Additionally, the distended bladder may be painful, especially in instances of acute urinary retention.

Hematuria, usually grossly visible, is also a mode of presentation for obstructive lesions. Whether this is initiated by trauma or some other cause once again is not clear. Certainly the abnormal, distended urinary tract is more easily traumatized; minimal trauma could then result in gross hematuria.

Children with infravesical obstruction may present with voiding disturbances. Occasionally an astute mother will notice that her child's stream is abnormal, although, as was pointed out, the urinary stream is not always decreased in infravesical obstruction, especially in its early stages. Polyuria may result from a superimposed nephrogenic diabetes insipidus. Another, albeit rarer, presentation is hypertension, detected only by the routine monitoring of blood pressure.

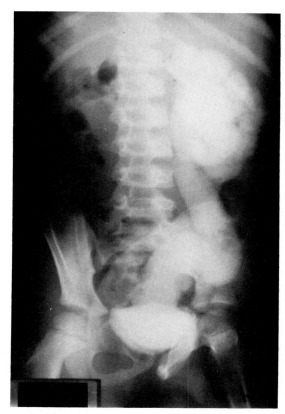

Figure 5-3. Excretory urogram delayed film at 24 hours. Early films showed very poor visualization of a hydronephrotic kidney, but this film clearly demonstrates hydroureteronephrosis with dilation to the ureterovesical junction.

RADIOGRAPHY

Urinary tract obstruction, once suspected, is most accurately diagnosed radiographically with excretory urography and voiding cystourethrography. Cystography is almost always necessary to complement urography for complete evaluation of the urinary tract in children. Often, renal function is poor, and delayed films are necessary for complete visualization and accurate assessment of the site of obstruction. If visualization is incomplete, imaging should continue for as long as 24 hours after injection (Fig. 5-3).

Radioisotope renal scanning is a more sensitive means of evaluating the obstruct-

ed or poorly functioning urinary tract. Delayed renal imaging is an excellent means of determining the site of obstruction, and, in addition, one can often determine the coexistence of reflux by obtaining delayed voiding films (the indirect isotope cystogram).

Occasionally, percutaneous antegrade pyelography or cystography will delineate the site of obstruction when conventional studies have failed to do so (Fig. 5-4). Additionally, if one suspects that the dilation of the urinary tract is nonobstructive, perfusion-pressure studies can be performed at the same time (Whitaker, 1973). Lastly, a newer, noninvasive means of establishing or refuting the presence of obstruction has been developed in which radionuclide transport is compared before and after the administration of furosemide (the Lasix-stimulated renal scan). If an obstruction is present, the radionuclide will clear

KIDNEY

Intrarenal Obstructions

Intrarenal obstructions may involve only a portion of the kidney. Such problems

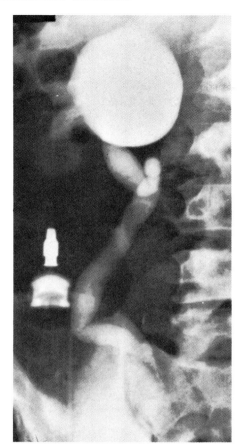

Figure 5–4. Sonographically guided percutaneous puncture and antegrade pyelogram. (From Harrison, J. H., Gittes, R. F., Perlmutter, A. D., et al.: Campbell's Urology, Vol. 1, 4th ed. Philadelphia, W. B. Saunders Co., 1979, p. 236.)

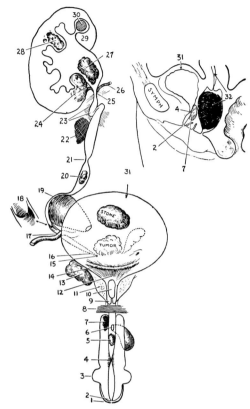

Figure 5–5. Potential sites of urinary tract obstruction: 1, phimosis, stenosis of prepuce, 2, stenosis of urethral meatus, 3, paraphimosis, 4, urethral stricture, 5, urethral stone, 6, urethral diverticulum, 7, periurethral abscess, 8, external sphincterospasm, 9, congenital valves of the posterior urethra, 10, hypertrophy of the verumontanum, diverticulum of utricle, 11, prostatic abscess or growths, 12, contracted bladder neck, median bar, 13, periprostatic abscess, 14, mucosal fold at bladder outlet, trigonal curtain, 15, stricture of ureteral meatus, ureterocele, 16, ureterovesical junction stricture, 17, vascular obstruction of lower ureter, 18, congenital ureteral valves, 19, ureteral obstruction by compression by vesical diverticulum, fecal overdistention of rectosigmoid, pelvic cyst, etc., 20, ureteral stone, 21, ureteral stricture, 22, periureteritis or tumor, 23, ureteral kink, periureteral fibrous bands, 24, renal tumor, 25, ureteropelvic junction stricture, 26, aberrant vessel obstruction of upper ureter, 27, pelvic stone, 28, renal tuberculosis (secondary obstructive lesions consequent thereto), 29, stricture of calyceal outlet, 30, calyceal stone, 31, neuromuscular vesical disease, 32, urethral compression by hematocolpometra of hydrocolpos. (From Campbell, M. F.: Clinical Pediatric Urology, Philadelphia, W. B. Saunders Co., 1951, p. 106.)

more slowly from the obstructed system than from the nonobstructed system (Koff, 1979) (see Chap. 2).

SPECIFIC SITES OF OBSTRUCTION

With these general remarks in mind, it would now be pertinent to consider specific sites of urinary tract obstruction seen in children. Obstruction may occur at any site from the calyx to the preputial meatus (Fig. 5–5). For organizational reasons alone, it will be most convenient to begin our journey down the urinary tract at its cephalad end and to work our way to its terminal caudal portion.

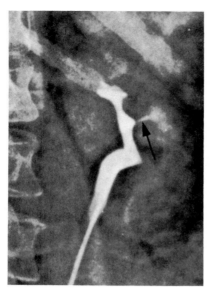

Figure 5–6. Infundibular stenosis produced by tuberculosis. (From Harrison, J. H., Gittes, R. F., Perlmutter, A. D., et al.: Campbell's Urology, Vol. 1, 4th ed. Philadelphia, W. B. Saunders Co., 1979, p. 565.)

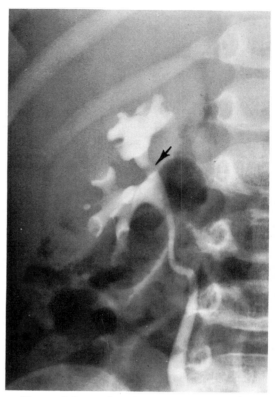

Figure 5–7. Hydrocalycosis due to vascular compression in asymptomatic two year old boy whose bladder was ruptured in a car accident. Excretory urogram shows dilatation of right upper calyx and infundibular compression by renal vessels (arrow). (From Kelalis, P. P., King, L. R., and Belman, A. B. : Clinical Pediatric Urology, Vol. 1. Philadelphia, W. B. Saunders Co., 1976, p. 236.)

most frequently occur in the infundibulum of a calyx. Infundibular stenosis frequently results from tuberculosis; its presence may produce further destruction of the calyx behind it (Lattimer and Wechsler, 1979) (Fig. 5–6). Calculi can similarly obstruct the infundibula. Fraley (1966) has described a condition in which the infundibulum is obstructed by a crossing vessel, usually with resultant pain (Fig. 5–7). Whether or not this lesion is truly of functional significance has never been demonstrated by urodynamic studies. Although not truly an obstructive lesion, calyceal diverticula present many of the problems posed by the other intrarenal obstructions (Fig. 5–8). Calyceal diverticula are visualized in 3.3 of 1000 pediatric excretory urograms (Timmons et al., 1975). Approximately one third are symptomatic. The etiology is probably congenital but could be acquired. The intrarenal lesions may cause pain, infection, or stones. If they are asymptomatic, no treatment is indicated. However, when they are symptomatic, relief can be achieved surgically by an infundibuloplasty or by ablation of that portion of the kidney.

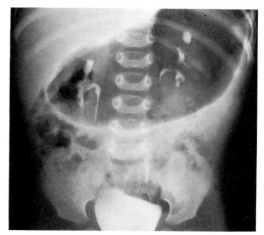

Figure 5–8. Calyceal diverticulum. (From Kelalis, P. P., King, L. R., and Belman, A. B.: Clinical Pediatric Urology, Vol. 1. Philadelphia, W. B. Saunders Co., 1976, p. 237.)

URETEROPELVIC JUNCTION OBSTRUCTION

The ureteropelvic junction is the most frequent site of supravesical obstructive uropathy in children. Anatomically, obstruction may be caused by an intrinsic narrowing of the ureter, angulation by a vessel crossing from the midline to the lower pole of the kidney, or angulation by kinks or bands between the ureter and the renal pelvis (Culp, 1967) (Fig. 5–9). At times there may be no obvious anatomic obstruction, but there is a functionally demonstrable obstructive area through which fluid is poorly transported (Murnaghan, 1958). Electron microscopy suggests that there is excessive collagen in the affected area (Hanna et al., 1976); this would explain such lesions.

For the moment, the embryogenesis of these lesions is unclear. Perhaps some of the problems result from intrauterine vascular accidents. Folds and valves may result from persistence of a fetal configuration (Fig. 5–10).

Presentation

Such lesions usually present during childhood; twenty-five per cent are detected in the first year of life (Williams and Kenawi, 1976). However, ureteropelvic junction obstruction may manifest at any age. The left side is obstructed more often than the right. Bilateral obstructions are seen in roughly 10 per cent of cases (Johnston et al., 1977). Children with ureteropelvic junction obstruction usually present in one of several manners.

Mass. A palpable mass is the most common mode of presentation in the infant. These masses are often quite large. Usually they are smooth, and often their fluid-filled nature is evident. They transilluminate. At times the mass may be so large that it extends across the midline.

Abdominal Pain. Pain in the abdomen is a frequent complaint of the child with ureteropelvic junction obstruction. Even though adults lateralize complaints well, most children do not; hence, the pain is usually stated to be periumbilical. The pain may be associated with nausea and vomiting and therefore may be confused with acute appendicitis. At times the pain may be intermittent, and in some instances the obstruction itself is intermittent—triggered by excessive fluid intake. Hydronephrosis may then be detectable only when the patient is symptomatic (Nesbit, 1956) (Fig. 5–11).

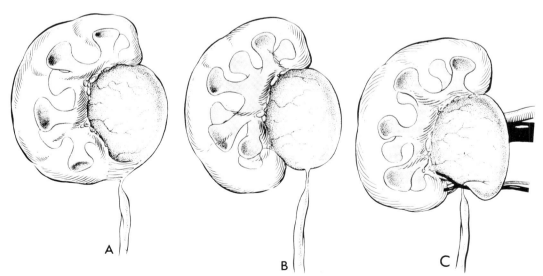

Figure 5–9. Ureteropelvic junction obstruction produced by *A*, fibrous bands, *B*, Intrinsic narrowing, and *C*, angulation. (From Eckstein, H. B., Hohenfellner, R., and Williams, D. I.: Surgical Pediatric Urology. Philadelphia, W. B. Saunders Co., 1977, pp. 125–126.)

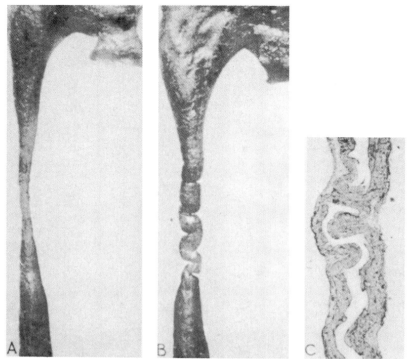

Figure 5–10. Embryologic considerations in the genesis of ureteral folds, kinks, and strictures. *A,* Cast of the ureter and the renal pelvis in a newborn. There is physiologic narrowing of the upper ureter below, which is the normal main spindle of the ureter. No ureteral folds are present. *B,* Cast of the ureter and the renal pelvis in the newborn. The ureteral folds proceed alternately from the opposite sides. *C,* Ureteral kinks that appear as muscular folds with axial offshoots of the loose adventitia. (Courtesy of Dr. Karl Ostling.) (From Campbell, M. F.: *In* Campbell, M. F., and Harrison, J. H.: Urology, Vol. 2, 3rd ed. Philadelphia, W. B. Saunders Co., 1970.)

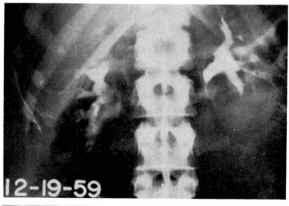

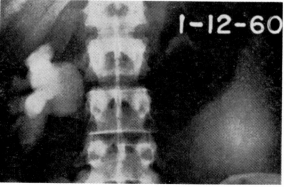

Figure 5–11. Intermittent right ureteropelvic junction obstruction. *A,* between attacks of pain and *B,* during an attack of pain. (From Ansell, J., and Patten, J. R. S.: N. Engl. J. Med., 267:447, 1962.)

Hematuria. The onset of hematuria, especially following minor trauma, often brings such a problem to attention. Urinary tract infection, on the other hand, is not very commonly a mode of presentation for ureteropelvic junction obstruction. When present, it raises the question of other problems, such as stones or reflux, compounding the problem. Minor degrees of reflux may be present in 40 per cent of children with ureteropelvic junction obstructions (Williams and Kenawi, 1976). Conversely, major degrees of vesicoureteral reflux may simulate ureteropelvic junction obstruction (pseudoureteropelvic junction obstruction) (Fig. 5–12). In the majority of these children, surgical revision of the ureteropelvic junction is not necessary. Repair of the reflux alone is corrective. Occasionally, however, a secondary pyeloplasty is required.

Laboratory Studies. Appropriate studies will document the presence or absence of hematuria, isosthenuria, and urinary tract infection. Disturbances of serum urea or creatinine concentrations would be expected only in solitary obstructed systems or in bilateral disease.

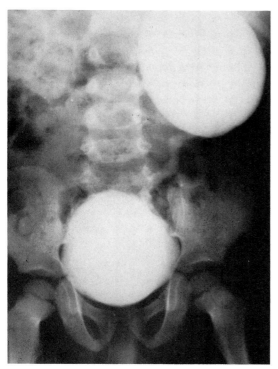

Figure 5–12. Cystogram with vesicoureteral reflux simulating ureteropelvic junction obstruction.

Excretory urography with delayed images and voiding cystourethrography will suggest the diagnosis in most instances. Occasionally, ultrasonography will initially suggest the diagnosis in the evaluation of an abdominal mass. Recently, antenatal ultrasonography has led to the earliest possible detection of such problems (Mendoza et al., 1979). In doubtful cases, percutaneous antegrade pressure flow studies or furosemide isotopic washout studies may be helpful for diagnosis. Retrograde or antegrade pyelography is usually not necessary for diagnosis but does help localize the site of obstruction and establishes the normalcy of the ureter distal to the obstruction.

Treatment

Once the diagnosis is established, the treatment is surgical repair. Delay in correction is particularly unacceptable in the neonate since development of the terminal nephrons continues at birth, and the potential for improving renal functional capabilities exists. Although many different procedures have been employed in the past, the most widely used procedure today is one in which the obstructive area is excised and the continuity of the dismembered ureteropelvic junction is reestablished (Fig. 5–13). The results of such a procedure are good to excellent in over 90 per cent of instances.

In adults, severely hydronephrotic kidneys are often removed. In children, however, renal recovery after relief of obstruction, especially in infancy, can be profound. For this reason, it is rare that we would recommend primary nephrectomy for such lesions in childhood. In those instances in which recovery does not occur, secondary nephrectomy can always be accomplished.

MEGACALYCOSIS

There are other causes for chronically dilated calyces aside from obstruction. The major problem of this type has been termed megacalycosis (Talner and Gittes, 1974) (Fig. 5–14). There is thought to be a congenital absence of the medulla so that the calyces appeared ballooned. It is usually a

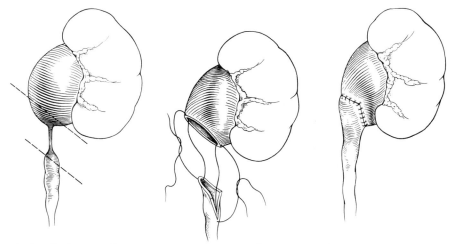

Figure 5–13. Technique of operative repair of ureteropelvic junction obstruction. (From Kelalis, P. P., King, L. R., and Belman, A. B.: Clinical Pediatric Urology, Vol. 1. Philadelphia, W. B. Saunders Co., 1976, p. 254.)

unilateral lesion. There are often an increased number of calyces. There does not seem to be a reduction in renal cortical substance. Johnston feels that this entity may represent instead the residuum of a previous obstruction that has spontaneously been relieved (Johnston, 1973). Children with this problem usually present with urinary tract infection. In any event, recognition of this entity as well as the demonstration of absence of obstruction by the Whitaker test or a diuretic renal scan is important because operative intervention in such an instance will not result in an improvement of either anatomy or function.

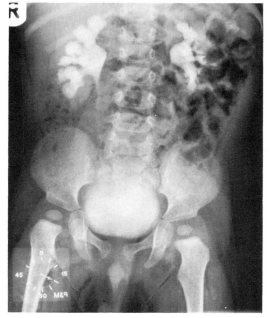

Figure 5–14. Megacalycosis of right kidney in a one year old boy. (From Johnston, J. H.: Megacalicosis: A burnt-out obstruction? J. Urol., *110*:344–346, 1973. © 1973, The Williams & Wilkins Co., Baltimore.)

URETERAL OBSTRUCTIONS

The ureter itself can be obstructed, although problems occurring along the course of the ureter are much less common than those occurring at either of its ends, i.e., the ureteropelvic or ureterovesical junction. Most of the obstructive lesions that affect the ureter itself are rare; they include valves, polyps, retrocaval ureters, and retroperitoneal fibrosis.

Ureteral Valves. Ureteral valves have been reported from time to time (Rizk et al., 1967) (Fig. 5–15); they must be differentiated from persistent fetal folds as well as from kinks and bends that result from tortuosity. In most instances, it would be helpful to prove urodynamically that the lesion seen is actually obstructive. Intrinsic congenital stenosis of the ureter occurs rarely and is usually located at the junction of the lower third and upper two thirds of the ureter. The embryogenesis of these valves and stenoses

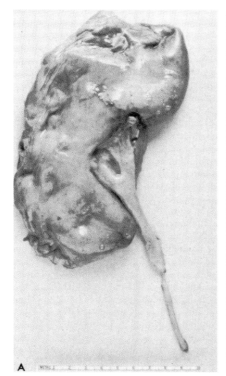 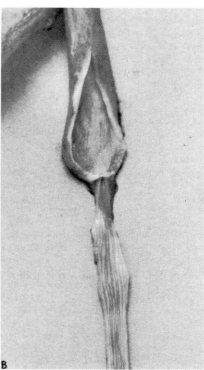

Figure 5–15. Congenital ureteral valve: *A,* Extended view. *B,* Long section showing greatly dilated ureter above the valve and normal size below. (From Simon, J. B., et al.: J. Urol., 74:336, 1955.)

is unclear. They usually present clinically with infection or hematuria and less often as a painful mass. The diagnosis is made radiographically, and the management requires surgical excision or repair.

Ureteral Polyps. The ureter in adults is sometimes obstructed by intrinsic tumors. These are almost always malignant. Such lesions have not been reported in children. However, a few cases of benign fibrous polyps obstructing the ureter in childhood have been reported (Colgan et al., 1973). They usually present as abdominal pain or masses (caused by hydronephrosis produced by the polyp). The benign nature of these lesions is to be stressed. The management is excision of the lesion and its base rather than a radical procedure such as might be appropriate for a malignancy.

Retrocaval Ureter. The retrocaval ureter is an uncommon anomaly that results from a vascular abnormality rather than a primary ureteral one. Because the vena cava in such cases derives from the subcardinal vein rather than the supracardinal vein as it

normally does, the ureter passes behind the inferior vena cava (Fig. 5–16). This anomaly occurs exclusively on the right side except in cases of situs inversus (Brooks, 1962). The anomaly is of significance only when hydronephrosis results from it.

The ureter in these cases passes behind the vena cava at approximately the junction of the upper third of the ureter with its lower two thirds. The ureter forms a rather characteristic S-shaped curve as a result of its abnormal course. Obstruction often occurs at this point, and it will be this obstruction that mandates treatment. Most patients present with pain or hematuria. It is of interest that despite its congenital origin, many patients with this problem will present in adult life (Kenawi and Williams, 1976). The preferred management when intervention is necessary is surgical and consists of ureteral division, repositioning, and reanastomosis.

Retroperitoneal Fibrosis. The ureter may also be obstructed by extrinsic lesions that involve the retroperitoneum. The most

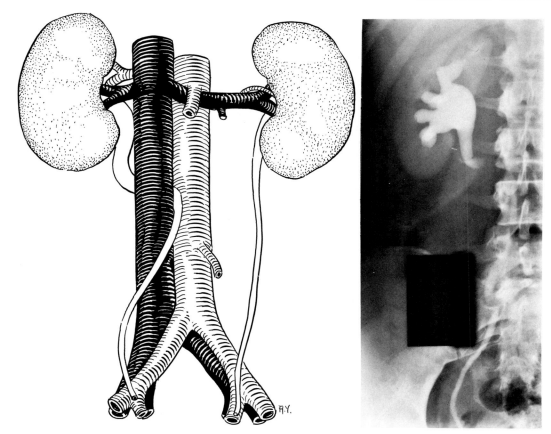

Figure 5–16.   Retrocaval ureter. *Left*, Drawing. (From Hollinshead, W. H.: Anatomy for Surgeons, Vol. 2, 2nd ed. New York; Harper and Row, 1971. © 1971 by Harper and Row, Inc. *Right*, Excretory urogram. (From Kelalis, P. P., King, L. R., and Belman, A. B.: Clinical Pediatric Urology. Vol. 1. Philadelphia, W. B. Saunders Co., 1976, p. 259.)

common of these is idiopathic retroperitoneal fibrosis. This uncommon problem of largely unknown etiology primarily affects adults. However, there are a few reports in children (Chan et al., 1979). These patients usually present with vague back pain and azotemia. A helpful laboratory finding is marked elevation of the erythrocyte sedimentation rate. On excretpry urography, the ureters, in addition to being obstructed, are pulled to the midline. The treatment is surgical relocation of the ureters so that they no longer traverse the fibrotic area. In less severe cases, corticosteroids may be effective as therapy.

Additionally, other forms of periureteral inflammation may result in ureteral obstruction. Such problems predominate on the right side and have been reported in both appendicitis and Crohn's disease (Kaplan and Keiller, 1974). Iatrogenic causes include lumbar-subarachnoid shunts for hydrocephalus (Sullivan et al., 1972) and Dwyer procedures for scoliosis (Silver and McMaster, 1977). In the non-iatrogenic forms of inflammation, ureteral obstruction will usually subside with resolution of the primary process. In the iatrogenic forms, scarring usually mandates operative intervention for resolution of the problem.

URETEROVESICAL JUNCTION OBSTRUCTION

Megaureter. The second most common site in which ureteral obstruction may occur is the area of the ureterovesical junction. The most frequently encountered problem in this location is megaureter. Megaureter can be defined as any ureter greater than 1 cm in diameter regardless of

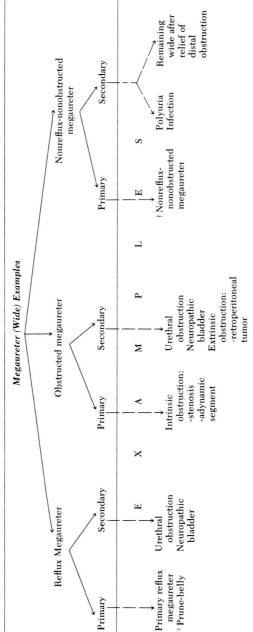

Megaureter — A Proposed Classification

Megaureter (Wide) Examples

Figure 5-17. From Report of Working Party to Establish an International Nomenclature for the Large Ureter. *In* Bergsma, D., and Duckett, J. W. (Eds.): Urinary System Malformations in Children. Birth Defects: Original Article Series, *13*, No. 5. New York, Alan R. Liss for The National Foundation–March of Dimes, 1977.
*Some conditions (e.g., prune-belly, ureteroceles, ectopic ureters, etc.) may appear under several other columns.
†As proved not to be obstructed.
Note: An occasional megaureter may show reflux and apparent obstruction.

the cause. Because the etiology of this problem is variable, multiple classifications have been proposed. Recently there has been general agreement upon a classification, and this schema is depicted in Figure 5–17. Megaureters may be produced by both obstruction and vesicoureteral reflux. Excluding that group in which voiding cystourethrography demonstrates the reflux, the pyelographic picture of all types of megaureters is similar and is not helpful in differential diagnosis. Conversely, the clinical setting in which the megaureter presents may indeed be helpful in differentiating one type from another.

The primary obstructed megaureter is the most frequently seen of the various types of megaureters. Megaureters are seen more frequently in children than in adults. The usual mode of presentation is urinary tract infection or hematuria. Primary megaureters are bilateral in 20 per cent of patients with megaureters. There is a male preponderance and the left side is more frequently involved than the right side (Williams and Hulme-Moir, 1970). An anatomic characteristic of most megaureters is that the lower ureter is usually proportionately more dilated than the upper ureter. Additionally, regardless of the degree of dilation, the ureter is straight rather than tortuous. The dilation may involve only the distal ureteral spindle, especially when first detected in adults (Fig. 5–18). In children especially, the dilation seen is often much greater than in adults; and in such children it is obvious that there is marked functional impairment of the ipsilateral kidney. If one observes primary obstructed megaureters fluoroscopically, peristalsis will be noted to be ineffective in the lower third of the ureters; beyond the dilated segment, the ureter tapers to a normal caliber as it enters the bladder (Fig. 5–19). As mentioned, cystography will not demonstrate vesicoureteral reflux; if cystoscopy is performed, the ureteral orifice will be seen to be normal. In addition, the ureteral orifice will accept at least a 3 or 4 French ureteral catheter; this is considered the normal caliber ureteral orifice for most prepubertal children.

Histologically, the findings in such

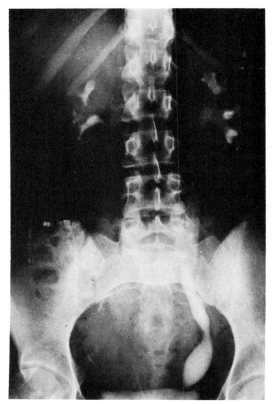

Figure 5–18. Intravenous urogram typical of primary megaureter. Fusiform distal ureteral dialatation with normal renal collecting system and proximal ureter. (From Kelalis, P. P., King, L. R., and Belman, A. B.: Clinical Pediatric Urology, Vol. 1. Philadelphia, W. B. Saunders Co., 1976, p. 275.)

cases have been quite variable, but electron microscopy suggests that the problem is similar to that of ureteropelvic junction obstruction (Hanna et al., 1976). It would appear that the distal ureteral segment is aperistaltic and acts as a functional obstruction. This occasionally can be graphically demonstrated in the course of an operative procedure. When the ureter has been dissected free from the bladder with this aperistaltic segment still attached, the ureter will remain dilated; there may be vigorous peristalsis proximally, but none will be noted in the normal-caliber segment. However, if the dilated ureter is then transected immediately above this normal-caliber aperistaltic segment, the ureter will immediately collapse, and a diuresis will ensue.

The treatment of primary obstructed megaureters is dictated largely by the de-

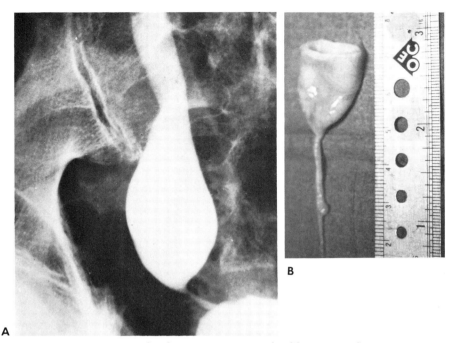

A

B

Figure 5–19. A, Excretory urography demonstrating normal caliber terminal ureter in a case of primary obstructed megaureter. (From McLaughlin, A. P. III, Pfister, R. C., Leadbetter, W. F., et al.: The pathophysiology of primary megaureter. J. Urol., *109*:805–811, 1973. © 1973, The Williams & Wilkins Co., Baltimore.) *B*, Operative specimen demonstrating the same pathologic anatomy.

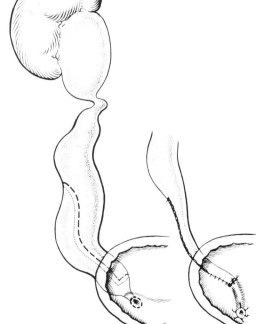

Figure 5–20. Operative repair of megaureter. (From Eckstein, H. B., Hohenfellner, R., and Williams, D. I.: Surgical Pediatric Urology. Philadelphia, W. B. Saunders Co., 1977, p. 215.)

gree of resultant hydronephrosis and whether or not infections or stones are complicating problems. Basically the aperistaltic segment is excised, and the affected dilated ureter reimplanted. Distal ureteral tailoring is usually necessary to achieve the proper ratio of submucosal tunnel length to ureteral diameter (Chap. 4) (Hendren, 1969) (Fig. 5–20).

In some infants, if an excretory urogram is performed following a severe infection, marked ureteral dilation, occasionally with calycectasis, will be seen. However, over the course of several weeks to months, this resolves with no therapy other than treatment of the primary infection. This phenomenon has been quite well documented by Makker and colleagues (1972). In the experimental animal, it has been shown that urinary tract infection, presumably by virtue of endotoxin, induces ureteral atonicity (Grana et al., 1965). This is the presumed mechanism of this phenomenon as well. Consequently, if one encounters an infant who has just had an infection and has marked ureteral dilation without vesicoureteral reflux, one should not

proceed immediately to operative intervention, as the problem may resolve with medical management alone. Certainly, though, careful follow-up is mandatory with repeat radiographic studies several weeks after control of infection.

Bladder Diverticula. Another common problem that is usually found at the ureterovesical junction is that posed by periureteral saccules or diverticula. These diverticula are usually developmental in origin, although they can be secondary to distal obstruction (Johnston, 1960). Most children with diverticula present between ages three to 10 years because of urinary tract infection. In many instances, these sacculations sufficiently distort the ureterovesical junction so that reflux is produced. In rare instances, the position of the diverticulum is such that reflux does not occur. Because of the size and position of a diverticulum, the ipsilateral ureter may become obstructed. Rarely, a bladder diverticulum is located in such a position that as the bladder fills, the diverticulum compresses the bladder neck against the pubis and thereby acts as an obstruction to bladder emptying.

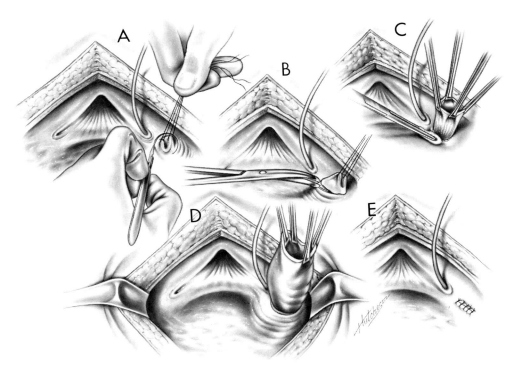

Figure 5–21. Transvesical diverticulectomy. (From Kelalis, P. P., King, L. R., and Belman, A. B.: Clinical Pediatric Urology, Vol. 1. Philadelphia, W. B. Saunders Co., 1976, p. 290.)

When infection or ipsilateral ureteral obstruction complicates diverticula, excision of the diverticulum is considered appropriate therapy (Fig. 5–21). Usually reimplantation of the ureter will be necessary in the course of such an undertaking.

BLADDER NECK OBSTRUCTION

Although today considered a "dirty word," bladder neck obstruction probably does rarely exist as a true entity in children. There is no question that this problem is seen in the young adult male; it is presumed that such lesions are congenital (Gute et al., 1968). If so, it is only reasonable to assume that these problems should occasionally be encountered in childhood as well. The whole issue is clouded by recent history. In the late 1950s and early 1960s, bladder neck obstruction was a very fashionable diagnosis in both boys and girls. Bladder neck obstruction was thought responsible for urinary tract infection and vesicoureteral reflux. Formal open vesical neck revisions and transurethral resections were performed for this diagnosis. It was subsequently recognized that most of these operations were not indicated and that bladder neck obstruction was not the frequent problem it was thought to be (Kaplan and King, 1970).

Nonetheless, there occasionally may be a child who does indeed have a bladder neck obstruction. The etiology of this problem when present may be either smooth muscle hypertrophy or fibroelastosis. Elastic tissue replacement seen in fibroelastosis may be a secondary phenomenon rather than a primary obstructive lesion, but this particular issue is as yet unsettled (Young, 1965).

In all likelihood, bladder neck obstruction, if it exists, is limited to males. It is a well-established fact that the endoscopic diagnosis of this problem in children is tenuous at best. This diagnosis is inferred from the presence of heavy trabeculation in the absence of any other lesion that can produce this finding. Shopfner (1967) has shown that bladder neck obstruction cannot be diagnosed radiographically. Presumably, however, one could establish the diagnosis

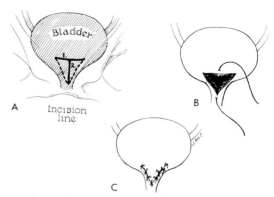

Figur 5–22. Operative technique of Y-V vesicourethroplasty. (From Kaplan, G. W., and King, L. R.: An evaluation of Y-V vesicourethroplasty in children. Surg. Gynecol. Obstet., *130*:1059–1066, 1970. Reproduced by permission of Surgery, Gynecology, and Obstetrics.)

using modern urodynamic techniques. If one could establish that a child voids with low to normal flow rates with high intravesical pressures and without urethral sphincter dyssynergia, one might then infer the diagnosis of bladder neck obstruction. Under such circumstances, Y-V plasty may then be an accepted therapeutic modality (Fig. 5–22).

Non-Neurogenic, Neurogenic Bladder. Another group of children has recently been identified and is discussed in Chapter 6. These are the children with the occult neuropathic bladder or the non-neurogenic neurogenic bladder. These children are usually male and present with day and night wetting, often with associated encopresis. They empty their bladders very poorly and may even have marked hydronephrosis. No obstructive or neurogenic lesions can be demonstrated. In all likelihood, these children have urethral sphincter dyssynergia, which may be primarily psychogenic in origin. Such children are best treated nonoperatively. The complications of this problem, however, do occasionally require temporary urinary diversion. It is unexplained but of interest that these children may sometimes improve spontaneously following puberty (Chaps. 6 and 7).

MÜLLERIAN DUCT CYSTS

Another rare lesion that may produce obstructive uropathy in boys is a müllerian

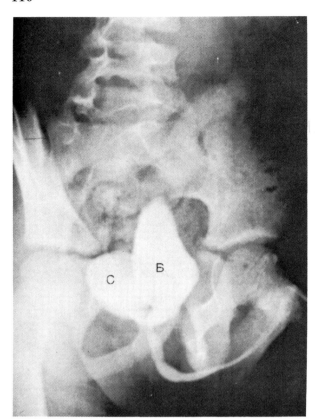

Figure 5–23. Voiding cystourethrography demonstrating a müllerian duct cyst. The bladder is labeled "B" and the cyst "C". (From Kaplan, G. W., et al.: Müllerian duct and seminal vesical cysts. *In* Bergsma, D., and Overett, J. W. (Eds.): Urinary System Malformations in Children. Birth Defects: Original Article Series, *13*, No. 5. New York, Alan R. Liss for the National Foundation-March of Dimes, 1977, p. 245.)

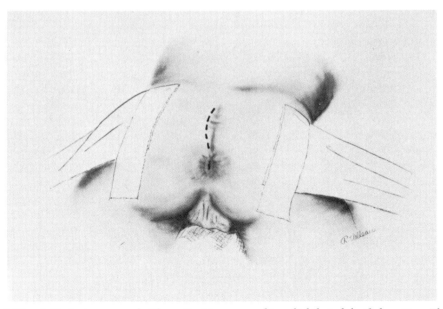

A

Figure 5–24. A, Posterior approach: The patient is prone and in a slightly jack-knifed position. The incision is indicated by dotted lines.

duct or seminal vesicle cyst (Schuhrke and Kaplan, 1978) (Fig. 5–23). These cysts are müllerian remnants that open into the urethra at the verumontanum. Small müllerian duct cysts are often seen in severe degrees of hypospadias and are usually of no clinical significance. When large, urine can pool and become stagnant, thereby set-ting the stage for urinary tract infection. In addition, because of size alone, such cysts may impinge on the bladder neck and act as an obstruction. When symptomatic these are best treated surgically. The easiest surgical approach to this problem, in our opinion, is a posterior parasacral approach (Fig. 5–24).

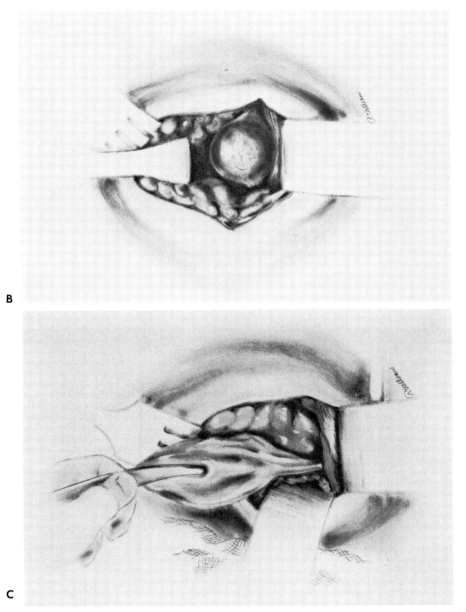

B

C

Figure 5–24 Continued. B, The coccyx has been amputated, and the rectum is retracted laterally. C, Denonvillier's fascia has been incised, and the lesion has been mobilized. (From Kaplan, G. W., et al.: Müllerian duct and seminal vesical cysts. *In* Bergsma, D., and Overrett, J. W. (Eds.): Urinary System Malformations in Children. Birth Defects: Original Article Series, *13*, No. 5. New York, Alan R. Liss for the National Foundation-March of Dimes, 1977, p. 244.)

POSTERIOR URETHRAL VALVES

The most frequently seen of the obstructive lesions of the boy's lower urinary tract is the one called posterior urethral valves. This name is a misnomer as these are really folds or a diaphragm that traverse the urethra from a point just distal to the verumontanum to the proximal limit of the membranous urethra (Fig. 5–25). Embryologically, valves occur presumably because there is failure of migration of the distal extent of the wolffian duct (Fig. 5–26).

Children with valves often present early in infancy but may present at any age. As a general rule, the more severely affected children present at the earliest ages. The mortality rate of children with valves presenting within the first month of life has in the past approached 50 per cent, presumably because in this group there is associated renal dysplasia (Kaplan, 1976). With modern therapy, many of these infants will survive but may later in childhood become candidates for dialysis and transplantation. Because of the profound nature of the obstruction produced, the prostatic urethra balloons, and the bladder neck hypertrophies. The bladder becomes heavily trabeculated and sacculated.

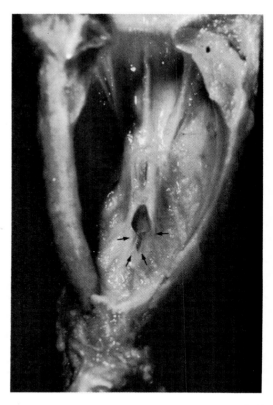

Figure 5–25. Autopsy specimen opened by unroofing rather than incising the anterior urethral wall. The valves are clearly seen to be an oblique diaphragm (arrows). (From Robertson, W. B., and Hayes, J. A.: Br. J. Urol., *41*:592–598, 1969. Reproduced by permission.)

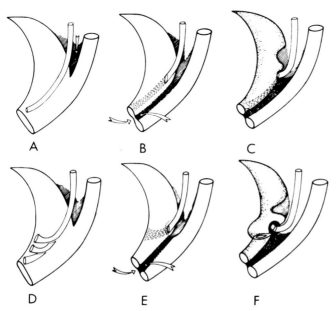

Figure 5–26. Development of posterior urethral valves. A–C, Development of the normal urethral crest. Migration of the orifice of the wolffian duct from its anterolateral position in the cloaca to the site of Müller's tubercle on the posterior wall of the urorectal septum, occurring synchronously with cloacal division. (Dots denote pathway of migration.) This pathway is swept laterally and posteriorly and remains as the normal inferior crest and the plicae colliculi. *D-F,* Abnormal anterior positions of the wolffian duct orifices and consequent abnormal migration of the terminal ends of the ducts, resulting in circumferential obliquely oriented ridges that comprise the valve. (Drawings are supplied through the courtesy of F. D. Stephens.)

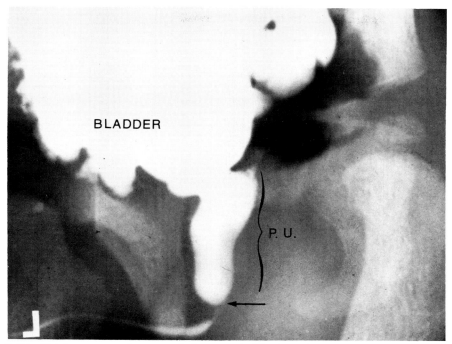

Figure 5-27. Voiding cystourethrogram of a four month old infant, showing posterior urethral valves (arrow). Note elongated prostatic urethra (PU) and trabeculated bladder. (From Kelalis, P. P., King, L. R., and Belman, A. B.: Clinical Pediatric Urology, Vol. 1. Philadelphia, W. B. Saunders Co., 1976, p. 312.)

Infants with valves may present with sepsis and profound electrolyte imbalance. Some present with abdominal masses or failure to thrive. Older children tend to present with voiding disturbances or infections. The diagnosis is made radiographically on voiding cystourethrography (Fig. 5–27). It is confirmed endoscopically (Fig. 5–28). Resuscitative measures are often necessary at first presentation and consist of treatment of the infection, fluid and electrolyte replacement to correct electrolyte imbalance, and drainage of the urinary tract. A small urethral catheter will often suffice for drainage for a few days. At times some temporary procedure to divert the urine may be necessary, such as vesicostomy or loop ureterostomy. In the majority of cases, fortunately, transurethral valve ablation can be carried out directly without the need for additional surgery (Fig. 5–29).

Most often, after resection of the valve, although the child has improved dramatically, the radiographic picture has not. In past years, the slow improvement in the amount of dilation was thought to be evidence of ongoing obstruction, and many reconstruc-

tive procedures were recommended. We can now perform urodynamic studies on the upper tract to prove or disprove the need for surgery when these concerns arise. In most instances, it will be found that such surgery is not indicated and that a nonoperative course may then be pursued. The radiographic appearance of the urinary tract may never achieve normality.

STRICTURES

Strictures of the urethra occur in children as well as in adults (Leadbetter and Leadbetter, 1962). Congenital strictures are rare. Trauma, either external or iatrogenic, is the most frequent cause of urethral stricture in childhood. The most frequent sites of stricture resulting from trauma are the membranous urethra following pelvic fractures, the bulbous urethra following straddle injuries, and the penoscrotal junction following instrumentation.

Occasionally, a congenital stricture can be treated by simple urethral dilation or transurethral incision with resultant rupture

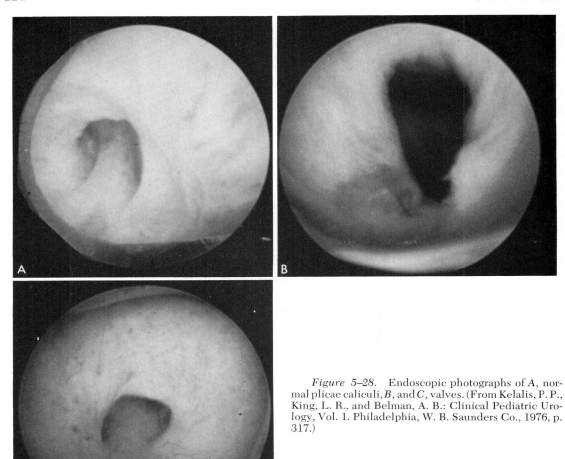

Figure 5–28. Endoscopic photographs of *A*, normal plicae caliculi, *B*, and *C*, valves. (From Kelalis, P. P., King, L. R., and Belman, A. B.: Clinical Pediatric Urology, Vol. 1. Philadelphia, W. B. Saunders Co., 1976, p. 317.)

Figure 5–29. Diagram representing engagement of valve leaflet with resectoscope loop. (From Kelalis, P. P., King, L. R., and Belman, A. B.: Clinical Pediatric Urology, Vol. 1. Philadelphia, W. B. Saunders Co., 1976, p. 318.)

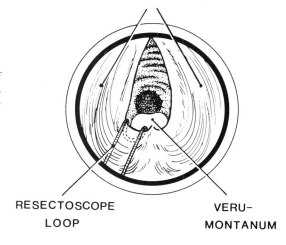

of the stricture. However, most traumatic strictures require formal repair for resolution. Although it may be appropriate to attempt a course of urethral dilation for relief of stricture, surgical repair is indicated if more than one or two dilatations are required. Otherwise the child is committed to the lifelong need for dilatation.

ANTERIOR URETHRAL VALVES

A rare but definitely obstructive lesion is a valve of the anterior urethra (Firlit and King, 1972). Although they may occur alone, these valves often are associated with a urethral diverticulum so that a distal lip is elevated into the urethral lumen as the diverticulum fills, producing an obstruction. These lesions can be quite difficult to diagnose. They are best visualized on urethrography. Voiding urethrography will demonstrate the obstruction, but retrograde urethrography may be necessary to show the diverticulum component. When these lesions are identified, they are best treated with endoscopic resection.

URETHRAL DIVERTICULA AND MEGALOURETHRA

Urethral diverticula are often seen as a complication of hypospadias repair and are usually manifest with infection and post-voiding dribbling. Such diverticula also rarely occur spontaneously. The treatment of these lesions when symptomatic is surgical excision.

This unusual lesion (Fig. 5–30) occurs presumably because there is a lack of corpus spongiosum in the affected area. It may best be thought of as a specialized diverticulum. Associated upper tract abnormalities (reflux and dysplasia) are common. Megalourethra also is often associated with the prune-belly syndrome. It is best treated by reducing the caliber of the enlarged area of the urethra.

MEATAL STENOSIS

Meatitis can be a vexing problem in the circumcised infant. In such instances, urinary obstruction may temporarily result from the formation of a crust over the meatus at the time. Whether or not meatal stenosis exists as a significant obstructive lesion in the otherwise normal penis at other times is open to serious question. Meatal stenosis has been blamed for all manner of urinary problems from wetting to anecdotal reports of severe hydronephrosis. Unfortunately, none of these cases has been well documented. There is no correlation between the visual size of the meatus and its caliber. Meatal stenosis can result in a cephalad

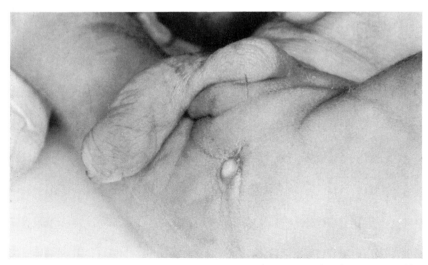

Figure 5–30.   Severe megalourethra. (From Kelalis, P. P., King, L. R., and Belman, A. B.: Clinical Pediatric Urology, Vol. 2. Philadelphia, W. B. Saunders Co., 1976, p. 625.)

deflection of the urinary stream but in our opinion results in little else in the way of abnormal function. Meatotomy is indicated to correct the course of the stream and to allow passage of instruments. Generally, the small meatus can be easily spread in the office with a tiny hemostat, disrupting the ventral web that has formed from previous episodes of meatitis. Hospitalization, a trip to the operating room, and general anesthesia with all its risks and expense are rarely required.

DISTAL URETHRAL STENOSIS

A very popular diagnosis in girls with vesicoureteral reflux, urinary tract infection, and voiding dysfunctions of all types is distal urethral stenosis (or its variant, meatal stenosis). The underlying thesis proposed by those utilizing this diagnosis is that the normal distal urethra, being fibrous, acts as a point of functional or anatomic obstruction. The normal urethral calibers in girls have been established in several studies (Immergut and Wahman, 1968; Graham et al., 1967). Interestingly, there is a negative correlation between urethral size and recurring infection; that is, girls with larger caliber urethras tend to become infected more frequently (Graham et al., 1967). Most controlled studies of urethral dilation or urethrotomy (procedures designed to eliminate the obstructive lesion) show these procedures to be no better than medication alone in the control of infection (Kaplan et al., 1973). Although of no apparent harm, urethral dilation cannot be supported as an effective tool in the management of lower urinary tract problems in girls. Urethrotomy, however, carries a small risk of producing incontinence and is, in our opinion, best avoided.

PHIMOSIS

Although definitely obstructive when present, this lesion is greatly overdiagnosed. In true phimosis, the orifice of the prepuce is so small that it obstructs the flow of urine. In most instances, what is thought to be phimosis in a child is merely the normal physiologic inability to retract the prepuce due to incomplete separation of the prepuce from the glans. In the physiologic variant, there is no balooning of the preputial sac during voiding, whereas in phimosis there is. Treatment of phimosis is best accomplished by circumcision.

REFERENCES

Belman, A. B., Kropp, K. A., and Simon, N. M.: Renal pressure hypertension secondary to unilateral hydronephrosis. N. Engl. J. Med., 278:1133, 1968.

Berlyne, G. M.: Distal tubular function in chronic hydronephrosis. Q. J. Med., 30:339, 1961.

Brooks, R. E., Jr.: Left retrocaval ureter associated with situs inversus. J. Urol., 88:484, 1962.

Chan, S. L., Johnson, H. W., and McLoughlin, M. G.: Idiopathic retroperitoneal fibrosis in children. J. Urol., 122:103, 1979.

Colgan, J. R., III., Skaist, L., and Morrow, J. W.: Benign ureteral tumors in childhood. J. Urol., 109:308, 1973.

Culp, O. S.: Management of ureteropelvic junction obstruction. Bull. N.Y. Acad. Med., 43:355–377, 1967.

Drew, J. H., and Acton, C. M.: Radiological findings in newborn infants with urinary infection. Arch. Dis. Child., 51:628, 1976.

Firlit, C. F., and King, L. R.: Anterior urethral valves in children. J. Urol., 108:972, 1972.

Fraley, E. E.: Vascular obstruction of superior infundibulum causing nephralgia: A new syndrome. N. Engl. J. Med., 275:1403, 1966.

Goodwin, W. E., and Kaufman, J. J.: The renal lymphatics. Urol. Surv., 6:305, 1956.

Gottschalk, C. W., and Mylle, M.: Micropuncture study of pressures in proximal tubules and peritubular capillaries of the rat kidney and their relation to ureteral and renal venous pressures. Am. J. Physiol., 185:430, 1956.

Graham, J. B., King, L. R., and Kropp, K. A.: The significance of distal urethral narrowing in young girls. J. Urol., 97:1045, 1967.

Grana, L., Kidd, J., Idriss, F., and Swenson, O.: Effect of chronic urinary tract infection on ureteral peristalsis. J. Urol., 94:652, 1965.

Gute, D. R., Chute, R., and Baron, J. A., Jr.: Bladder neck revision for obstruction in men. J. Urol., 99:744, 1968.

Hanna, M. K., Jeffs, R. D., Sturgess, J. M., and Barkin, M.: Ureteral structure and ultrastructure. Part II. Congenital ureteropelvic junction and obstruction and primary obstructive megaureter. J. Urol., 116:725, 1976.

Hendren, W. H.: Operative repair of megaureter in children. J. Urol., 101:491, 1969.

Immergut, M. A., and Wahman, G. E.: The urethral caliber of female children with recurrent urinary tract infections. J. Urol., 99:187, 1968.

Johnston, J. H.: Vesical diverticula without urinary obstruction in children. J. Urol., 84:535, 1960.

Johnston, J. H.: Megacalicosis: A burnt out obstruction? J. Urol., 110:344, 1973.

Johnston, J. H., Evans, J. P., Glassberg, K. I., and Shapiro, S. R.: Pelvic hydronephrosis in children: A review of 219 personal cases. J. Urol., *117*:97, 1977.

Kaplan, G. W.: Posterior urethra. *In* Kelalis, P. P., King, L. R., and Belman, A. B.: Clinical Pediatric Urology, Vol. 1. Philadelphia, W. B. Saunders Co., 1976.

Kaplan, G. W., and Keiller, D. L.: Ureteral obstruction after appendectomy. J. Pediatr. Surg., 9:559, 1974.

Kaplan, G. W., and King, L. R.: An evaluation of Y-V vesicourethroplasty in children. Surg. Gynecol. Obstet., *130*:1059, 1970.

Kaplan, G. W., Sammons, T. A., and King, L. R.: A blind comparison of dilation, urethrotomy, and medication alone in the treatment of urinary tract infection in girls. J. Urol., *109*:917, 1973.

Kenawi, M. M., and Williams, D. I.: Circumcaval ureter. Br. J. Urol., *48*:183, 1976.

Kerr, W. S., Jr.: Effect of complete ureteral obstruction for one week on kidney function. J. Appl. Physiol., 6:762, 1954.

Koff, S. A., Thrall, J. H., and Keyes, J. W., Jr.: Diuretic radionuclide urography: Non-invasive method for evaluating nephroureteral dilatation. J. Urol., *122*:451, 1979.

Lattimer, J. K., and Wechsler, M.: Genitourinary tuberculosis. *In* Harrison, J. H., Gittes, R. F., Perlmutter, A. D., et al.: Campbell's Urology, Vol. 3, 4th ed. Philadelphia, W. B. Saunders Co., 1979.

Leadbetter, G. W., Jr., and Leadbetter, W. F.: Urethral strictures in male children. J. Urol., 88:409, 1962.

Lorentz, W. B., Jr., Labiter, W. E., and Gottschalk, C. W.: Renal tubular permeability during increased intrarenal pressure. J. Clin. Invest., *51*:484, 1972.

Marker, S. P., Tucker, A. S., Izant, R. J., Jr., and Heymann, W.: Nonobstructive hydronephrosis and hydroureter associated with peritonitis. N. Engl. J. Med., 287:535, 1972.

Malvin, R. L., Kutchai, H., and Ostermann, T.: Decreased nephron population resulting from increased ureteral pressure. Am. J. Physiol., *207*:835, 1964.

Mayor, G., Genton, N., Torrado, H., and Guignard, J.: Renal function in obstructive nephropathy: Long-term effect of reconstructive surgery. Pediatrics, 56:740, 1975.

Melicow, M. M., and Uson, A. C.: Palpable abdominal masses in infants and children: A report based on a review of 653 cases. J. Urol., *81*:705, 1959.

Mendoza, S. A., Griswald, W. R., Leopold, G. R., and Kaplan, G. W.: Intrauterine diagnosis of renal anomalies by ultrasonography. Am. J. Dis. Child., *133*:1042, 1979.

Murnaghan, G. F.: The dynamics of the renal pelvis and ureter with special reference to congenital hydronephrosis. Br. J. Urol., 30:321, 1958.

Nesbit, R. M.: Diagnosis of intermittent hydronephrosis. J. Urol., 75:767, 1956.

O'Donnell, B., Vella, L., and Maloney, M.: The measurement of lower urinary tract obstruction in infants and children. J. Pediatr. Surg., 2:518, 1967.

O'Grady, F., and Cattell, W. R.: Kinetics of urinary tract infection. II. The bladder. Br. J. Urol., 38:156, 1966.

Rizk, G. K., Melhem, R. E., and Azoury, B. S.: Congenital ureteral valves. Br. J. Radiol., *40*:544, 1967.

Ruse, J. G., and Gillenwater, J. Y.: Pathophysiology of ureteral obstruction. Am. J. Physiol., *225*:830, 1973.

Schuhrke, T. D., and Kaplan, G. W.: Prostatic utricle cysts (Müllerian duct cysts). J. Urol., *119*:765, 1978.

Selkurt, E. E.: Effect of ureteral blockade on renal blood flow and urinary concentrating ability. Am. J. Physiol., *205*:286, 1963.

Shopfner, C. E.: Roentgenological evaluation of bladder neck obstruction. Am. J. Roentgenol. Radium Ther. Nucl. Med., *100*:162, 1967.

Silber, I., and McMaster, W.: Retroperitoneal fibrosis with hydronephrosis as a complication of the Dwyer procedure. J. Pediatr. Surg., *12*:255, 1977.

Sullivan, M. J., Barcowsky, L. N., and Lackner, L. H.: A urological complication of lumbar subarachnoid shunt. Am. J. Dis. Child., *123*:597, 1972.

Talner, L. B., and Gittes, R. F.: Megacalyces: Further observations and differentiation from obstructive disease. Am. J. Roentgenol. Radium Ther. Nucl. Med., *121*:473, 1974.

Timmons, J. W., Jr., Malek, A. S., Hattery, R. R., and DeWeerd, J. H.: Caliceal diverticulum. J. Urol., *114*:6, 1975.

Vaughan, E. D., Jr., Sweet, R. E., and Gillenwater, J. Y.: Peripheral renin and blood pressure changes following complete unilateral ureteral occlusion. J. Urol., *104*:89, 1970.

Vaughan, E. D., Jr., Sweet, R. E., and Gillenwater, J. Y.: Unilateral ureteral occlusion: Pattern of nephron repair and compensatory response. J. Urol., *109*:979, 1973.

Weaver, R. G.: Resorptive patterns and pressures in hydronephrosis with a clinical application. J. Urol., *100*:112, 1968.

Wedge, J. J., Grosfeld, J. L., and Smith, J. P.: Abdominal masses in the newborn: 63 cases. J. Urol., *106*:770, 1971.

Whitaker, R. H.: Methods of assessing obstruction in dilated ureters. Br. J. Urol., *45*:15, 1973.

Williams, D. I., and Hulme-Moir, I.: Primary obstructive mega-ureter. Br. J. Urol., *42*:140, 1970.

Williams, D. I., and Kenawi, M. M.: The prognosis of pelviureteric obstruction in childhood. Europ. Urol., 2:57, 1976.

Young, B. W.: Elastic components of the vesical neck and urethra in childhood. Invest. Urol., 3:20, 1965.

Chapter Six

URINARY INCONTINENCE (INCLUDING ENURESIS)

One way to gain the full attention of physicians responsible for the care of children is to promise a reliable treatment for enuresis. Failure to arrive at a simple solution to this problem cannot be blamed upon lack of effort. Throughout history, in virtually every culture, a variety of remedies and approaches have been offered as the best means of curing the child who wets. The ultimate solution, when everything else fails, and the consideration that must be given when interpreting the effectiveness of all forms of therapy, is the simple fact that the problem is virtually always self-limiting. With that in mind, careful consideration must be given the propriety of extensive, invasive, and risky maneuvers in either the evaluation or treatment of enuresis.

It is worthwhile to remind ourselves periodically that enuresis is a symptom. Like many relatively nonspecific symptoms, it may have any number of underlying causes as its basis. Enthusiastic proponents of each medical discipline involved in the care of patients who wet occasionally overemphasize the importance a single etiologic factor plays in the genesis of this problem. The usual result of such "tunnel vision" is that one specific therapeutic regimen is suggested as the only solution. Unfortunately, no single treatment plan has proved unequivocally effective when subjected to prospective clinical evaluation on a matched patient basis.

DEFINITION OF TERMS

Enuresis means the involuntary loss of urine without specific implications as to time of day. Although most children who present with poor urinary control are night wetters, there are a significant number of children who also wet during the day and a few who wet only during the day. Boys outnumber girls in the night wetting category, whereas in our experience, girls outnumber boys in the group with daytime problems either alone or coupled with nocturnal symptoms.

The age at which one labels a child as enuretic varies in different cultures. One might say that enuresis begins when the family perceives the wetting as a problem — in which circumstance we have seen children as early as 24 months of age. For a universal definition, criteria must be established as to age and the number of episodes of wetting per week or month for one to qualify as an enuretic. Some authors suggest that one episode per month is abnormal. We will be more liberal and will define the nocturnal enuretic as a child over five years of age who is wet at least one night per week. Nevertheless, occasionally a child who wets only once a month may seek help if that episode creates a problem in the home.

The child who never attains dryness is labeled as a primary enuretic, whereas the child who is dry for periods of time and then begins to wet is called a secondary enuretic. Again, one must establish a period of sustained dryness to define secondary enuresis; it is suggested that at least six months of dryness elapse before the child is considered a secondary enuretic.

Lack of daytime urinary control often presents itself at an earlier age than bed wetting because being wet may interfere with activities outside the home. Some schools, for example, find children who are non–toilet-trained unacceptable for registration. Pressure by other family members or intrusive friends may precipitate secondary conflicts in the child's parents, contributing to underlying feelings of failure in this area. Child beatings may even result. We must, therefore, be more attuned to greater potential problems in the diurnal enuretic and consider earlier therapeutic or investigative measures than in the pure night wetter.

INCIDENCE

Because no single definition as to what comprises enuresis has been universally accepted, it is difficult to arrive at conclusive data as to its incidence. DeJonge (1973), in an extensive review, noted the incidence of nocturnal enuresis at age five to be between 4 per cent and 20 per cent, depending on definition. At age eight years, almost 30 per cent of children wet the bed if nocturnal enuresis is defined as wetting as seldom as once per month, an overly restrictive definition. At age 10, 2 to 5 per cent still wet the bed occasionally. Of the total, about

two thirds of bedwetters are primary enuretics and have never achieved a significant period of dryness (Starfield, 1972).

In virtually every study of children under age 12 years, the ratio of boys to girls with nocturnal enuresis is between 3:2 and 2:1. Although it is known that 15 to 20 per cent of night wetters also have some difficulty with daytime control (Forsyth and Redmond, 1974), little differentiation is made in this area between girls and boys.

Less is reported regarding the ultimate achievement of urinary control in those few adolescents who still wet. Statistics from the American Armed Services during World War II indicate that approximately 1 per cent of adult men have some difficulty with nocturnal urinary control (Thorne, 1944). This is approximately the same incidence noted in children at 15 years and, if correct, suggests that the prognosis for achieving urinary control in that older group of wetters is poor.

ETIOLOGY

There is no single underlying cause for either nocturnal or diurnal enuresis. Since a purely organic pathologic condition does not generally limit itself to time of day, some impressions can be gained as to etiology by accurately determining when wetting occurs.

ORGANIC PATHOLOGY

Some classical causes exist which, although rarely presenting as enuresis alone, are readily amenable to diagnosis and, in many, treatment. One of the most obvious of these is neurogenic disease. One should be particularly suspicious of the wet child who also has poor stool control and a gait abnormality. Acquired pathologic conditions, such as cord tumors, may present as secondary enuresis and should be suspected in the child with progressive symptoms. Occasionally a child with meningomyelocele and a balanced bladder may develop enuresis if the spinal cord is tethered and becomes stretched with body growth, resulting in a change in bladder innervation.

Additionally, the pediatric urologist should always be looking for the girl with an ectopic ureteral orifice in the vagina presenting with paradoxical incontinence. Unless infected, these children have regular bladder emptying habits; however, they also dribble urine continuously in between voiding. They are never completely dry. The extraurinary ureter positioned outside the control of the bladder sphincter mechanism puts out urine constantly with resultant continuous wetting.

Another group of girls have postmicturition dribbling from the vagina (Kelalis et al., 1973). These girls void with their legs squeezed together. Urine that has accumulated in the vagina then dribbles out as they stand, soiling their panties. Treatment simply requires having them void with their legs apart and pausing before getting off the toilet.

There are some clinicians who suggest that virtually every child with enuresis has some obstructive abnormality (Mahoney, 1971; Arnold and Ginsberg, 1974). Stenosis of the urethral meatus or valvular obstruction of the posterior urethra in boys, or narrowing of the meatus or distal urethra in girls is thought to be the underlying cause for the child's wetting. Increasing the diameter of the urethra by dilatation, internal urethrotomy, and various forms of meatotomy have been offered as cures. Unfortunately, no prospective control has been performed to our knowledge that verifies the need for or the efficacy of these maneuvers. In view of the rate of spontaneous resolution of enuresis and the failure of long-term follow-up studies to determine recurrence rates following urethral manipulation, the burden of responsibility is upon those proponents of invasive therapeutic measures to demonstrate that these are justified.

One definable cause of wetting that is readily diagnosable by simple, noninvasive techniques is urinary tract infection. Culture of a clean voided urine sample should always be performed in the child who does not toilet train when expected or who begins wetting anew. Urinalysis itself is not sufficient.

Recent evidence suggests that the incidence of urinary tract infections in preschool children is equal to that in school-age children (Chap. 3). Bladder irritability from infection in the 18 to 36 month range, an age at which the cerebral inhibitory centers are learning to effect bladder control, may well disrupt the natural progression to dryness (Yeates, 1973). Evidence supporting the effects of chronic urinary tract infection on urinary control is seen in

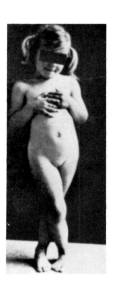 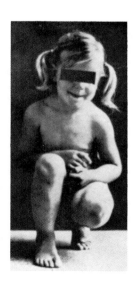 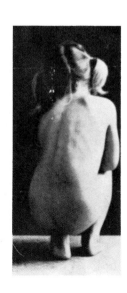

Figure 6–1. Typical posturing of child with the urge syndrome, characterized by an unpredictable urge to void, often associated with urge incontinence. To avoid wetting, the child assumes a posture that provides for external urethral compression, usually by squatting onto one heel until the urgency disappears. Urge incontinence is often associated with diurnal or nocturnal enuresis and is often associated with chronic infection. For some children the syndrome appears to be an abnormality of micturition. (From DeJonge, G. A.: The urge syndrome. *In* Kolvin, I., MacKeith, R. C., and Meadow, S. R. (Eds.): Bladder Control and Enuresis. London, W. Heinemann Medical Books Ltd., 1973, pp. 66–69.)

those patients with severe chronic bladder infection (cystitis follicularis). A significant proportion have urgency and urgency incontinence that persist long after sustained control of infection has been achieved and even beyond the point when visible changes no longer are present on the bladder mucosa (Belman, 1978). These girls will squat, often sitting on their heel, in an effort to maintain control. Typical of the age, however, is the fact that when the bladder spasm responsible for this discomfort passes, the child often will not go to the bathroom and may later become wet. This has been labeled the "urge syndrome" by Vincent (1966) (Fig. 6–1).

It has come to our attention that a large number of children with daytime dribbling also have severe constipation problems. Often these are the same children who have frequently recurring lower urinary tract infections. Attention should be paid to the bowel habits of this group, and digital rectal examination becomes an important step in those with constipation, stool soiling, or when a distended descending colon is palpable. The finding of Mikkelsen and colleagues (1979), that 11 of 40 enuretic children studied had some degree of associated encopresis confirms our clinical observation.

DEVELOPMENTAL DELAY

Developmental delay or a learning disability, is one of the suspected causes of diurnal enuresis. Parents often refer to this as laziness on the part of the child. Children who fit into this category can best be described as having either sensory or inhibitory failure (Yeates, 1973).

Children with sensory failure seem to have no understanding of the voiding process. When asked if they have to urinate, they invariably respond negatively, yet they may be wet moments later with little or no realization of that fact. Like all problems in medicine, the extreme cases represent only a small segment of the whole. In this group, the ability to sense bladder filling usually exists when the child concentrates on being

dry. However, when playing or otherwise involved, the same child may not recognize the need to void. This adds fuel to their home problems since their parents may interpret the wetting as willful disobedience. Understandably, then, they are usually dry when they see the consultant.

The other group falling into this category are those who recognize the necessity to urinate but cannot inhibit the impending bladder contraction. These children have tremendous urgency and urgency incontinence. They literally knock people over trying to get to the bathroom in an effort to stay dry. Many become so frustrated with their inability to control this urge that they give up and are reduced to continuous wetness. It may then become difficult to differentiate them from the group with a sensory deficit.

Studies in adult (postpubertal) enuretics (Torrens and Collins, 1975) suggest that this type of patient has a degree of uninhibited bladder contractions. The end result may be a disturbance in the subcortical arousal center through which bladder messages pass, or the problem may represent a failure of subconscious inhibition. It may well be that such adults constitute a group of individuals who never achieve voluntary control as we know it but who learn to initiate a timed voiding schedule in recognition of their sensory-inhibitory neurologic deficit.

BLADDER CAPACITY

Children who wet the bed are often labeled as having "small bladders." Troup and Hodgson must be credited with their study in 1971 that revealed that these patients do indeed have a functionally limited bladder capacity that is decreased as much as 50 per cent when compared to peers. Urinary frequency in such children is two to four times greater than normal. This is true both day and night even in those patients who wet only at night. Under anesthesia, however, the bladders of all are able to accept a volume normally anticipated for their size. This phenomenon may be sensory, with a limitation of tolerance of the individual for bladder filling, probably on a habitual basis.

SLEEP FACTORS

Many nocturnal enuretics can be categorized as being deep sleepers. Arousal studies have demonstrated an apparently greater depth of sleep in bed wetters (Boyd, 1960; Bostock, 1958). Most parents will agree that it is difficult to awaken the child who wets at night.

EEG studies in nocturnal enuretics until recently were interpreted to indicate that night wetting occurs in deep, non-REM (rapid eye movement) sleep. Urination was reported to occur between deep sleep and REM sleep or during predream sleep (Broughton, 1968). The explanation offered was that the stimulus of a full bladder during an arousal state resulted in an exaggerated physiologic response (Starfield, 1972).

More recently, Kales and colleagues (1977) reported that night wetting is not confined to slow wave sleep (non-REM) but rather occurs in each of the sleep stages. This has been corroborated by Mikkelsen and coworkers (1979). Additionally, Kales and associates noted that the frequency of wetting during any specific stage of sleep is proportional to the total time spent in that particular stage.

ALLERGY

Periodically one is asked whether allergies contribute to bed wetting. Siegel and coworkers (1976) studied 234 upper-class white children and were unable to substantiate a relationship between allergy and either enuresis or urinary tract infection. Kaplan and colleagues (1977) found that serum IgE levels in enuretics were no different from controls.

GENETIC FACTORS

An increased familial incidence of bed wetting has been demonstrated (Bakwin,

1961). Additionally, there is a stastically significant increase in the incidence of wetting in identical twins as opposed to fraternal twins (Bakwin, 1973). There is also an increased incidence of enuresis in children when both parents have a history of enuresis.

PSYCHIATRIC CAUSES

Just as some urologists would have us believe that enuresis is purely mechanical, some psychiatrists would have us believe that enuresis is always based on some emotional disorder. There is no doubt that many enuretic children have emotional problems, particularly as they grow older. In some, to be sure, this is the primary cause. Others, however, develop their psychopathology in response to their wetting and the stresses it provokes. Reviews along this line seem to indicate a correlation between emotional deprivation and enuresis, noting an increased incidence of enuresis in urban lower socioeconomic groups (Oppel et al, 1968).

Half of the sample of 40 enuretics studied by Mikkelsen and associates (1979) received a diagnosis of a psychiatric disorder. However, no specific psychopathologic pattern was noted that could be correlated with enuresis.

Those dealing with patients on a referral basis may well overinterpret the incidence of associated psychological disturbances since they are dealing with a selected population. Nevertheless, ın a series of studies by Rutter and colleagues (1973), no specific correlation seems to exist in males, who are primarily night wetters, but a "moderately strong association" was noted in girls, who were, for the most part, diurnal enuretics. Kolvin and Taunch (1973) suggest that primary enuresis is by and large a physiologic abnormality, whereas secondary enuresis is primarily psychiatric in origin.

It is difficult for us to appreciate on a purely organic basis how a child can achieve total urinary control for six months and then become enuretic. Could transient emotional stress start the wetting cycle and then, even with resolution of the psychopathology, could the wetting perpetuate itself? Similarly, could unrecognized or transient urinary tract infection or cystitis be the trigger mechanism?

NON-NEUROGENIC, NEUROGENIC BLADDER (DETRUSOR-SPHINCTER DYSSYNERGIA)

Recently an unusual group of children have been recognized who do appear to have an underlying emotional cause for their enuresis (Hinman and Baumann, 1973;

Allen, 1977). Boys appear to be affected more often than girls. They wet both day and night and almost always have encopresis as well. It would appear, for reasons not at all clear, that these children shut off their external urinary sphincter (voluntary sphincter or urogenital diaphragm) during the act of voiding, that is, while their bladders are actively contracting. The result is that these children void with a "stuttering" urinary stream and, more importantly, they have periods of extremely high intravesical pressure. The result is bladder thickening and trabeculation and, in some, either vesicoureteral reflux or urterovesical obstruc-

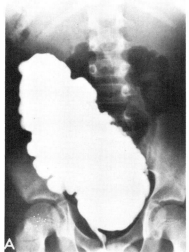 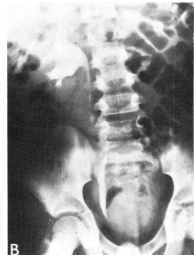 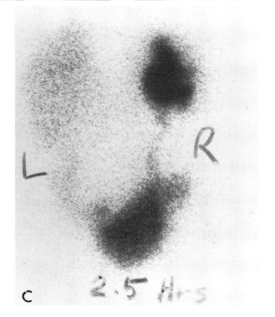

Figure 6–2. A, Cystogram in boy with non-neurogenic, neurogenic bladder demonstrating large capacity and severe trabeculation. B, Excretory urogram reveals nonvisualization on the left. C, Renal scan reveals virtual nonfunction on the left and fullness on the right collecting system. This child required an indwelling tube for drainage while undergoing psychotherapy.

tion (Fig. 6–2) secondary to the bladder changes. Radiographically the urinary tract in these children cannot be differentiated from those typically described as "neurogenic," yet no underlying neurologic abnormality can be localized (Chap. 7), hence, the label non-neurogenic, neurogenic bladder. This problem is also referred to as voiding dyssynergia because of an apparent lack of coordination between the bladder and voluntary sphincter.

The diagnosis should be entertained when seeing a child with enuresis and encopresis with or without a history of urinary tract infection. Cystography is essential to evaluate the bladder in this group, and complete urodynamic evaluation is generally helpful (see next section).

The underlying cause of this problem is likely emotional. Toilet phobias or familial stress at a time when toilet training is occurring may interfere with the ability to relax the external sphincter. The pathophysiology of the associated encopresis is also unclear, as most of these children are not severely constipated. There appears to be poor understanding and control of the entire urogenital diaphragm, including the anal sphincter.

EVALUATION OF THE ENURETIC PATIENT

Careful attention to the history is essential to determine if a specific underlying cause might be responsible for the child's problem. As a rule, those children who are purely nocturnal enuretics should not be subjected to *radiographic evaluation* or other studies unless an abnormality is found on physical examination or a positive urine culture is noted (Cutler et al., 1978). Eight hundred and thirty radiographic studies reported by Forsyth and Redmond (1974) demonstrated potentially significant findings in only 2 per cent. In none was an absolute cause for the wetting established. Those children with significant urinary tract pathology are most likely excluded earlier, having been brought to medical attention with urinary tract infection or other specific

complaints (Stannard and Lebowitz, 1978). On the other hand, the child over five years who wets both day and night should have, at the very least, an excretory urogram with a good voiding film. A case may be made for obtaining a separate voiding cystourethrogram in boys for better clarification, and, of course, a complete study should be done in each patient with culture-documented urinary tract infection (Chap. 3).

Although physical examination is rarely rewarded with a clue as to the etiology, it should be thoroughly performed. Eight hundred such patients subjected to detailed neurologic examination revealed no specific underlying cause (Forsyth and Redmond, 1974). Although it has been suggested that urethral meatal obstruction is a significant cause of enuresis in boys, this has not been objectively substantiated. The visual appearance of the meatus is not indicative of its calibrated size (Litvak et al., 1976), and there appears to be no relationship between meatal size and secondary changes of the bladder or kidneys.

Cystoscopic evaluation should be considered only in those children with an abnormal urinary radiograph. Routine endoscopy and urethral calibration cannot be justified in terms of anesthetic risk and patient cost in the child whose only problem is enuresis.

Complete *urodynamic evaluation*, including simultaneous cystometrics, anal sphincter or urogenital diaphragm electromyography, and urine flow studies, have been helpful in clarifying the pathologic state in some of those patients with a non-neurogenic, neurogenic bladder. These studies are performed by inserting a small suprapubic catheter into the bladder percutaneously and EMG wires into the anal sphincter (Cook et al, 1977). Our preference is to set all this up at the time of endoscopic evaluation under general anesthesia. The study is carried out the next day after the child has recovered from the anesthesia and after urethral irritation has subsided. Sterile saline is infused through the suprapubic catheter. A side arm measures intravesical pressure, anal sphincter electromyographic activity is recorded, and urine flow is measured simultaneously (Firlit et al., 1978;

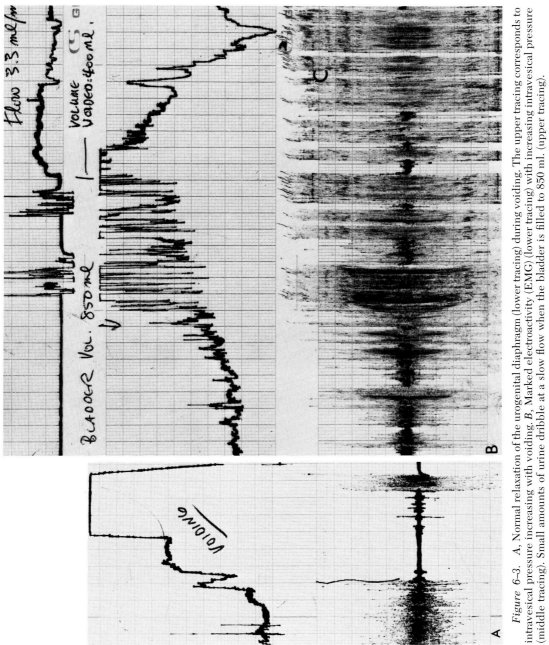

Figure 6-3. A, Normal relaxation of the urogenital diaphragm (lower tracing) during voiding. The upper tracing corresponds to intravesical pressure increasing with voiding. B, Marked electroactivity (EMG) (lower tracing) with increasing intravesical pressure (middle tracing). Small amounts of urine dribble at a slow flow when the bladder is filled to 850 ml. (upper tracing).

Allen and Bright, 1978). The three-channel record then documents whether there is normal external sphincter relaxation during bladder contraction (Fig. 6–3A) or whether there is dyssynergia (Fig. 6–3B). Bladder emptying can then be determined by checking residual urine either by subtraction of voided volume from that infused or by direct drainage from the suprapubic catheter.

There is definitely a role for *psychiatric evaluation* in some enuretics. Those with a non-neurogenic, neurogenic bladder may belong in this category as may any other child who exhibits psychopathologic behavior in other developmental areas besides wetting. Kolvin and Taunch (1973) suggest that the child with primary nocturnal enuresis has an organic pathologic condition, while those who have secondary wetting have an underlying psychological problem. Although this may be a simplistic differentiation, it helps to cue the primary physician to a possible underlying cause.

The approach we recommend for the child with purely nocturnal enuresis and no history of urinary tract infection is an in-depth evaluation of patient and family by the primary physician before any further studies are carried out. In the majority there is little indication of serious disorders, and family counseling and a directed approach will be all that are required. Occasionally enuresis is a cry for help, particularly in the child who wets during the day and night. These children may be candidates, after organic pathologic conditions are ruled out, for psychiatric evaluation.

TREATMENT

The best treatment for any problem is prevention. Brazelton (1962) published the lowest incidence of nocturnal enuresis on record — 1.4 per cent at five years of age. This was apparently achieved by establishing a supportive educational program with the parent in advance of toilet training.

When one reviews any treatment modality, the spontaneous rate of cure must be recognized. Werry and Cohrssen (1965) noted a 10 per cent favorable response in an untreated control group in their study, while Forsyth and Redmond, in a long-term follow-up study reported in 1974, found that the spontaneous remission rate is 14 per cent in children ages five to nine and 16 per cent in both the 10 to 14 and 15 to 19 age groups. Troup (1978) reported a 50 to 60 per cent cure rate at five years in the group previously evaluated (Troup and Hodgson, 1971) for functional bladder capacity. Treatment in this group included increased fluids, prolonging the interval between voiding, and administration of anticholinergics — all relatively nonspecific modalities.

Blackwell and Currah (1973) reviewed pharmacologic treatment and found no objective data to support the use of stimulants, MAO inhibitors, tranquilizers, anticonvulsants, diuretics, anticholinergics, or pituitary snuff. More recently, however, excellent success has been reported with intranasal vasopressin. It effects a diminished urine output at night and dryness has been achieved in approximately 50 per cent of patients. In one group, wetting did not recur after cessation of treatment (Birkasóva, et al. 1978); however, in another group, recurrence was the rule (Tuvemo, 1978). Additionally, a recent controlled study reported success with the potent anticholinergic oxybutynin when given four times daily in 31 of 36 children who had not responded to imipramine (Buttarazzi, 1977).

Many studies have been carried out using the various tricyclic antidepressants (imipramine, nortriptyline, desipramine, and amitriptyline) demonstrating a 20 to 40 per cent positive response to treatment (McKendry et al. 1975; Forsyth and Merrett, 1969; Kales et al., 1977). The exact mechanism of the effect of imipramine (Tofranil), the most commonly used drug in this group, remains poorly understood. It may exert a primary stimulating effect on the bladder outlet (Mahoney et al., 1973) as well as diminishing activity of the detrusor mechanism (Labay and Boyarsky, 1973). Bladder capacity itself has reportedly increased during its use (Hägglund and Parkkulainen, 1965). Shaffer and colleagues (1978) evaluated the effect of a pure alpha adrenolytic drug in an effort to see if stimulation of bladder neck trigonal muscle contractility is the means by which these drugs work. There was no significant dryness in the group treated with a pure alpha stimulator.

It is thought that the tricyclic antidepressants exert their primary effect by changing sleep patterns. However, since the timing of the enuretic episode does not seem to be affected by the drug, it seems unlikely that the changes in sleep stages are of significance (Rapaport et al., 1979). Kales and coworkers (1977) concluded that imipramine does not produce dryness by affecting sleep patterns but by increasing bladder capacity early in the night when sleep is deepest and when most primary enuretics wet. In their study, bladder control was adequate in the final third of the night, when sleep is lightest.

Responsiveness to treatment with imipramine on an individual basis cannot be predicted with standard dosage schedules. A distinct correlation appears to exist between tricyclic plasma levels and enuretic control (Rapaport et al., 1979). Additionally, in some, side effects of restlessness and irritability may limit its usefulness. A new, slow release, nighttime product has been effective in older children, in whom doses of 75 mg or more may be required to achieve dryness (Tofranil pm).

Those who have had clinical experience with the tricyclic antidepressants in the management of enuresis are aware of a significant "escape" from treatment. This has been corroborated by Rapaport and associates (1979) in their clinical study. However, even in those who escape, imipramine may be effective when used occasionally. We recommend its use intermittently in those situations when staying dry is important, such as when sleeping over at someone's house or when going to camp.

Behavior modification by means of mechanical awakening devices has achieved more popularity in England than in the United States. The response to this form of treatment has been consistently reported as being greater than with any other single form of therapy. The system is based on the completion of an electrical circuit with contact with urine resulting in ringing of a bell, flashing of a light, or with some, administration of a mild shock. (We do not endorse this last type.) Although the financial investment in this form of therapy is not great, it requires a sustained family commitment for success. Often the soundly sleeping patient himself is not awakened by the device; however, the remainder of the family may be. The patient then must be awakened as soon as the alarm goes off and must be made to complete urination in the bathroom. Since wetting often occurs multiple times during the night in children, this cycle may be repeated more than once per night. Ultimately the patient himself will become awakened by the bell and within 6 to 12 weeks is conditioned to recognize the significance of a detrusor contraction when asleep. The response rate has been reported as high as 100 per cent by Mowrer and Mowrer (1938), but a more realistic figure would probably be 60 to 80 per cent in those who continue therapy. The relapse rate is 10 to 30 per cent (Turner and Young, 1966). One of the major problems is that many families abandon this form of therapy before success is realized.

Emotional side effects of this intrusive form of therapy are apparently uncommon. Skin ulcerations from low-current burns have been noted and should be guarded against by careful skin care and caution when setting up the device.

It appears that bladder filling tolerance in enuretics is also diminished (Troup and Hodgson, 1971). Some encourage increasing daytime fluid intake rather than fluid deprivation and suggest that the patient attempt to progressively prolong intervals between trips to the bathroom. There is no evidence that oral fluid deprivation, other than in rare cases, affects the incidence of night wetting. However, as mentioned earlier, nasal vasopressin is effective in reducing bed wetting, apparently by reducing nocturnal urine production.

Those children who have daytime urgency incontinence or severe frequency may be aided by the use of anticholinergics to increase their physiologic bladder capacity. Propantheline, 7.5 to 15 mg three times daily or oxybutynin chloride, 5 mg two to four times daily, have proved effective.

Children with the urge syndrome (p. 121) often are helped most with anticholinergic medication. Those with a sensory-inhibitory deficit may achieve significant dryness with a timed voiding schedule alone (every two to three hours) or in conjunction with an anticholinergic. Unfortunately, it is very difficult for younger children to abide by schedules, and being constantly reminded to void by their parents often becomes a point of conflict.

Patients with detrusor-sphincter dyssynergia (non-neurogenic, neurogenic bladder) have reportedly responded favorably to hypnotism (Hinman and Baumann, 1973). Diazepam (Valium) has also been said to be effective by reducing voluntary muscle activity at the level of the external sphincter (Cook et al., 1977). Retraining of the actual voiding act is an important part of the treatment process and may be as effective as drug therapy alone. This is very difficult to achieve, however, and temporary urinary diversion may rarely be necessary to preserve renal function.

In those in whom constipation plays a significant role, a 10-day course of enemas to empty the large bowel and allow it to regain muscular tonus, the long-term intake of a high-fiber diet (bran) and a lubricant (mineral oil), and regular toilet habits for bowel movements are highly recommended. We suggest the child spend 10 minutes on the toilet after either breakfast or dinner daily.

The relationship between constipation, encopresis, and enuresis cannot be overstressed. Many patients with encopresis and enuresis require associated psychiatric evaluation and support, but no measure along these lines will be effective unless the constipation itself is controlled. It is difficult to understand how this cycle is initiated, but some children become voluntary stool retainers possibly secondary to painful bowel movements early in childhood associated at times with problems such as fissure in ano. The results, a constant bolus of impacted stool in the rectal ampulla around which soft stool passes, will never resolve independently. Restoration of normal muscle tone by emptying the bowels with enemas, however psychologi-cally distasteful, often cannot effectively be accomplished by other means. Institution of normal stool habits may lead to an improvement in both urinary control and psychological well-being.

REFERENCES

Allen, T. D.: The nonneurogenic, neurogenic bladder. J. Urol., *117*:232, 1977.

Allen, T. D., and Bright, T. C., III.: Urodynamic patterns in children with dysfunctional voiding problems. J. Urol., *119*:247, 1978.

Arnold, S. J., and Ginsberg, A.: Radiographic and photoendoscopic studies in posterior urethral valves in enuretic boys. Urology, *4*:145, 1974.

Bakwin, H. G.: Enuresis in children. J. Pediatr., *58*:806, 1961.

Bakwin, H.: The genetics of enuresis. *In* Kolvin, I., MacKeith, R. C., and Meadow, S. R. (eds.): Bladder Control and Enuresis. Philadelphia, J. B. Lippincott Co., 1973.

Belman, A. B.: The clinical significance of cystitis cystica in girls: Results of a prospective study. J. Urol., *119*:661, 1978.

Birkásová, J., Birkás, O., Flynn, M. J., and Court, J. H.: Desmopressin in the management of nocturnal enuresis in children: A double blind study. Pediatrics, *62*:970, 1978.

Blackwell, B., and Currah, J.: The psychopharmacology of nocturnal enuresis. *In* Kolvin, I., MacKeith, R. C., and Meadow, S. R. (Eds.): Bladder Control and Enuresis. Philadelphia, J. B. Lippincott Co., 1973.

Bostock, J.: Exterior gestation, primitive sleep, enuresis and asthma. Med. J. Aust., *149*:185, 1958.

Boyd, M. M.: The depth of sleep in enuretic school children and non-enuretic controls. J. Psychosom. Res. *4*:274, 1960.

Brazelton, T. B.: A child oriented approach to toilet training. Pediatrics, *29*:121, 1962.

Broughton, R.: Sleep disorders: Disorder of arousal? Science, *159*:1070, 1968.

Buttarazzi, P. J.: Oxybutynin chloride (Ditropan) in enuresis. J. Urol., *118*:46, 1977.

Cook, W. A., Firlit, C. F., Stephens, F. D., and King, L. R.: Techniques and results of urodynamic evaluation of children. J. Urol., *117*:346, 1977.

Cutler, C., Middleton, A. W., Jr., and Nixon, G. W.: Radiographic findings in children surveyed for enuresis. Urology, *11* 480, 1978.

DeJonge, G. A.: Epidemiology of enuresis: A survey of the literature. *In* Kolvin, I., MacKeith, R. C., and Meadow, S. R. (Eds): Bladder Control and Enuresis. Philadelphia, J. B. Lippincott Co., 1973.

Firlit, C. F., Smey, P., and King, L. R.: Micturition urodynamic flow studies in children. J. Urol., *119*:250, 1978.

Forsyth, W. I., and Merrett, J. D.: A controlled trial of imipramine and mortriptyline in the treatment of enuresis. Br. J. Clin. Pract., *23*:210, 1969.

Forsyth, W. I., and Redmond, A.: Enuresis and spontaneous cure rate: Study of 1,129 enuretics. Arch Dis. Child., *49*:259, 1974.

Häggland, T. B., and Parkkulainen, K. V.: Enuretic children treated with imipramine (Tofranil): A cystometric study. Ann. Paediatr. Fenn., *11*:53, 1965.

Hinman, F., and Baumann, F. W.: Vesical and ureteral damage from voiding dysfunction in boys without neurologic or obstructive disease. J. Urol., *109*:727, 1973.

Kales, A., Kales, J. D., Jacobson, A., et al.: Effects of imipramine on enuretic frequency and sleep stages. Pediatrics, *60*:431, 1977.

Kaplan, G. W., Wallace, W. W., Orgel, H. A., and Miller, J. R.: Serum immunoglobulin E and incidence of allergy in a group of enuretic children. Urology, *10*:428, 1977.

Kelalis, P. P., Burke, E. C., Stickler, G. B., and Hartman, G. W.: Urinary vaginal reflux in children. Pediatr., *51*:941, 1973.

Kolvin, I., and Taunch, J.: A dual theory of nocturnal enuresis. *In* Kolvin, I., MacKeith, R. C., and Meadow, S. R. (Eds.): Bladder Control and Enuresis. Philadelphia, J. B. Lippincott Co., 1973.

Labay, P., and Boyarsky, S.: The effect of imipramine on the bladder musculature. J. Urol., *109*:385, 1973.

Litvak, A. S., Morris, J. A., and McRoberts, J. W.: Normal size of the urethral meatus in male children. J. Urol, *115*:736, 1976.

Mahoney, D. T.: Studies of enuresis. I. Incidence of obstructive lesions and pathophysiology of enuresis. J. Urol., *106*:951, 1971.

Mahoney, D. T., Laverte, R. O., and Mahoney, J. E.: Studies of enuresis. VI. Observations on sphincter augmenting effect of imipramine in children with urinary incontinence. Urology, *1*:317, 1973.

McKendry, J. B. J., Stewart, D. A., Kharma, F., and Netley, C.: Primary enuresis: Relative success of three methods of treatment. Can. Med. Assoc. J., *113*:953, 1975.

Mikkelsen, E. J., Rapaport, J. L., Nee, L., et al: Childhood enuresis. I. Sleep patterns and psychopathology. Arch. Gen. Psychiatr., *37*:1139, 1980.

Mowrer, O. H., and Mowrer, W.M.: Enuresis — a method for its study and treatment. Am. J. Orthopsychiatry, *8*:436, 1938.

Oppel, W. C., Harper, P. A., and Rider, R. V.: The age of attaining bladder control. Pediatrics, *42*:614, 1968.

Rapaport, J. L., Mikkelsen, E. J., Zavadil, A., et al.: Childhood enuresis. II. Psychopathology, plasma tricyclic concentration and antienuretic effect. Arch. Gen. Psychiatr., 37:1146, 1980.

Rutter, M., Yule, W., and Graham, P.: Enuresis and behavioral deviance: Some epidemiological considerations. *In* Kolvin, I., MacKeith, R. C., and Meadow, S. R. (Eds.): Bladder Control and Enuresis. Philadelphia, J. B. Lippicott Co., 1973.

Shaffer, D., Hedge, B., and Stephensen, J.: Trial of an alpha-adrenolytic drug (indoramin) for nocturnal enuresis. Dev. Med. Child. Neurol., *20*:183, 1978.

Siegel, S., Rawitt, L., Sakoloff, B., and Siegel, B.: Relationship of allergy, enuresis, and urinary infection in children 4 to 7 years of age. Pediatrics, *57*:526, 1976.

Stannard, M. W., and Lebowitz, R. L.: Urography in the child who wets. Am. J. Roentgenol., *130*:959, 1978.

Starfield, B.: Enuresis: Its pathogenesis and management. Clin. Pediatr., *11*:343, 1972.

Thorne, F. C.: The incidence of nocturnal enuresis over 5 years. Am. J. Psych., *100*:686, 1944.

Torrens, M. J., and Collins, C. D.: Urodynamic assessment of adult enuretics. Br. J. Urol., *47*:433, 1975.

Troup, C. W.: Nocturnal functional bladder capacities in enuretic children. Society of Pediatric Urologists Newsletter, p. 25, 1978.

Troup, C. W., and Hodgson, N. B.: Nocturnal functional bladder capacity in enuretic children. J. Urol., *105*:129, 1971.

Turner, R. K., and Young, G. C.: CNS stimulant drugs and conditioning treatment of nocturnal enuresis. A long-term follow-up study. Behav. Res. Ther., *4*:225, 1966.

Tuvemo, T.: DDAVP in childhood nocturnal enuresis. Acta Paediatr. Scand., *67*:753, 1978.

Vincent, S. A.: Postural control of urinary incontinence. Lancet, *2*:631, 1966.

Werry, J. S., and Cohrssen, J.: Enuresis: An etiological and therapeutic study. J. Pediatr., *67*:423, 1965.

Yeates, W. K.: Bladder function in normal micturition. *In* Kolvin, I., MacKeith, R. C., and Meadow, S. R. (Eds.): Bladder Control and Enuresis. Philadelphia, J. B. Lippincott Co., 1973.

Chapter Seven

NEUROGENIC BLADDER

Urinary tract dysfunction resulting from deranged neurologic innervation will account for a significant number of children seen by the pediatric urologist. Myelomeningocele and other congenital abnormalities of the spinal cord are the most frequent causes of neurogenic vesical dysfunction in childhood. Other examples of congenital lesions that may result in similar problems are sacral agenesis or dysgenesis, the tethered cord syndrome, and diastematomyelia.

Spinal cord trauma can result in injury to the nerve supply to the bladder as well as to the extremities, such as paraplegia and quadriplegia. Tumors of the spine or pelvis may also affect bladder innervation. While the sacral nerve roots may be directly involved by tumor, surgical extirpation of the tumor may unavoidably result in iatrogenic neurogenic vesical dysfunction. Although neurogenic vesical dysfunction follows abdominoperineal resection of the rectum for carcinoma in many adults, such an occurrence is unusual after operations for imperforate anus or Hirschsprung's disease in children (Belman and King, 1972).

Another group of diseases that commonly result in bladder dysfunction in adults but rarely in childhood are the systemic neuropathies, such as diabetes, lues, and multiple sclerosis. It is of interest, similarly, that although stroke patients may have urinary incontinence on a neurogenic basis, such a problem is only infrequently seen in children with cerebral palsy or profound mental retardation (Shapiro).

PHYSIOLOGY

Prior to discussing specific voiding problems with which children present, it will be helpful to review some basic neuroanatomic and neurophysiologic concepts. This review will be, of necessity, brief and perhaps dogmatic, but it is hoped that it will facilitate an understanding of the material that follows.

To the uninitiated, voiding is often thought to be a voluntary act in the same sense that movement of an extremity is voluntary. This is not the case, and a better concept would be that of an involuntary reflex that is modified by volition. Anatomically, there are alternating areas in the cerebral cortex that either facilitate or inhibit the urge to void (Tang and Ruch, 1956). Fibers from these cortical centers pass through the spinal cord in the lateral spinothalamic tracts to the "sacral micturition center," the ganglia of the second, third, and fourth sacral nerve roots (Bors and Porter, 1970). At this anatomic level, there is an intact reflex arc. Efferent fibers pass through the parasympathetic fibers in the pelvic ganglia and supply the detrusor and proximal urethra. Additionally, there are somatic fibers that pass through the pudendal nerve and supply the musculature of the pelvic floor. Afferent fibers return to the sacral spinal cord segments by these same routes (Bors and Porter, 1970). It was long thought that the sympathetic nervous system played no role in voiding, but recent information contradicts this view. There are sympathetic motor and sensory fibers predominantly in the area of the bladder neck and proximal urethra (Homsy, 1967). Their exact role is not clear, but pharmacologic manipulation of the alpha- and beta-adrenergic system have measurable effects on voiding. Blockade of the beta receptors facilitates voiding, whereas stimulation of the alpha system promotes continence.

The bladder fills gradually at a rate determined by urine production. Normally there is very little rise in intravesical pressure during filling (McClellan, 1939). In the adult, the urge to void is first recognized at an intravesical volume of 100 to 150 ml, but this urge can be inhibited by the cerebral cortex. The normal bladder capacity in the adult is 450 to 500 ml. Age-related or size-related bladder capacities have not been established for children but are definitely below this figure. When bladder capacity is reached or when the desire to void occurs and cerebral inhibition is withdrawn, intravesical pressure rises quickly to 50 to 60 cm H_2O. Simultaneously, the pelvic floor relaxes, the vesical neck opens, and the detrusor contracts, resulting in voiding to complete emptying. Note that there is no need for the Valsalva maneuver or increased intra-abdominal pressure in this mechanism.

In infants, several physiologic differences from the previous schema have been noted. Firstly, bladder capacity is much less than in the adult; it approximates 60 ml (Muellner, 1960). Secondly, voiding does not usually empty the bladder completely (Osborne and DuMont, 1977). Thirdly, uninhibited bladder contractions at volumes below capacity have been noted cystometrically (Linderholm, 1966). Between the toddler stage and ages four to five years, bladder capacity seems to triple or quadruple, voiding to complete emptying is routinely seen, and uninhibited contractions are considered abnormal (Muellner,

1960). This maturation of bladder function is thought to play a role in normal toilet training but is incompletely understood.

Much of the understanding, or lack thereof, of neurogenic bladder dysfunction derives from the interpretation of cystometry in adults with traumatic paraplegia and other well-defined neurologic states. Cystometry is the measurement of intravesical pressure in response to filling. Several characteristic cystometrographic patterns have been recognized and correlated with known neuropathic states. The normal cystometric pattern follows the normal filling and emptying sequence already described (Fig. 7–1). When there is a lesion of central inhibition, bladder capacity is normal as is sensation, but detrusor contractions of increasing intensity (called uninhibited contractions) are seen. If such contractions exceed 50 to 60 cm H_2O, pressure incontinence of urine may occur. This cystometric pattern may be seen in patients with strokes or multiple sclerosis and occurs normally in infancy and early childhood (Fig. 7–2).

When there are isolated lesions of the sacral sensory nerves, bladder sensation is decreased, and capacity may be increased; detrusor contractile strength may be similarly decreased. The resulting cystometrogram has been termed hypotonic or atonic depending on its degree (Fig. 7–3). This pattern has been observed in the spinal shock phase of traumatic paraplegia, in lues, and in diabetic neuropathy.

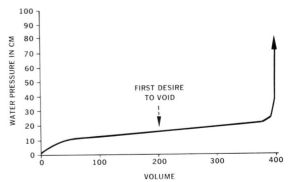

Figure 7–1. Normal cystometrogram. (From Kaplan, G. W., and O'Conor, V. J.: Care of the bladder in spinal cord injuries. *In* Ruge, D. (Ed.): Spinal Cord Injuries. Springfield, Ill., Charles C Thomas, 1969, p. 128.)

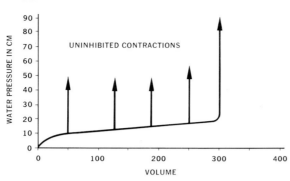

Figure 7–2. Uninhibited neurogenic bladder. (From Kaplan, G. W., and O'Conor, V. J.: Care of the bladder in spinal cord injuries. *In* Ruge, D. (Ed.): Spinal Cord Injuries. Springfield, Ill., Charles C Thomas, 1969, p. 128.)

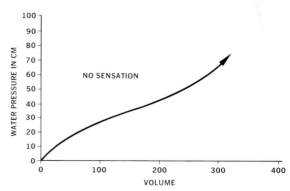

Figure 7–4. Lower motor neuron bladder. (From Kaplan, G. W., and O'Conor, V. J.: Care of the bladder in spinal cord injuries. *In* Ruge, D. (Ed.): Spinal Cord Injuries. Springfield, Ill., Charles C Thomas, 1969, p. 128.)

Should there be an isolated lesion of the sacral motor supply to the bladder, such as after removal of a pelvic tumor, the bladder will contract by virtue of its inherent myogenic stretch reflex. The response to filling will be virtually a straight line rise in intravesical pressure without inhibition of this pressure rise (Fig. 7–4). When capacity is reached, the bladder will contract but will usually not empty to completion.

If there is a lesion that affects the spinal cord between the sacral ganglia and the cerebral cortex, another characteristic pattern emerges. Sensation is diminished to absent, bladder capacity is reduced, and the rise in pressure in response to filling is less than that seen in lesions of sacral motor

supply but is steeper than normal. Uninhibited bladder contractions may also be seen (Fig. 7–5).

Additionally, other phenomena occur when there is a lesion of the nerve supply in this area. Because the pelvic floor musculature may be affected via the pudendal nerve, one of two situations may pertain. The pelvic floor may be so lax that incontinence results, or, conversely, the pelvic floor may be constantly tonic, and obstruction to the flow of urine may occur because of a relative imbalance between the detrusor and the pelvic floor. Obviously, any true obstructive lesion, such as a urethral stricture, could magnify such problems.

Because the detrusor is weakened,

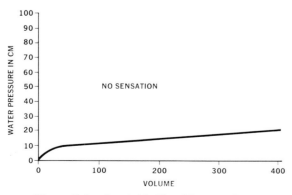

Figure 7–3. Atonic bladder. (From Kaplan, G. W., and O'Conor, V. J.: Care of the bladder in spinal cord injuries. *In* Ruge, D. (Ed.): Spinal Cord Injuries. Springfield, Ill., Charles C Thomas, 1969, p. 128.)

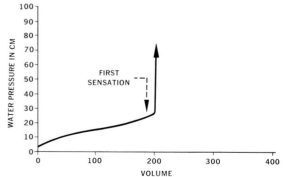

Figure 7–5. Upper motor neuron bladder. (From Kaplan, G. W., and O'Conor, V. J.: Care of bladder in spinal cord injuries. *In* Ruge, D. (Ed.): Spinal Cord Injuries. Springfield, Ill., Charles C Thomas, 1969, p. 128.)

paraureteral sacculation of the bladder may result (see Fig. 4–1). This can produce either vesicoureteral reflux or occasionally ureteral obstruction. Additionally, the incompletely emptied bladder loses one of its bacterial defense mechanisms and is more vulnerable to urinary infection.

When the detrusor is ineffective, the upper urinary tract may be affected. In the face of incomplete vesical emptying, ureterectasis and hydronephrosis may result. In some instances, this is presumably due to high intravesical pressures that prevent efficient ureteral emptying, whereas in others it is due to the direct transmission of intravesical pressure to the ureter via the mechanism of vesicoureteral reflux. Regardless of how this occurs, when intravesical pressure (and thereby intrapelvic pressure) is elevated, renal blood flow (and hence urine formation) is reduced.

Continence is achieved when intravesical pressure is less than infravesical resistance. Hence, should the vesical neck opening pressure be low or should resistance at that "external sphincter" be less than detrusor pressure (momentarily or continuously), incontinence will result.

CLINICAL IMPLICATIONS

Neurogenic bladder dysfunction is of importance for at least three reasons. Firstly, it can greatly affect longevity. Patients with myelomeningocele who survive the first two years of life and then die prematurely usually do so from renal failure (Smith, 1965). It has been well shown that adult traumatic paraplegics have a shortened life span, again largely the effect of renal insufficiency (Nyquist and Bors, 1967). Secondly, neurogenic dysfunction affects urinary continence and thereby sociability, an important factor in the growing child's development. Thirdly, male patients with neurogenic bladder dysfunction often have associated sexual dysfunction — impaired erectile potency, ejaculatory capability, and fertility — which creates problems during adolescence and adult life (Comarr, 1971).

CLASSIFICATION

There have been many attempts at classification of neurogenic bladder dysfunction, none of which is completely satisfactory clinically, either prognostically or therapeutically. Standard classifications based largely on cystometric findings (i.e., autonomous, automatic, hypotonic, and uninhibited) seem somewhat artificial. Bors' classification (1957) (upper motor neuron, lower motor neuron, complete, incomplete, sensory, motor, and mixed) is of utility in traumatic paraplegia but is of little utility with myelomeningocele patients because these patients fall largely into the mixed category. For pragmatic reasons, it seems most efficacious at present to classify patients on their ability to store urine, the ability to empty the bladder, the presence or absence of sensation, the resistance of the pelvic floor, and the presence or absence of uninhibited detrusor contractions.

ETIOLOGY

TRAUMA

Although uncommon, traumatic paraplegia or quadriplegia is seen in childhood. Following injury, there is a period of "spinal shock" lasting for variable periods of time from a few hours to several months during which the bladder is areflexic. Following this, bladder function will follow a predictable pattern of recovery depending on the level of the lesion.

In traumatized patients, there are several goals of therapy. In the initial stages (spinal shock), the bladder must be kept empty by indwelling catheterization or, preferably, emptied regularly by intermittent catheterization to prevent vesical overdistention and compounding of long-term management problems. Additionally, a very high fluid intake should be stressed to prevent stone formation.

Once bladder reflexes have recovered (as shown by cystometry), a catheter-free state with continence is the goal of therapy. Approximately 90 per cent of the time this goal can be achieved (Comarr, 1965). Often this requires continued clean intermittent catheterization, but, in many instances, even this is unnecessary, as the bladder can be "triggered" by nonspecific stimuli such as suprapubic tapping or stroking of the thigh. If a voiding reflex can be provoked, it is important that voiding occur to a residual of 10 to 20 per cent of vesical capacity; otherwise, renal deterioration often occurs. If such is not the case, pharmacologic or surgical intervention may be necessary to achieve this goal.

A common misconception is that traumatic paraplegics are "asexual." Such is far from true (Comarr, 1971). Female paraplegics can be sexually active and are fertile. Male paraplegics have erections and are potentially potent. Fertility is often impaired owing to retrograde ejaculation but often can be achieved by artificial insemination. As many of the modalities employed to achieve a "balanced urinary tract" (that is, bladder emptying to 10 to 20 per cent of capacity with each voiding) may interfere with sexual function, this factor must be taken into account when such intervention is contemplated.

As was stated earlier, most children do not develop neurogenic vesical dysfunction following abdominoperineal surgery for congenital lesions. However, there is a high incidence of sacral dysplasia in children with imperforate anus, and this may lead to neurogenic vesical dysfunction (Belman and King, 1972). After the extirpation of large pelvic tumors in childhood, we have seen temporary or permanent neurogenic vesical dysfunction from injury to the pelvic plexuses.

TUMORS

Tumors of the spinal cord or occult congenital lesions of the cord may present initially with urinary dysfunction. Early recognition may limit the degree of neurologic damage and significantly influence the prognosis. The secondary onset of urinary incontinence following toilet training, particularly if associated with incontinence of stool, suggests the need for neurologic

evaluation. Unfortunately, the discovery of such tumors is often delayed because of the subtlety of their presentation leading to irreversible nerve damage.

NON-NEUROGENIC, NEUROGENIC BLADDER

In recent years, there has been recognized a group of children without a definable neurologic lesion who present with daytime and nighttime urinary incontinence, usually accompanied by encopresis (Hinman and Baumann, 1973). These children empty their bladders poorly. The bladder on cystography and cystometrography has many characteristics of a neurogenic lesion. There is often rather astounding hydronephrosis (Fig. 7–6). Boys are affected much more commonly than girls. The natural history of this problem is completely unknown, but there have been some instances of death from renal failure (Allen, 1977). The problem has been termed the occult neuropathic bladder or the non-neurogenic, neurogenic bladder.

The etiology of this problem is unclear. Some workers feel that there is some intrinsic abnormality in the nerve supply to the bladder although to date there has been no demonstration thereof (Kamhi et al., 1971). Others have suggested that it may be an intrinsic abnormality in the bladder musculature, but, once again, no definite evidence has been forthcoming. Some feel that these problems are secondary to constipation. While it is true that bowel problems often coexist, even with relief of the bowel problems many of these children do not improve. It is most likely that this is a primary psychiatric disturbance. There has been success with short-term psychotherapy and bladder training or with hypnotherapy to relieve these problems (Hinman, 1974). An observation supporting an underlying emotional cause is the fact that some children with this problem will improve spontaneously.

The diagnosis, for the moment, is largely one of exclusion. The urinary incontinence that these children manifest is of an overflow type. There often are associated problems with urinary tract infection. Upper tract changes, when present, are often rather dramatic. Vesicoureteral reflux may or may not be part of the problem. If the bladder is emptied for some prolonged period, upper tract dilatation does improve, thereby establishing that the site of the lesion is at the bladder neck or below.

On voiding cystourethrography the bladder assumes a "Christmas tree" shape similar to that seen in bladders with neurogenic dysfunction. No obstructive lesions can be demonstrated from the bladder neck distally. On careful neurologic examination, no neurologic lesions have been demonstrated. Myelography and computerized tomography of the spine have failed to uncover lesions of the spinal cord to account for the clinical picture.

It has been demonstrated by Hinman (1974) that direct attacks on the urinary tract surgically in these children are fraught with hazard and are frequently destined to failure. Although surgery may be indicated for relief of ureterovesical obstruction, which is felt to be secondary, or for the relief of vesicoureteral reflux, if at all possible, invasive procedures should be delayed until such time as the child voids normally. Allen and associates (1977) have utilized bladder training, attempting to teach the children to relax the perineal floor as they void. Hinman (1974) has used hypnotherapy to accomplish the same result. In some children

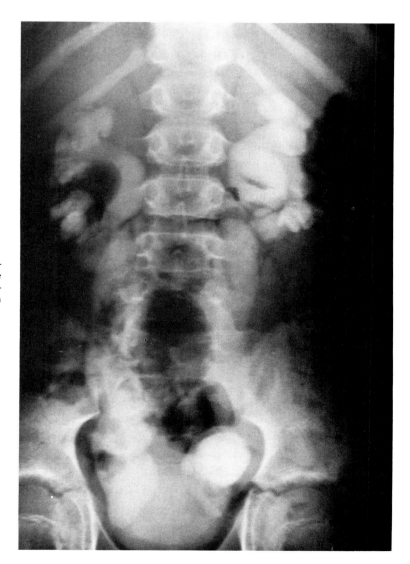

Figure 7–6. Intavenous urogram from a nine year old male with a non-neurogenic neurogenic bladder who presented with day and night wetting.

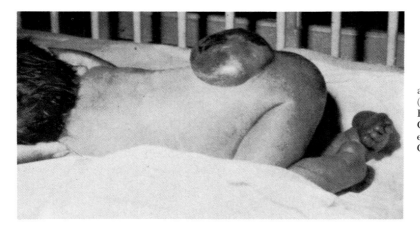

Figure 7–7. Newborn with an intact myelomeningocele. (From Harrison, J. H., Gittes, R. F., Perlmutter, A. D., et al.: Campbell's Urology, Vol. 2, 4th ed. Philadelphia, W. B. Saunders Co., 1979, p. 1783.)

with this problem, the upper tract is at such risk that the only alternative is urinary diversion (Also see Chap. 6).

MYELOMENINGOCELE

Myelomeningocele (Fig. 7–7) is the most common cause of neurogenic vesical dysfunction in childhood. Recent experience suggests that these patients are best handled by a multidisciplinary team that includes a pediatrician as coordinator, a urologist, a neurosurgeon, an orthopedic surgeon, and a host of paramedical personnel (Fig. 7–8). Experience has also shown that not every child born with a myelomeningocele can be expected to develop into a self-sufficient, relatively unencumbered adult member of society (Shurtleff et al., 1975). Utilizing retrospective data, several authorities have developed criteria to indicate at birth which patients might achieve this goal and, hence, would best be treated aggressively and to indicate which patients are best left untreated (Lorber, 1971; Stein et al., 1974). There are great philosophical differences among authorities regarding the validity of these criteria, and, for the moment, the issue of treatment versus nontreatment of selected patients is quite unsettled.

Myelomeningocele is best defined as a developmental defect of the spinal column

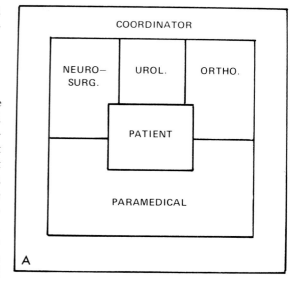

PARAMEDICAL DISCIPLINES

GENETIC COUNSELING
SOCIAL WORKER
FINANCIAL COUNSELOR
EDUCATIONAL EVALUATOR
PHYSICAL THERAPY
ORTHOTIST
OCCUPATIONAL THERAPY
REHABILITATION NURSES
ENTEROSTOMAL THERAPY

Figure 7–8. *A,* Schema of the interrelationship of personnel and patient in the multidisciplinary approach to the patient with myelomeningocele. *B,* Paramedical personnel used in the "team" approach to patients with myelomeningocele. (From Harrison, J. H., Gittes, R. F., Perlmutter, A. D., et al.: Campbell's Urology, Vol. 2, 4th ed. Philadelphia, W. B. Saunders Co., 1979, p. 1784.)

that manifests itself by a failure of fusion between the arches of the vertebrae, with protrusion and dysplasia of the spinal cord or its membranes (Smith, 1965). Perhaps a better but more pragmatic definition is Nash's description (1956) of a "paraplegic incontinent cripple . . . snatched from the jaws of death in the neonatal months, only to be delivered over to the tragedy of an expanding head, or to a life of social exclusion and the fumes and filth of double incontinence and trophic ulcers."

The preceding remarks are not to be interpreted as unduly pessimistic but as realistic. Actually anyone, regardless of specialty, undertaking the care of these patients is best advised to adopt as optimistic an attitude as possible. Firstly, one often misjudges the developmental prognosis (both overestimation and underestimation) at birth. It could be tragic to allow the urinary tract to deteriorate on the assumption that a patient might not develop mentally only later to have a patient of normal intellect in renal failure. Secondly, there are great but intangible psychological benefits to both family and patient that accrue when a positive therapeutic approach is adopted. Even if the family itself should elect withholding active treatment of the patient, the parents must be continually supported psychologically. Under such circumstances, the physicians must be prepared to periodically reconsider the nontreatment decision in order to avoid a child surviving with progressive neurologic, urologic, or orthopedic deterioration.

Incidence

The incidence of myelomeningocele is approximately 1 to 2 per 1000 live births in the United States and as high as 4 per 1000 live births in Ireland (Smith, 1965). The etiologic event leading to myelomeningocele occurs between the 18th and 28th day of gestation, but the causes for this event are unknown. A few years ago it was suggested that a potato blight was an etiologic factor, accounting for the increased incidence in some areas of the British Isles; this theory has not been confirmed (Duckett and Raezer, 1976). There are no other exogen-

ous or economic factors that seem to predict its occurrence other than a familial one. It is established that the incidence of myelomeningocele rises to approximately four per cent if there is already one affected member of a family and to approximately 20 to 25 per cent if there are two or more affected family members (Duckett and Raezer, 1976).

Myelomeningoceles are most frequently lumbosacral in position (42 per cent), with thoracolumbar (27 per cent) and sacral (21 per cent) lesions being slightly less common. Thoracic and cervical lesions are distinctly less common (10 per cent) and usually result in less severe motor and urologic deficits because the spinal cord itself is less often dysplastic than in the lower level lesions.

Natural History

It is difficult to work with large numbers of myelomeningocele patients without some appreciation of the natural history of the overall problem. Prior to the institution of aggressive and prompt neurosurgical treatment, 68 per cent of affected patients died. After the adoption of an aggressive approach (closure of the defect promptly after birth and shunting procedures for hydrocephalus, should it become clinically manifest), the mortality rate dropped to 34 per cent (Smith, 1965). In Lorber's series (1971), 83 per cent of the patients had hydrocephalus by ventriculography; admittedly, not all of these patients required shunting procedures. Most deaths occurred in the first two years of life and were neurosurgical in nature (such as hydrocephalus and meningitis). Deaths occurring after age two were usually renal in etiology.

As is so often the case, a child with one congenital abnormality often has multiple anomalies; myelomeningocele is no exception to this dictum, as approximately one third of patients have other congenital anomalies. Roberts (1961) studied patients with myelomeningocele at autopsy and found an 18 per cent incidence of other anomalies of the urinary tract alone, exclusive of any hydronephrosis that might be secondary to a neurogenic bladder. Fusion anomalies, such as horseshoe kidney, were most common, with cystic disease next; even renal agenesis was not uncommon. Exstrophy and cloacal exstrophy occur more frequently with myelomeningocele than in the general population. According to Forbes (1972) renal dysplasia occurred in 12 per cent of myelomeningocele patients at autopsy compared to a nil incidence in his control autopsies.

The obvious implications of these data are that renal functional potential may already be decreased at birth. The exact incidence of renal functional impairment at birth is unknown but may approximate 10 per cent (Smith, 1965). In a series of patients studied by Chapman and colleagues in 1969, 75 per cent of myelomeningocele patients at age four had already developed a urinary tract infection, 100 per cent had abnormal cystograms, 25 per cent had vesicoureteral reflux, and 30 per cent had abnormal excretory urograms. Bucy (1971) has suggested that such changes in the upper urinary tract in myelomeningocele patients are totally age-related and cannot be related to the level of the lesion. Many would disagree, but there are no good data to support this difference of opinion.

Of those children surviving after aggressive neurosurgical treatment, only nine per cent are without any disability. The disabilities in 38 per cent of patients are moderately severe. These are obvious and consist of mental retardation, musculoskeletal impairment, urinary and fecal incontinence, trophic skin problems, and sexual difficulties (Shurtleff et al., 1975). In a survey of the status of a group of myelomeningocele patients surviving into adult life, a significant minority were mentally retarded, especially those with lesions above the L2 level (Shurtleff et al., 1975). Urinary incontinence was common in patients who had not undergone urinary diversion, as were urinary tract infections, calculi, and hydronephrosis. Urinary incontinence often led to a low self-image. One third of the patients were active sexually; potential fertility was present in patients of both sexes but existed more frequently in females (Shurtleff et al., 1975).

Ericsson and others (1970) have attempted to determine which factors would best predict eventual urinary and fecal continence in patients with myelomeningocele. Some series have stated that only three per cent of myelomeningocele patients will eventually have normal urinary control (Shurtleff et al., 1975; Harlowe et al., 1965); perhaps these few patients actually have meningoceles rather than myelomeningoceles. Patients with high sacral lesions and a unilateral orthopedic deficit seem most likely to achieve true continence. Forty-six per cent of the patients in Ericsson's series were partially continent. This partial continence usually evolved at about age four. These patients did have some sense of bladder filling and could initiate a urinary stream without voluntary increasing intra-abdominal pressure. Fecal continence seems to bear no relation to the level of the lesion; the most favorable prognostic sign is normal anal sphincter tone on rectal examination. There seems to be no correlation with the anal cutaneous reflex. If true continence is to develop, it usually develops at age two to three years. Fecal pseudocontinence usually develops at about age seven (Ericsson, 1970).

ROUTINE UROLOGIC EVALUATION

As one attempts to assess patients with neurogenic bladder dysfunction, a careful history of the voiding pattern is quite helpful. Constant dribbling suggests that the bladder remains relatively empty and that the pelvic floor is lax. Intermittent dribbling suggests a degree of overflow incontinence in which the pelvic floor resistance is greater than the propulsive force of the detrusor. Voiding in a stream occurs when the pelvic floor can relax at a time when either the detrusor contracts or intra-abdominal pressure increases, leading to propulsion of urine. The former is usually a steady stream, whereas the latter is usually intermittent. This is not to infer, however, that the bladder then completely empties. In a few patients, there will be continence but with frequency and precipitate voiding. The ability to voluntarily interrupt the stream suggests some control over the muscles of the pelvic floor. The presence of a sense of fullness or a sense of voiding are helpful in assessing capacity for continence.

Bowel control should be assessed to determine the frequency and character of stool, whether or not there is a sense of fullness, and an ability to control loose stools.

On physical examination it is important to note any other congenital abnormalities, such as imperforate anus or exstrophy, for their possible effects on overall prognosis and management. Physical signs suggesting renal developmental malformation, such as ear abnormalities, should be sought. The

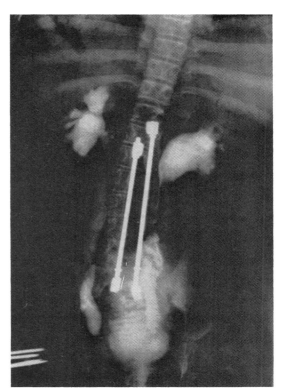

Figure 7–10. Intravenous urogram of a 12 year old boy followed elsewhere with yearly urograms. These remained normal until he entered puberty, when hydronephrosis developed. (From Harrison, J. H., Gittes, R. F., Perlmutter, A. D., et al.: Campbell's Urology, Vol. 2, 4th ed. Philadelphia, W. B. Saunders Co., 1979, p. 1788.)

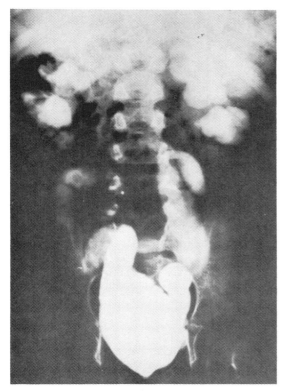

Figure 7–9. Intravenous urogram of an 11 year old boy with a myelomeningocele. His only muscular defect was bilateral pes cavus. He presented for control of his urinary incontinence. His blood urea nitrogen (BUN) and serum creatinine levels were 55 mg. per 100 ml. and 4.5 mg. per 100 ml., respectively, at that time. (From Harrison, J. H., Gittes, R. F., Perlmutter, A. D. et al.: Campbell's Urology, Vol. 2, 4th ed. Philadelphia, W. B. Saunders Co., 1979, p. 1788.)

abdomen is palpated for renal enlargement or fusion and bladder enlargement. One should attempt to express the bladder manually to determine the status of the pelvic floor musculature. Rectal examination is mandatory, and special attention is paid to the presence or absence of anal sphincter tone, the presence and strength of the bulbocavernous reflex (contraction of the anal sphincter in response to tapping or squeezing the glans penis or clitoris), and the amount of stool in the rectal ampulla. During neurologic examination, cutaneous reflexes (abdominal, cremasteric, dartos, and anal) are tested as well. The normal infant's bladder cannot be expressed by the Credé maneuver (i.e., by forceful manual suprapubic compression of the bladder). In the patient with neurogenic vesical dysfunction, either of two patterns exists: the bladder is not palpable but can be expressed very easily, or the bladder is palpable but is difficult to express. Anal paralysis and perineal anesthesia indicate that bladder function will be abnormal.

We wish to emphasize that even those myelomeningocele patients whose only involvement seems to be a minor foot disturbance usually also have disturbed bladder function. Some children with minimal orthopedic involvement may, unfortunately, have disproportionately severe urologic dysfunction (Fig. 7–9). Smith (1965) observed in longitudinal studies that patients tended to change their voiding patterns with age, tending to go from total dribbling incontinence at birth to urinary retention with overflow incontinence at puberty, especially in boys (Fig. 7–10).

LABORATORY ASSESSMENT

Laboratory studies that are helpful in assessment are urinalysis, urine culture, blood urea nitrogen, serum creatinine, and creatinine clearance. A word of caution is necessary in the interpretation of elevated blood urea nitrogen levels. We have seen several myelomeningocele patients with chronically elevated blood urea nitrogen levels as well as normal serum creatinine and creatinine clearances and normal intravenous pyelograms. The cause for this disparity has not yet been elucidated. Urine cultures, when positive, must have been reliably obtained (catheterized or aspirated) to have any validity.

RADIOGRAPHIC EVALUATION

Regularly scheduled radiographic evaluation of these children is an essential part of their care. Whereas in the normal child, once it is established that the urinary tract is anatomically normal, repeat urinary tract radiographs are rarely required. This is not true of the child with a neurogenic bladder. Body growth coupled with a tethered spinal cord may lead to a change in bladder innervation with deterioration of urinary tract function. Additionally, the poorly innervated bladder is functionally partially obstruct-

ed and over a period of time may decompensate.

Excretory urography is essential to assess the anatomic and functional status of the upper urinary tract. Upper tract problems have been reported more frequently in patients with constant dribbling than in those with overflow incontinence for reasons that, for the moment, are unclear (Ericsson et al., 1971). It is to be emphasized, however, that the experience of both authors has been the converse, that is, that those patients who dribble (have a lax pelvic floor) are less likely to develop hydronephrosis. Hydronephrosis is found at some time in about 50 per cent of untreated patients; it is most common in patients who have reflux (Smith, 1965).

Voiding cystourethrography can be quite helpful in assessment, although it is reserved for instances in which either the excretory urogram is abnormal or specific information is required that can only be obtained with this study. Some authors prefer to use it routinely, but the fear of introducing infection into an abnormal bladder that is not periodically emptied (such as by intermittent catheterization) would seem to us to outweigh the benefit to be gained in most routine assessments of patients with neurogenic bladder dysfunction, and for this reason we tend to delay voiding cystourethrography until it is indicated. The bladder wall can vary from thin to thick. The bladder configuration is frequently elongated (the "Christmas tree bladder") (Fig. 7–11). Trabeculation is often present, even in thin-walled bladders, perhaps induced in some instances by chronic infection; trabeculation seems to occur more frequently in higher-level lesions. Vesicoureteral reflux is seen in as many as 50 per cent of patients but is less common in the neonate, suggesting that infection or relative obstruction may have some role in its genesis (Ericsson et al., 1971).

Endoscopy tends to confirm the findings of the studies just mentioned but is rarely required for routine assessment. Trabeculation is seen slightly more frequently endoscopically than radiographically. The ureteral orifices can be evaluated for their competence and for the presence of para-

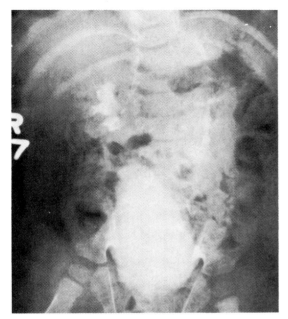

Figure 7–11. Urogram of a patient with a myelomeningocele, demonstrating vesical elongation and narrowing — the "Christmas tree" configuration. (From Harrison, J. H., Gittes, R. F., Perlmutter, A. D., et al.: Campbell's Urology, Vol. 2, 4th ed. Philadelphia, W. B. Saunders Co., 1979, p. 1789.)

ureteral saccules in those patients in whom reflux or obstruction are a problem. The bladder neck in patients with neurogenic vesical dysfunction is usually patulous endoscopically regardless of its radiographic appearance (admittedly, a subjective impression).

THERAPEUTIC GOALS

The goals of urologic management of children afflicted with neurogenic vesical dysfunction can best be categorized as (1) maintenance and preservation of renal function and protection from urinary infection, (2) social urinary continence and bowel control, and (3) preservation of sexual activity. In order to achieve these goals, the urologist should be involved at birth or at diagnosis and through the remainder of the patient's life (DeSantis and Lattimer, 1974). A stylized surveillance pattern should be established and rigidly adhered to. The recommendations of the American Academy of Pediatrics (Klauber et al., 1979) for myelomeningocele are that a blood urea nitrogen, serum creatinine, urinalysis, and urine culture as well as an excretory urogram should be obtained shortly after birth. Voiding cystourethrograms are not advised as routine procedures. Excretory urography should then be performed approximately yearly to age three and then every other year. Urinalysis should be performed at six-month intervals to age three, then yearly (Ridlon et al., 1975). Our personal approach has been a bit tighter than this in that excretory urograms are also obtained at six months of age. Our patients are seen at three-month intervals through the first few years of life and at six-month intervals thereafter. Urinalysis, urine culture, blood urea nitrogen, and serum creatinine are determined at each of these visits. A similar program is desirable for other neurogenic vesical dysfunction patients.

UROLOGIC MANAGEMENT

Urinary tract infection is aggressively sought. When identified and documented by suprapubic aspiration, catheterization, or a freshly expressed specimen, it has been vigorously treated. Some authors have suggested that asymptomatic bacteriuria with myelomeningoceles is of no consequence, and yet in Mebust's series, two thirds of his asymptomatic patients went on to develop clinical pyelonephritis (Mebust et al., 1969).

Manual expression of the bladder (Credé maneuver) has been recommended by others as routine for all these children (Smith, 1965). It has been our practice not to utilize this maneuver as a routine, as it is futile in many patients and potentially harmful in those patients with vesicoureteral reflux, especially when associated with urinary tract infection. Furthermore, we have seen no patient achieve continence with this maneuver alone.

In those patients who do not have severe problems with recurring infection and who do not manifest hydronephrosis, no

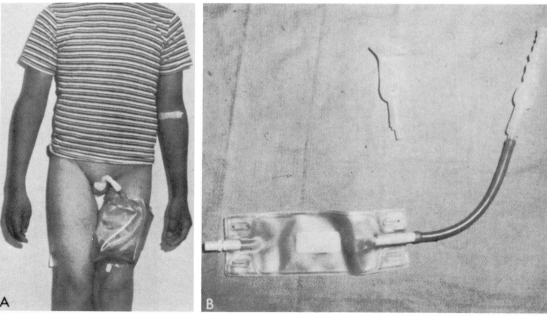

Figure 7–12.   An eight year old boy with a myelomeningocele who has been fitted with an external collecting device that he manages independently. *B,* Close-up view of the components of the external collecting device we are currently using. (From Harrison, J. H., Gittes, R. F., Perlmutter, A. D., et al.: Campbell's Urology, Vol. 2, 4th ed. Philadelphia, W. B. Saunders Co., 1979, p. 1790.)

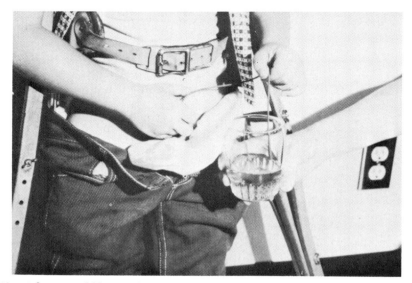

Figure 7–13.   A five year old boy performing self-catheterization. He is dry between catheterizations. (From Schoenberg, H. W., Shah, J. P., and Gregory, J. G.: Pharmacologic modification of therapeutic measures used in managing the neurogenic bladder. *In* Bergsma, D., and Duckett, J. W. (Eds.): Urinary System Malformations in Children. New York, Alan R. Liss for the National Foundation-March of Dimes, Birth Defects, Original Article Series, *13*(5):123, 1977.)

early active intervention has been employed. However, at about age five, prior to entering school, the concern for *urinary continence* becomes significant. Males were formerly fitted with an external collection device (Fig. 7–12), although in recent years both boys and girls have been started on an intermittent catheterization program in an effort to achieve this goal. Clean intermittent catheterization has favorably altered the management of the neurogenic bladder. Children and parents can be easily taught the technique (Fig. 7–13). Hydronephrosis can often be resolved, and continence frequently can be achieved when the bladder is periodically emptied with catheterization (Rabinovitch, 1974) (Fig. 7–14). Although many patients on intermittent catheterization will have bacteriuria, this does not seem to be harmful. Kass and colleagues (1981) reviewed the records of 255 children managed with clean intermittant catheterization over a 10-year period. Although bacteriuria was present in 56 per cent, fresh renal damage was noted in only 26 per cent.

Largely as a result of employing intermittent catheterization, supravesical diversion is currently employed only when other modalities have proved unsuccessful.

Infants who have developed hydronephrosis can also be managed quite successfully by temporary *cutaneous vesicostomy* (Fig. 7–15). Our experience with this procedure has been uniformly successful (Cohen et al., 1978). Once vesicostomy has been performed, the child is left in diapers until an appropriate time to consider social continence, at which time the vesicostomy is closed and intermittent catheterization employed. Although Shochat and Perlmutter (1972) and Johnston (1968) have found it of benefit in infant females, both "super" dilation of the urethra and internal urethrotomy have not proved beneficial in our experience. Additionally, this may lower bladder outlet resistance limiting the success of intermittent catheterization.

In boys an alternative to promote vesical emptying is *transurethral external sphincterotomy* (Koontz et al., 1972). This

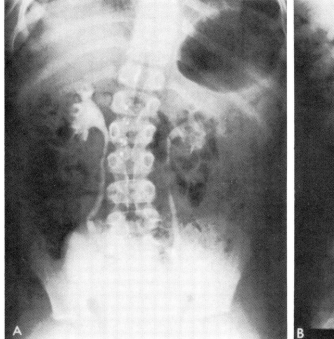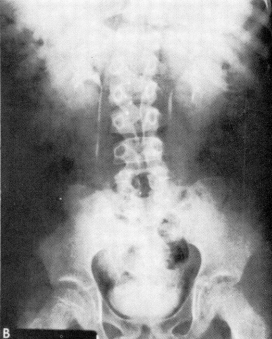

Figure 7–14. A, Intravenous urogram of a seven year old girl, demonstrating bilateral early hydronephrosis. B, Intravenous urogram of the same patient five months after instituting intermittent catheterization. (From Harrison, J. H., Gittes, R. F., Perlmutter, A. D., et al.: Campbell's Urology, Vol. 2, 4th ed. Philadelphia, W. B. Saunders Co., 1979, p. 1792.)

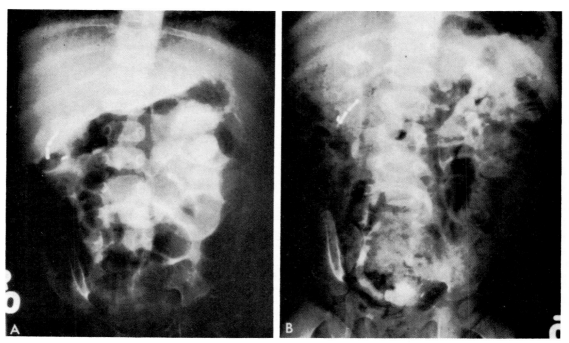

Figure 7–15. *A,* Intravenous urogram of a six month old girl with hydronephrosis and urinary infection. *B,* Intravenous urogram of the same patient three months after cutaneous vesicostomy. (From Harrison, J. H., Gittes, R. F., Perlmutter, A. D., et al.: Campbell's Urology, Vol. 2, 4th ed. Philadelphia, W. B. Saunders Co., 1979, p. 1781.)

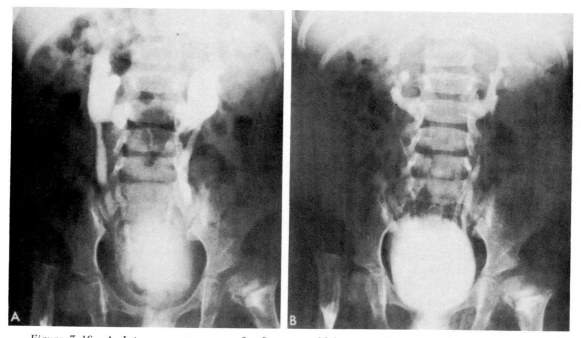

Figure 7–16. *A,* Intravenous urogram of a five year old boy with bilateral hydronephrosis. (Note the horeseshoe kidney.) *B,* Intravenous urogram of the same patient four months following transurethral external sphincterotomy. (From Harrison, J. H., Gittes, R. F., Perlmutter, A. D., et al.: Campbell's Urology, Vol. 2, 4th ed. Philadelphia, W. B. Saunders Co., 1979, p. 1792.)

has been utilized with success in incontinent boys by substituting dribbling incontinence for overflow incontinence (Fig. 7–16). A condom catheter is then utilized to collect the almost continuous flow of urine.

In patients in whom intermittent catheterization or sphincterotomy has been unsuccessful in relieving hydronephrosis, *supravesical diversion* may then be necessary (Ferguson and Geist, 1971). Other maneuvers, such as transurethral resection of the bladder neck and Y-V plasty, have been directed toward weakening the bladder neck in hopes of promoting improved vesical emptying. Inasmuch as it is the pelvic floor that produces the "obstruction," these procedures seem to have very little basis in theory or fact and, for that reason, are now rarely utilized (Kaplan and King, 1970). Pudendal neurectomy and pudendal blocks have been largely avoided in boys because of their interference with sexual function (Stark, 1969). Selective *sacral rhizotomy*, which produces a flaccid bladder that is

amenable to intermittent catheterization, has been successfully utilized to control incontinence in some girls with spastic bladders (Manfredi and Leal, 1958). Thus, even in this type of patient, supravesical diversion can often be avoided. *Indwelling catheters* have frequently led to recurrent pyelonephritis, vesical and renal calculi, and increased bladder irritability and are now no longer recommended for long-term control of incontinence (Fig. 7–17).

Pharmacologic agents are of benefit in achieving dryness in some patients, either alone or as an adjunct to intermittent catheterization. Imipramine, by virtue of its anticholinergic and beta-adrenergic blockade, decreases bladder contractility and increases bladder outlet resistance, leading to continence in some patients (Cole and Fried, 1972). Phenoxybenzamine (Krane and Olsson, 1973) and diazepam have not thus far proved beneficial in our patients despite their theoretical utility. It is possible that the voluntary muscle relaxant dan-

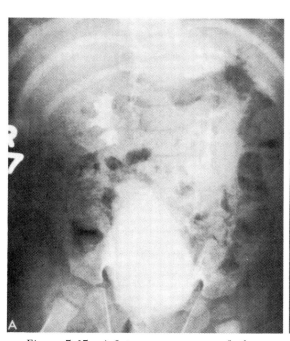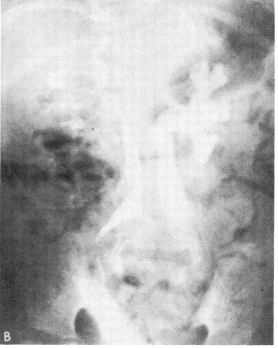

Figure 7–17. *A*, Intravenous urogram of a three year old girl with recurring pyelonephritis but normal upper urinary tracts. *B*, Intravenous urogram of the same patient six months after the institution of indwelling Foley catheter drainage. Both renal calculi and hydronephrosis had developed in the interim. (From Harrison, J. H., Gittes, R. F., Perlmutter, A. D., et al.: Campbell's Urology, Vol. 2, 4th ed. Philadelphia, W. B. Saunders Co., 1979, p. 1793.)

trium may prove of some utility in improving bladder emptying, but to date there is no experience with this modality in children (Murdock and Krane, 1976). Anticholinergics, such as propantheline and oxybutynin to reduce bladder contractions, and alpha stimulators, such as ephedrine and phenylpropanolamine, have proved useful adjuncts to intermittent catheterization in some patients (Diokno and Lapides, 1973).

Artificial urinary sphincters may have some promise, but their exact roles are as yet undetermined (Scott et al., 1973). Conversely, implantable and external bladder pacemakers to date have not proved of value in children (Katona and Eckstein, 1974).

Bowel control should be an achievable goal in all patients and can be accomplished by manipulating the diet and using suppositories or enemas on a regular basis if necessary. Colostomy should never be utilized to achieve fecal continence, as this merely substitutes an abdominal stoma for a perineal one. We currently advocate initiating a bowel regimen at age three years in those patients who have not spontaneously achieved bowel control by that time.

There are, unfortunately, very little data yet regarding the sexual ability of patients with congenital forms of neurogenic vesical dysfunction. Many have been quite sheltered and are slow to develop normal sexual interests and behavior. More attention should be paid to sexuality and related aspects in the future. Certainly any procedure that might irreversibly interfere with sexual function or procreative ability is best avoided.

REFERENCES

Allen, T. D.: The non-neurogenic neurogenic bladder. J. Urol., *117*:232, 1977.

Belman, A. B., and King, L. R.: Urinary tract anomalies associated with imperforate anus. J. Urol., *108*:823, 1972.

Bors, E.: Neurogenic bladder. Urol. Surv., 7:177, 1957.

Bors, E., and Porter, R. W.: Neurosurgical considerations in bladder dysfunction. Urol. Int., 25:114, 1970.

Bucy, J. G.: Patterns of urological disease in patients with myelomeningocele. J. Urol., *106*:541, 1971.

Chapman, W. H., Shurtleff, D. B., Eckert, D. W., and Ansell, J. S.: A prospective study of the urinary tract from birth in myelomeningocele. J. Urol., *102*:363, 1969.

Cohen, J. S., Harbach, L. E., and Kaplan, G. W.: Cutaneous vesicostomy for temporary urinary diversion in infants with neurogenic bladder dysfunction. J. Urol., *119*:120, 1978.

Cole, A. T., and Fried, F. A.: Favorable experiences with imipramine in the treatment of neurogenic bladder. J. Urol., *107*:44, 1972.

Comarr, A. E.: Management of the traumatic cord bladder today. Urol. Int., *20*:1, 1965.

Comarr, A. E.: Sexual concepts in traumatic cord and cauda equina lesions. J. Urol., *106*:375, 1971.

DeSantis, P. N., and Lattimer, J. K.: Management of myelomeningocele: Plea for earlier urologic consultation. Urology, 3:421, 1974.

Diokno, A. C., and Lapides, J.: Oxybutinin: A new drug with analgesic and anticholinergic properties. J. Urol., *108*:307, 1973.

Duckett, J. W., Jr., and Raezer, D. M.: Neuromuscular dysfunction of the urinary bladder. *In* Kelalis, P. P., King, L. R., and Belman, A. B (Eds.): Clinical Pediatric Urology. Philadelphia, W. B. Saunders Co., 1976.

Ericsson, N. O., Hellstrom, B., Nergardh, A., and Rudhe, U.: Factors promoting urinary and anal continence in children with myelomeningocele. Acta Paediatr. Scand., 59:491, 1970.

Ericsson, N. O., Hellstrom, B., Nergardh, A., and Rudhe, U.: Micturition urethrocystography in children with myelomeningocele: A radiologic and clinical investigation. Acta Radiol. Diagn., *11*:321, 1971.

Fergusson, D. E., and Geist, R. W.: Pre-school urinary tract diversion for children with neurogenic bladder from myelomeningocele. J. Urol., *105*:133, 1971.

Forbes, M.: Renal dysplasia in infants with neurospinal dysraphism. J. Pathol., *107*:13, 1972.

Harlowe, S. E., Merrill, R. E., Lee, E. M., Turman, A. E., and Trapp, J. D.: A clinical evaluation of the urinary tract in patients with myelomeningocele. J. Urol., 93:411, 1965.

Hinman, F.: Urinary tract damage in children who wet. Pediatrics, 54:145, 1974.

Hinman, F., and Baumann, F. W.: Vesical and ureteral damage from voiding dysfunction in boys without neurologic or obstructive disease. J. Urol., 109:727, 1973.

Homsy, G. E.: The dynamics of the ureterovesical and vesico-urethral junctions. Invest. Urol., 3:1, 1967.

Johnston, J. H.: The neurogenic bladder in the newborn infant. Paraplegia, 6:157, 1968.

Kamhi, I. B., Horowitz, M. I., and Kovetz, A.: Isolated neurogenic dysfunction of the bladder in children with urinary tract infection. J. Urol., *106*:151, 1971.

Kaplan, G. W., and King, L. R.: Results of Y-V vesicourethroplasty in children. Surg. Gynecol. Obstet., *130*:1059, 1970.

Kass, E. J., Koff, S. A., Diokno, A. C., and Lapides, J.: The significance of bacilluria in children in long-term intermittent catheterization. J. Urol., 1981.

Katona, F., and Eckstein, H. B.: Treatment of neurogenic bladder by transurethral electrical stimulation. Lancet, *1*:780, 1974.

Klauber, G. T., et al.: Action Committee on Myelodysplasia, Section on Urology, American Academy of Pediatrics: Current approaches to evaluation and management of children with myelomeningocele. Pediatrics, 63:663, 1979.

Koontz, W. W., Jr., Smith, M. J. V., and Currie, R. J.:

External sphincterotomy in boys with myelomeningocele. J. Urol., 108:649, 1972.

Krane, R. J., and Olsson, C. A.: Phenoxybenzamine in neurogenic bladder dysfunction. I. A theory of micturition. J. Urol., 110:650, 1973.

Linderholm, R. E.: The cystometric findings in enuresis. J. Urol., 96:718, 1966.

Lorber, J.: Results of treatment of myelomeningocele. An analysis of 524 unselected cases, with special reference to possible selection for treatment. Dev. Med. Child. Neurol., 13:279, 1971.

Manfredi, R. A., and Leal, J. F.: Selective sacral rhizotomy for the spastic bladder syndrome in patients with spinal cord injuries. J. Urol., 100:17, 1958.

McClellan, F. C.: The Neurogenic Bladder. Springfield, IL., Charles C Thomas, 1939.

Mebust, W. K., Foret, J. D., and Valk, W. L.: Fifteen years experience with urinary diversion in myelomeningocele patients. J. Urol., 101:177, 1969.

Muellner, R. S.: Develoment of urinary control in children. J.A.M.A., 172:1256, 1960.

Murdock, M., Murdock, M. M., Sax, D., and Krane, R. J.: The use of dantrium in external sphincter dyssynergia. Urology 8:133, 1976.

Nosh, D. F. E.: Congenital spinal palsy. Br. Med. J., 3:133, 1956.

Nyquist, R. H., and Bors, E.: Mortality and survival in traumatic myelopathy during 14 years from 1946–1965. Paraplegia, 5:22, 1967.

Osborne, J., Du Mont, G., Beecroft, M., and Ayres, A. B.: Bladder emptying in neonates. Arch. Dis. Child., 52:896, 1977.

Rabinovitch, H. H.: Bladder evacuation in the child with myelomeningocele. Urology, 3:425, 1974.

Ridlon, H. C., Markland, C., Govan, D. E., Leadbetter, G., Price, S., Schoenberg, H., and Perlmutter, A. D.: Myelomeningocele: Suggested minimal urological evaluation and surveillance. Pediatrics, 55:477, 1975.

Roberts, J. B. M.: Congenital anomalies of the urinary tract and their association with spina bifida. Br. J. Urol., 33:309, 1961.

Scott, F. B., Bradley, W. E., Timm, G. W., and Kotharl, D.: Treatment of incontinence secondary to myelodysplasia by an implantable prosthetic urinary sphincter. South. Med. J., 66:987, 1973.

Shapiro, S. A.: Personal communication.

Shochat, S. J., and Perlmutter, A. D.: Myelodysplasia with severe neonatal hydronephrosis: The value of urethral dilatation. J. Urol., 107:146, 1972.

Shurtleff, D. B., Hayden, P. W., Chapman, W. H., Broy, A. B., and Hill, M. L.: Myelodysplasia. Problems of long-term survival and social function. West. J. Med., 122:199, 1975.

Smith, E. D.: Spina bifida and the total care of myelomeningocele. Springfield, IL, Charles C Thomas. 1965.

Stark, G.: Pudendal neurectomy in management of neurogenic bladder in myelomeningocele. Arch. Dis. Child., 44:698, 1969.

Stein, S. C., Schut, L., and Ames, M. D.: Selection for early treatment in myelomeningocele: A retrospective analysis of various selection procedures. Pediatrics, 54:553, 1974.

Tang, P. L., and Ruch, T. C.: Localization of brain stem and diencephalic areas controlling the micturition reflex. J. Comp. Neurol., 106:213, 1956.

Chapter Eight

URINARY DIVERSION

This is not a surgical text. However, it is felt that a short discussion outlining the various forms of temporary and permanent urinary diversion employed in clinical practice would be helpful. Our purpose is to offer a reference source identifying the indications for and the applicability of the various procedures currently in use.

TEMPORARY URINARY DIVERSION

INTUBATED TEMPORARY DIVERSION

Intubated diversion has a singular advantage, ease of reversal. This, however, is also one of its definite drawbacks. The inadvertent dislodging of an essential drainage tube, such as a nephrostomy tube, constitutes an emergency. The urinary tract tends to seal rapidly in such instances, and reinsertion might then require a secondary operative procedure. Additionally, catheters encrust or plug with debris, thereby requiring periodic changing. However, the most negative aspect of this form of drainage is the chronic bacteriuria associated with a foreign body in the urinary tract; this bacteriuria may constitute a threat to life in some children. Nevertheless, situations arise in which intubated diversion for several months to years becomes necessary. Nephrostomy drainage following a failed surgical procedure may be necessary to maintain function until healing has occurred and postoperative induration has resolved prior to a secondary attempt at surgical repair. Additionally, suprapubic cystostomy drainage may be the only means of management available in a patient following severe pelvic trauma or may be the most practical means of caring for the quadriplegic.

Nephrostomy

The insertion of a tube directly through the renal parenchyma into the kidney is a time-honored form of urinary diversion. Its usefulness in the acute situation, when it may be the only practical means of controlling sepsis or relieving obstruction and preventing significant renal loss, cannot be overemphasized. Two forms of operative nephrostomy drainage are currently employed: the use of a mushroom or Foley catheter (Fig. 8–1) and the loop nephrostomy (Fig. 8–2). Experience suggests that the loop nephrostomy may be the more stable and is particularly suitable when the necessity for diversion may become protracted.

Percutaneous Nephrostomy

Recent advances in imaging have made it possible to insert a temporary drainage tube directly into the kidney under fluoroscopic or ultrasonographic control. Small catheters can be inserted into the dilated

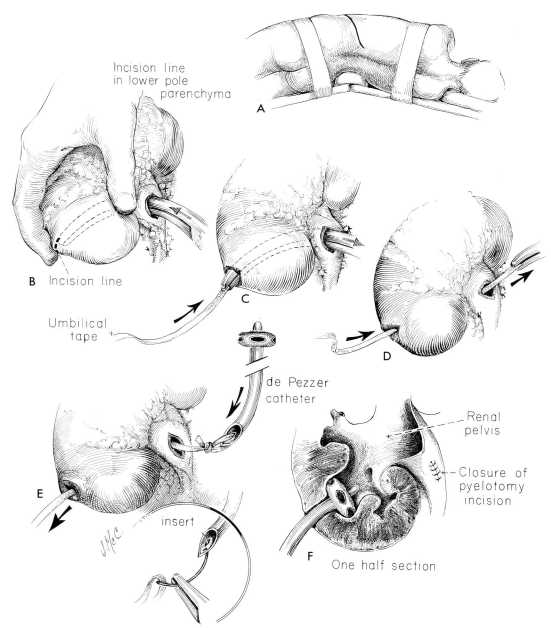

Incision line
in lower pole
parenchyma

A

B Incision line

Umbilical
tape

C

D

de Pezzer
catheter

E

insert

J.McC.

Renal
pelvis

Closure of
pyelotomy
incision

F One half section

Figure 8–1. Technique for nephrostomy in the absence of significant calycectasis. (From King, L. R., and Belman, A. B.: A technique for nephrostomy in the absence of calicectasis. J. Urol., *108*:518, 1972. © 1972, The Williams & Wilkins Co., Baltimore.)

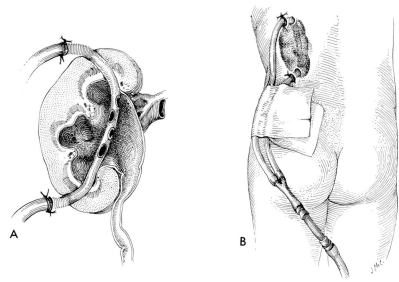

Figure 8–2. *A*, Loop nephrostomy using upper and lower calyces for exit of Silastic tubing. *B*, Tubing is stabilized to the patient with sutures and tape. (From Kelalis, P. P., King, L. R., and Belman, A. B.: Clinical Pediatric Urology, Vol. 1. Philadelphia, W. B. Saunders Co., 1976, p. 430.)

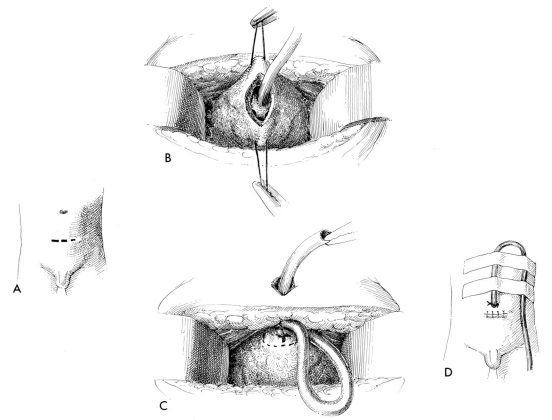

Figure 8–3. Suprapubic cystostomy. (From Kelalis, P. P., King, L. R., and Belman, A. B.: Clinical Pediatric Urology, Vol. 1. Philadelphia, W. B. Saunders Co., 1976, p. 431.)

collecting system with ease, allowing stabilization of a sick child prior to definitive surgery. Additionally, once a tract is established it is often possible to change such tubes to a more permanent type without an operation. Percutaneous nephrostomy is inappropriate, however, for the collecting system that is not significantly dilated, as may occur in acute obstruction.

Pyelostomy

The insertion of a tube directly into the renal pelvis rather than through the renal parenchyma is a form of diversion seldom used. The medial position of the renal pelvis and absence of any substance to stabilize the drainage tube makes this an extremely tenuous procedure.

Intubated Ureterostomy

The insertion of a tube into the ureter either in its intact state or through the stoma of a cutaneous ureterostomy is suitable for short-term drainage (days). Ureteritis with ultimate fibrosis of the ureter precludes this as a long-term form of intubated diversion.

Ureteral Stent

Ureteral catheters (in situ) can be placed endoscopically or during open surgery. Drainage of a kidney by a ureteral catheter alone is rarely employed in the pediatric population. Occasionally, however, such as in the unusual situation of an obstructive stone, bypassing the point of obstruction by this means is extremely effective. On the other hand, ureteral stents inserted at the time of open surgery are often employed temporarily to aid drainage during the postoperative period.

Suprapubic Cystostomy

A tube inserted through the lower abdominal wall directly into the bladder may function for years as a means of diversion and has historically served a vital role in the management of obstruction (Fig. 8–3). Current care, however, is directed toward definitive primary repair with very few circumstances in which semipermanent drainage of this type becomes necessary. We particularly advise against the use of cystostomy in infants and small children for periods longer than a few weeks. Chronic infection associated with a degree of ureterovesical obstruction secondary to the tube itself can cause serious renal damage in this most susceptible age group. Additionally, calculus formation is a real risk since stasis of some urine at the bladder base is guaranteed in this situation.

Trocar (Percutaneous) Cystostomy

This form of cystostomy is a product of modern technology and allows the insertion of various tubes into the bladder percutaneously by means of a disposable trocar device. This is useful as a temporary measure, such as following mild urethral trauma or postoperatively following hypospadias repair.

Urethral Catheterization

An indwelling urethral catheter must be considered a form of urinary diversion. Its applicability for the short-term (days to weeks) drainage of bladder urine in specific situations serves an important role. Although the introduction of silicone-impregnated catheters has reduced problems secondary to inflammation, urethritis leading to urethral strictures and urethrocutaneous fistulae remains a serious potential complication when employed long-term.

NONINTUBATED TEMPORARY DIVERSION

The direct anastomosis of the urinary tract to the skin offers the advantage of drainage without the necessity for an indwelling foreign body. If stasis can be prevented, bacilluria generally will not be associated with parenchymal infection. In many cases, the urine will be sterile. Unfortunately, reversal of all these procedures requires an additional operation for reconstruction. This is justifiable in the situation in which diversion may be necessary for several months if an intubated form of diversion can thus be avoided.

Loop Cutaneous Ureterostomy

The direct anastomosis of a knuckle of ureter to the skin is conceptually comparable to the loop colostomy (Fig. 8–4). Loop ureterostomy recently served an important function as a means of stabilizing the urinary tract, especially in infants with posterior urethral valves. Although primary valve resection has become the acceptable approach in the management of the majority of these children, occasionally a nonintubated form of high diversion is necessary, particularly if uncontrollable urinary tract infection is a problem.

There are a few variations on the same theme of high ureteral diversion, including the Y-ureterostomy (Fig. 8–5). These procedures are efforts to maintain some flow of urine into the bladder so that it will not be totally functionless. Irreversible bladder contracture after loop ureterostomy has been reported by Lome and colleagues (1972). This has been thought to occur as the end result of the combination of loss of the need for bladder function in association with pyocystis and may be preventable if some urine continues to flow down the distal ureter into the bladder.

A distinct disadvantage of high cutaneous diversion is the impracticality of fitting a urine collection device over the stoma. Diapers are often secured around the midabdomen for this purpose; however, as the child grows, keeping clothes dry becomes an increasingly more difficult problem.

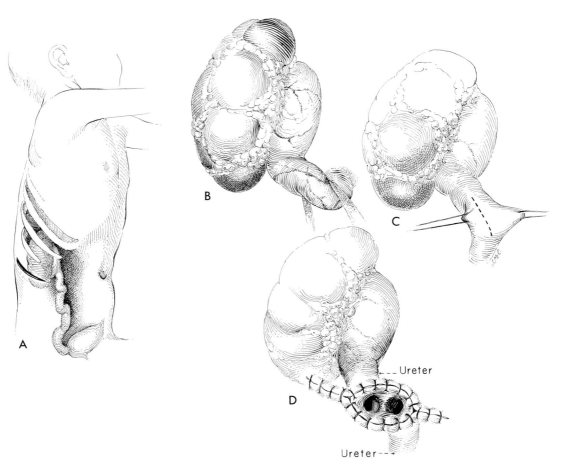

Figure 8–4. Loop ureterostomy. (From Kelalis, P. P., King, L. R., and Belman, A. B.: Clinical Pediatric Urology, Vol. 1. Philadelphia, W. B. Saunders Co., 1976, p. 434.)

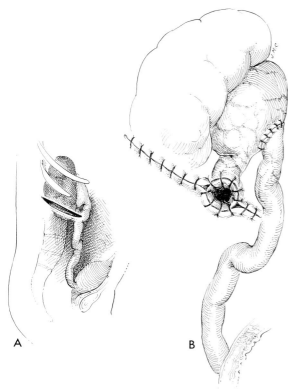

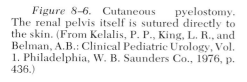

Figure 8–5. Y-Ureterostomy. This form of urinary diversion allows some urine to drain into the bladder, thus avoiding total defunctionalization. (From Kelalis, P. P., King, L. R., and Belman, A. B.: Clinical Pediatric Urology, Vol. 1. Philadelphia, W. B. Saunders Co., 1976, p. 435.)

Cutaneous Pyelostomy

The direct anastomosis of the massively dilated renal pelvis to the skin is an excellent means of high diversion (Fig. 8–6). Maintaining a urinary collecting device with this procedure is also difficult, and its applicability is limited to the child with significant pyelectasis. Its advantage rests in avoiding the use of the ureter as well as the ease of its reversal. It is applicable in infants with massive hydronephrosis in whom a definitive repair is not desirable, such as the very small, premature infant with a ureteropelvic junction obstruction or the very sick baby with posterior urethral valves.

End Ureterostomy

The direct anastomosis of the ureter to the skin can serve as either a temporary or permanent form of urinary diversion (Fig. 8–7). With the stoma placed in the lower abdominal quadrant, it is possible to apply a drainage bag in this group.

Some clinicians feel that ureterostomy provides poor drainage because peristalsis is usually decreased or absent in the mas-

Figure 8–6. Cutaneous pyelostomy. The renal pelvis itself is sutured directly to the skin. (From Kelalis, P. P., King, L. R., and Belman, A.B.: Clinical Pediatric Urology, Vol. 1. Philadelphia, W. B. Saunders Co., 1976, p. 436.)

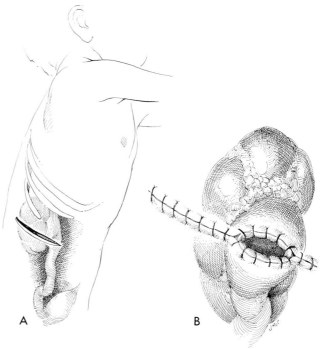

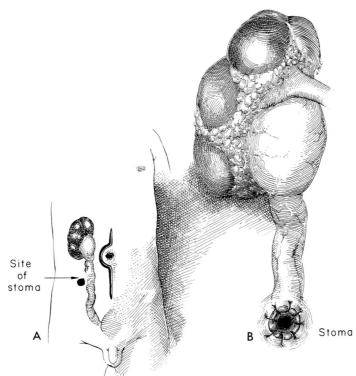

Site
of
stoma

A

B   Stoma

Figure 8–7. End ureterostomy. The anterior approach is preferred for accurate stomal location. (From Kelalis, P. P., King, L. R., and Belman, A. B.: Clinical Pediatric Urology, Vol. 1. Philadelphia, W. B. Saunders Co., 1976, p. 437.)

sively dilated ureter. However, it has been our experience that once obstruction is relieved, drainage is adequate. Nevertheless, low-pressure stasis may persist for a period of weeks until ureteral tone returns (if indeed it can return) to a more normal state.

Vesicostomy*

The direct anastomosis of the dome of the bladder to the skin, which allows continuous drainage of urine, is a simple and efficient way to deal with selected problems. Although definitive care of any medical problem is the preferred approach, situations occasionally arise that require a deferring tactic. Small babies with infravesical obstruction, massive reflux in the infant in whom infection cannot be controlled and in whom ureteral reimplantation is felt to be inadvisable, and the child with a poorly emptying neurogenic bladder who cannot be managed with intermittent catheteriza-

tion are situations in which cutaneous vesicostomy may be applicable (Fig. 8–8). This procedure is not appropriate for children with supravesical obstruction, such as ureterovesical junction obstruction.

Special care other than careful attention to the surrounding skin is not necessary. A urinary collection device need not be applied, as an ordinary diaper fits over the suprapubic stoma.

A final advantage of this procedure is the ease with which it can be performed. The abdominal location of the infant's bladder makes it possible to carry out this procedure under local anesthesia in the severely ill child.

PERMANENT URINARY DIVERSION

Permanent urinary diversion in children is being employed very infrequently these days. Other means of management of the neurogenic bladder, including intermittent catheterization and artificial sphincter devices, as well as nonablative surgery in

---

*Vesicostomy, a tubeless diversion, should not be confused with cystostomy, which requires some form of drainage tube.

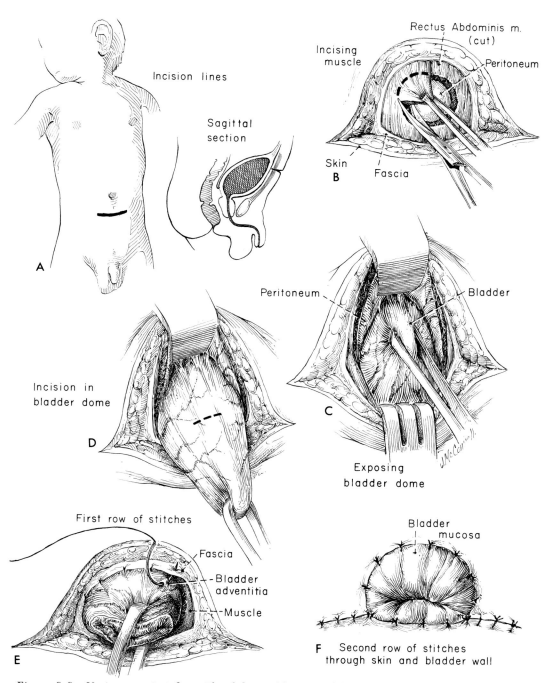

Figure 8–8. Vesicostomy in infants. The abdominal location of the bladder allows direct anastomosis of the dome to the skin. (From Belman, A. B., and King, L. R.,: Vesicostomy: Useful means of reversible urinary diversion in selected infants. Urology, *1*:208–213, 1973.)

the management of lower genitourinary sarcoma has made the necessity for urinary diversion a rarity in children.

CUTANEOUS DIVERSION

Cutaneous Ureterostomy, Transureteroureterostomy

The anastomosis of a single ureter to the skin with end-to-side transureteroureterostomy of the contralateral ureter (Fig. 8–9) is applicable only when one ureter is significantly dilated (1 cm). Ease and rapidity of performance as well as the opportunity to avoid multiple intraperitoneal anastomoses makes this an attractive alternative to diversionary procedures utilizing bowel. Permanent end-cutaneous ureterostomy is

not widely employed, probably because of concern for chronic bacilluria and the risk of stomal stenosis. The tendency to stomal stenosis can be minimized by choosing only dilated ureters for this operation.

Ileal Conduit

The most common form of urinary diversion utilized has been the ileal conduit. The ileal conduit was introduced by Bricker in 1950 and was thought to be the answer to the problems associated with urinary diversion. It has now been in use long enough to offer an opportunity for objective scrutiny. Although withstanding the test of time fairly well, at least 10 per cent of patients with a previously normal upper urinary tract have demonstrated signs of renal deterioration

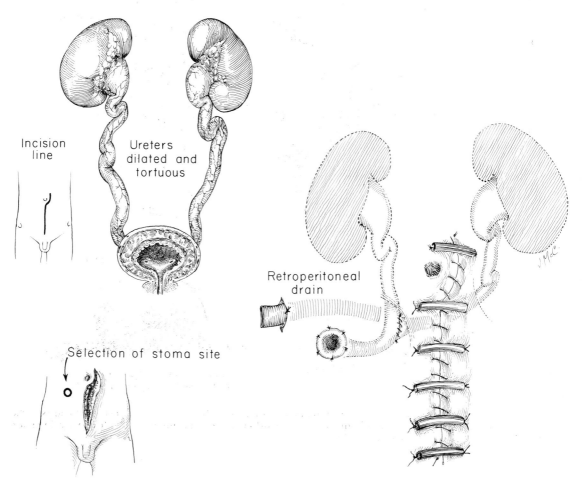

Figure 8–9. Transureteroureterostomy — cutaneous ureterostomy. (From Kelalis, P. P., King, L. R., and Belman, A. B.: Clinical Pediatric Urology, Vol. 1. Philadelphia, W. B. Saunders Co., 1976, p. 446.)

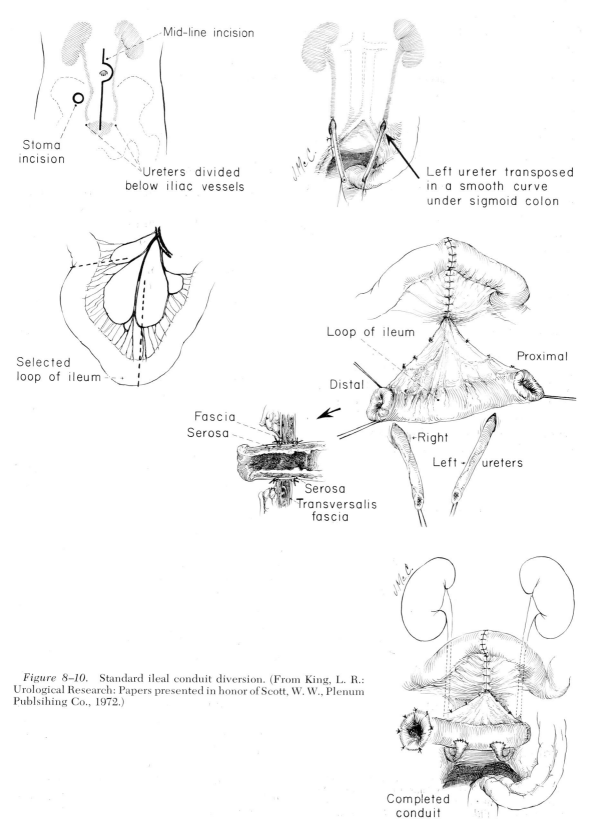

Figure 8–10. Standard ileal conduit diversion. (From King, L. R.: Urological Research: Papers presented in honor of Scott, W. W., Plenum Publsihing Co., 1972.)

(Smith, 1972; Shapiro et al., 1975). This suggests that the ileal conduit may not be the most ideal form of diversion in children who otherwise might be expected to survive for many years.

The procedure involves using an isolated segment of ileum (no longer in continuity with the intestinal tract) to convey urine from the ureters to the skin (Fig. 8–10). The ureters are anastomosed to the isolated ileal segment in an end-to-side fashion. The ileum should serve as a conduit, not as a reservoir, so the term "ileal bladder" is incorrect and "ileal conduit" is more accurate. It has been suggested that reflux of mucus and bacteria in a system that may not drain freely at all times may be responsible for the renal deterioration that has been observed (Kelalis, 1974).

Sigmoid (Colon) Conduit

The colon conduit is similar to the ileal conduit but offers a reliable means of avoiding reflux into the upper urinary tract. It is technically possible to create an antireflux submucosal tunnel in the colon, whereas this is very difficult in the ileum (Fig. 8–11). Another advantage includes a

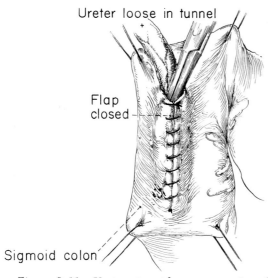

Figure 8–11. Ureterosigmoidostomy; creation of the antireflux ureterosigmoid anastomosis. (From Scott, R. (Ed.): Current Controversies in Urologic Management. Philadelphia, W. B. Saunders Co., 1972.)

larger bowel diameter and, therefore, a wider stoma and a decreased chance for stomal stenosis. The long-term effects on renal function comparing ileal conduit and colon conduit diversion are anxiously awaited.

NONCUTANEOUS URINARY DIVERSION

Ureterosigmoidostomy

Only one form of internal urinary diversion is popular in this country. Ureterosigmoidostomy, the anastomosis of the ureters to the intact colon, is applicable only occasionally in children. Normal bowel control and a nondilated upper urinary tract are prerequisites for this procedure. Therefore, only children with bladder exstrophy and malignancy in which the rectum is neurogenically normal can be considered as candidates for this procedure.

The advantage of ureterosigmoidostomy is obviously that of urinary control by the patient without the necessity for an external appliance. However, total control is achieved only by a few, and many stain when they do not empty the colon frequently. Additionally, electrolyte abnormalities with excessive reabsorption of chloride and urea result in a degree of metabolic acidosis in the majority. Excretion of the excessive chloride requires endogenous potassium, resulting in hypokalemia, which, when severe, may cause weakness. Normal kidney function compensates. However, in those with underlying renal disease, severe electrolyte problems may result. Chronic acidosis may contribute to retarded body growth (Spence, 1966).

The most disturbing consequence of ureterosigmoidostomy is the possibility of carcinoma developing at the site of the ureterointestinal anastomosis anywhere from seven to 46 years after diversion (Shapiro et al., 1979). The true incidence of this occurrence is unknown at this time. Those with this form of diversion should have annual urinary tract radiographs or sigmoidoscopy with visualization of the ureteral orifices to detect early ureterointestinal obstruction. How soon after the surgical procedure this should be instituted is unknown; however, routine evaluation should probably begin 10 to 15 years after diversion.

URINARY UNDIVERSION

Within the past several years, it has been recognized that urinary diversion was carried out in a number of individuals who now would be managed differently. Therefore, a self-limiting pool of patients exist who are candidates for undiversion. The ideal candidates are those in whom bladder function is normal, i.e., boys with posterior urethral valves or those diverted because of difficulty in the management of vesicoureteral reflux. Pioneering efforts in this area have been made primarily by Hendren (1974).

Obviously it becomes necessary first to evaluate the urinary tract in these individuals, paying attention to bladder emptying capability and the renal functional status. In a few patients, undiversion may not meet with success, in which case rediversion may become necessary. However, with proper selection the results have generally been quite satisfactory, in spite of what often becomes very tedious but inventive surgery.

Some centers are advocating urinary undiversion in children with neurogenic disease. Urinary control is then managed by clean intermittent catheterization or, in some instances, by insertion of an artificial sphincter mechanism. This is probably reasonable to consider in selected individuals.

REFERENCES

Bricker, E. M.: Bladder substitution after pelvic evisceration. Surg. Clin. North Am., 30:1511, 1950.

Hendren, W. H.: Urinary tract refunctionalization after prior urinary diversion in children. Ann. Surg., 180:494, 1974.

Kelalis, P. P.: Urinary diversion in children by the sigmoid conduit: Its advantages and limitations. J. Urol., 112:666, 1974.

Lome, L. G., Howat, J. M., and Williams, D. I.: The temporarily defunctionalized bladder in children. J. Urol., 107:469, 1972.

Shapiro, A., Berlatzky, Y., Pfeffermann, R., et al.: Carcinoma of colon after ureterocolic anastomosis. Urology, 13:617, 1979.

Shapiro, S. R., Lebowitz, R., and Colodny, A. H.: Fate of 90 children with ileal conduit urinary diversion a decade later: Analysis of complications, pyelography, renal function and bacteriology. J. Urol., 114:289, 1975.

Smith, E. D.: Followup studies on 150 ileal conduits in children. J. Pediatr. Surg., 7:1, 1972.

Spence, H. M.: Ureterosigmoidostomy for exstrophy of the bladder: Results in a personal series of thirty-one cases. Br. J. Urol., 38:36, 1966.

Chapter Nine

GENITAL ABNORMALITIES IN THE MALE

CLINICAL EMBRYOLOGY

Some understanding of fetal development is helpful when dealing with congenital abnormalities, particularly as it refers to the overall significance of any one particular problem. The purpose of this embryologic introduction is to give practical direction to the clinician faced with a patient with genital abnormalities.

Although wolffian duct development begins extremely early in fetal life with the origin of the pronephros, significant sexual differentiation does not become obvious until five to six weeks of gestation, when the genital tubercle appears and gonadal development begins. Further differentiation is dependent upon the presence or absence of the Y chromosome and its effect on gonadal differentiation. An antigen from the Y chromosome (H–Y antigen) stimulates formation of the testes (Wachtel, 1977). The testes produce androgen, which in turn is responsible for the development of male internal and external genitalia even if multiple X chromosomes are present (such as in Klinefelter's syndrome). On the other hand, in the absence of a Y chromosome, normal female sex development passively occurs because the testes are responsible not only for stimulation of masculine development

through the production of fetal testosterone but also for the regression of the müllerian system. This effect is distinctly ipsilateral. An appreciation of this fact is helpful in understanding many apparent clinical contradictions (Chap. 11). If there is a loss of one X chromosome, there is abnormal gonadal development but recognizable female genital development (XO–Turner's syndrome).

Under normal circumstances, characteristic external genital development progresses after the sixth week. However, the ability to recognize the actual gender of the fetus is delayed until the end of the first trimester, during which time there is phallic growth in the male, development and fusion of the labioscrotal folds, and formation of the urethra from the ventral urethral folds.

ABNORMAL HORMONAL STIMULATION

Increasingly, evidence suggests that stimulation of the male fetus with synthetic progestational agents in the first trimester doubles the risk of hypospadias (Aarskog, 1979). The biochemical basis appears to be an antiandrogenic effect. This is ironic because this same class of drugs also has the capability of masculinizing the female fetus.

Inadequate testosterone stimulation, on the other hand, is probably the underlying cause for all forms of incomplete penile and urethral abnormalities, with the various forms of hypospadias representing a spectrum of hormonal pathologic conditions (Aarskog, 1970; Jones and Scott, 1971). Milder forms of hypospadias are likely the result of early cessation or decrease in fetal testosterone stimulation; more severe forms of incomplete formation of the male genitalia may be the result of abnormal androgen synthesis or its inability to act at the cellular level, both of which can be inherited traits (Wilson et al., 1974). The most severe form of androgen inactivity is represented by the testicular feminization syndrome, in which the phenotype is female although normal intra-abdominal testes are present and no müllerian remnants remain (müllerian inhibiting substance is active). Testosterone is produced and is circulated, but phallic and scrotal development are completely lacking owing to the inability of the end organ to incorporate the hormone into an active cellular stimulant (Chap. 11).

HYPOSPADIAS

As pediatric urologists, one of our most gratifying therapeutic contributions is the ability to repair congenital genital abnormalities. Early recognition of the problem and its emotional overtones and proper direction by the primary physician are all-important initial steps in what might otherwise become a tragic misadventure.

Hypospadias is a common anomaly with an incidence of 8 in every 1000 male births. Fortunately, 87 per cent (7.1 in every 1000 births) are of the mild glanular or coronal variety; the remainder (0.8 per 1000 male births) are more severe. Only 3 per cent are of the penoscrotal type (Sweet et al., 1974). Examination of the genitalia should include assessment of the penis as to its position, size, corporal and preputial development, and meatal position. Evaluation of scrotal development is most opportune in the perinatal period when exogenous (maternal) gonadotropin stimulation has provoked both scrotal and labial hypertrophy. Poor unilateral development suggests ipsilateral failure of testicular descent. When neither testis is descended, the entire scrotum may appear hypoplastic.

Hypospadias should be considered a syndrome with a triad of developmental pathologic manifestations. The term itself refers only to the abnormal meatus (Gr. *hypo*, under, + Gr. *spadon*, a rent). The prepuce is also abnormal with failure of its development ventrally, and the phallus itself often has a ventral curvature accentuated by erection called chordee. Therefore, when describing the problem clinically, it is advisable to refer to both the meatal position and degree of chordee, since these are the two variables. Ventral foreskin development is almost uniformly absent when the glanular urethra fails to form (in epispadias the prepuce fails to form dorsally). One may therefore see glanular or coronal hypospadias without chordee, chordee without hypospadias or with only glanular hypospadias, distal shaft hypospadias with moderate chordee, midshaft hypospadias with severe chordee, or other variations (Fig. 9–1). Communications can be markedly enhanced by referring to these anatomic landmarks rather than "degrees" of hypospadias.

Severity of chordee is oftentimes difficult to assess, primarily because the hooded dorsal prepuce gives an appearance of exaggerated ventral phallic curvature. One should concentrate on an imaginary line drawn along the ventral aspect of the shaft and glans while holding the penis straight by the prepuce. In younger boys it is permissible to stimulate an erection for verification.

Neonatal Evaluation

At the time of initial assessment, the question of circumcision always arises. The rule of thumb should be to withhold circumcision in any child with abnormal genitalia

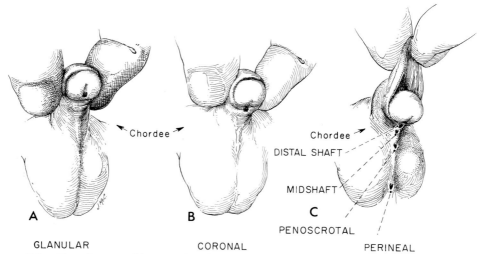

Figure 9–1. Classification of hypospadias based on anatomic location of the urethral meatus. Associated chordee is best described in terms of its severity: mild, moderate, or severe. (From Kelalis, P. P., King, L. R., and Belman, A. B.: Clinical Pediatric Urology, Vol. 1. Philadelphia, W. B. Saunders Co., 1976, p. 577.)

until a surgeon experienced in the repair of genital abnormalities has first had a chance to evaluate the patient. In the milder forms of hypospadias (coronal and glanular) with no chordee, excision of the hooded prepuce may be carried out, although the usual clamp techniques are probably hazardous in these children since ventral skin is lacking, and the risk of urethral damage is increased.

GENETIC EVALUATION

Genetic evaluation for all children with genital abnormalities is probably not justifiable. Buccal smear as a routine certainly cannot be condemned, however, since it is a noninvasive, relatively reliable, inexpensive test. More extensive evaluation in those with penile hypospadias (versus penoscrotal or perineal) and descended testes would also not appear to be indicated unless a familial variant is being considered. Certainly complete evaluation, including karyotyping, is indicated in those in whom the phenotype is truly ambiguous. Additionally, since some of these are inherited problems, genetic counseling is advised for the more complex variants.

Recent data (Bauer et al., 1979) indicate that a sibling of a child with hypospadias has a 14 per cent chance of also having hypospadias. A multifactorial mode of inheritance has been thought to be responsible for uncomplicated hypospadias. Page (1979) cites evidence to suggest that an autosomal dominant sex-limited inheritance may at times be responsible.

ASSOCIATED ABNORMALITIES

As outlined embryologically, completion of development of the male external genitalia occurs relatively late, toward the twelfth fetal week. The most significant step in the development of the urinary tract, on the other hand, is the budding of the ureters from the wolffian duct, an event that takes place somewhere around the fifth week. The question of the necessity for routine radiographic evaluation of the urinary tract is commonly brought up when faced with the child with hypospadias. Most of us have been taught that the presence of one genitourinary abnormality strongly suggests the possibility that others may also exist. If, however, we look at this problem developmentally, reason suggests that routine excretory urography and cystography are not necessary. Cystoscopy is certainly not indicated simply because a child has hypospadias.

Although reports suggest a variety of anomalies of the urinary tract in 5.5 to 33 per cent of those with hypospadias (Neyman and Schirmer, 1965), the true incidence appears to be little different from that in the general population. Additionally, the majority of the abnormalities found, such as renal malrotation, have not been of clinical significance, (Felton, 1959; McArdle and Lebowitz, 1975). Regardless, some authorities continue to suggest that an excretory urogram should be performed in all boys with hypospadias (Fallon et al., 1976).

We would agree that the child with any other objective reason for radiographic evaluation, such as an associated culture-documented urinary tract infection, should have radiographs. In the remainder one might consider an abdominal ultrasound study as a noninvasive, uncomplicated means of assuring the absence of significant renal maldevelopment.

There is, however, a 16 per cent incidence of cryptorchidism and inguinal hernias in boys with hypospadias (Ross et al., 1959). If there is indeed a hormonal etiology to hypospadias, the presence of abnormal testes in some of these boys, manifested by failure of descent, is not surprising.

Chordee

Chordee, as part of the clinical complex of hypospadias, may be the most significant deterrent to normal heterosexual function. The severity of chordee generally relates to the degree of hypospadias. It therefore follows that patients with glanular or coronal hypospadias may have negligible ventral curvature. Overall, clinically significant chordee can be found in 35 per cent of patients with hypospadias (Sweet et al., 1974).

Erectile tissue (corpus spongiosum) surrounds the normal urethra throughout its phallic course. With foreshortened urethral development, rudimentary spongiosum splays dorsolaterally from the hypospadiac meatus, often in the form of thickened fibrous bands. Normal ventral penile expansion associated with growth and exaggerated by tumescence is limited by these bands. Additionally, penile skin is normally flexible with little subcutaneous tissue and no significant attachment to the underlying fascial layers. In the absence of normal urethral development, this flexibility is often lost. There is tethering of the ventral penis by inflexible skin as well as adherence of this skin to the underlying abnormal urethra, that is, the portion deficient in corpus spongiosum. Either or both of these problems may be the underlying cause for chordee, and its correction is an essential precursor to hypospadias repair.

SURGICAL APPROACH TO HYPOSPADIAS AND CHORDEE

Technical advances over the past century, accentuated in the recent decade primarily because of a better understanding of the problem and improved surgical techniques, have led to marked progress in the field. The goal of surgical correction is to construct a functional penis that allows direction of the urinary stream while standing, is straight on erection, and is capable of sufficient depth of penetration for insemination and fertilization if the testes are able to produce normal spermatozoa. All this should be achieved while maintaining a normal-appearing, cosmetically pleasing phallus.

TIMING OF SURGERY

There is no ideal age for genital surgery, although t is preferable to perform the more simple procedures before the age of six months if possible. In some centers, definitive one-stage repairs are being successfully undertaken prior to six months of age. On the other hand, the more complex situation in which formal urethroplasty is required might best be postponed until age three years for the one-stage repair or might be broken into two widely separated procedures if a multistage approach is indicated. According to a report of the Action Committee on Surgery on the Genitalia of Male Children (Section on Urology, American Academy of Pediatrics, 1975), the least desirable time for elective genital surgery is between six months and three years. Nevertheless, there are no studies to support any strong recommendation as to proper age, and, therefore, the advice of the qualified surgeon should be followed.

It is ideal, however, for the family to have the child evaluated as an infant by an appropriately adept surgeon in the field. Questions will arise that can be answered only by that physician, and the timing of surgery may then be worked out. Too often the primary physician, out of lack of information on the subject, will postpone evaluation until the child is "older." The surgeon is then confronted with a prepubertal or already pubertal adolescent with increased psychosexual awareness referable to genital surgery as well as the increased incidence of wound infection in the presence of pubic hair and the risk of suture breakdown from uncontrollable erections.

Since this is not a surgical text, detailed descriptions of procedures will not be presented. However, in the interest of clarity, some diagrams are published to aid in conceptualization of some of the repairs currently in use.

GLANULAR TO CORONAL HYPOSPADIAS WITHOUT CHORDEE

The child with a coronal or glanular meatus, no chordee, and a hooded prepuce basically has a functional penis that is abnormal only in appearance. Once it is definitely established that urethral lengthening is not necessary and that the penis is truly straight, removal of the hooded prepuce and dorsal meatoplasty,* if indicated, can be performed at an early age. Since only the existing dorsal skin is removed, circumcision with a clamp is not recommended, as the ventral tissue overlying the urethra may be extremely thin and the risk of urethral injury may be considerable. A free-hand procedure under anesthesia at about four to six months not only is effective but also allows time to elapse after birth to be sure that more extensive repair is not necessary.

---

*The urethral meatus in boys with hypospadias truly may be small. If that is the case, enlargement of this meatus by incising the outer lip of tissue dorsally is recommended. Cutting back of the urethra (ventrally) exaggerates the hypospadias.

CHORDEE WITHOUT SIGNIFICANT HYPOSPADIAS

The urethral meatus is located in a position adequate for function in the majority of boys with hypospadias. Some of these, however, have chordee sufficient to require correction. An awareness of the relationship between the adherent ventral skin and chordee led Allen and Spence (1968) to demonstrate that freeing of this skin alone without urethral transection would release the chordee in many cases (Fig. 9–2). The dorsal prepuce may then be transposed ventrally to cover the resultant defect. This is a relatively simple procedure usually requiring only a day or two of hospitalization. It usually can be accomplished at six months of age and need not be delayed until three years. Surgical risk is minimal, the only significant complication being inadvertent tearing or transection of the thinned distal urethra.

Horton and Devine (1973) described two additional causes for chordee without hypospadias resulting in tethering of the urethra. In some cases it is possible to straighten chordee without transecting the urethra; however, in many a two-staged operation or a more extensive single-stage reconstructive procedure may be necessary (Fig. 9–3).

REPAIR OF HYPOSPADIAS

The time-honored procedures for the complete reconstruction of the penis involve a multistaged approach. Classically, the first stage is to straighten the penis (release chordee). The hooded prepuce is transposed ventrally to cover the resultant skin defect and to place skin in a position accessible for construction of the urethra, which is generally carried out no earlier than six months later. Various modifications of this type of repair exist; however, the majority incorporate the two important steps illustrated in Figure 9–4.

More recently, several single-stage procedures have been perfected that have added a great deal of flexibility to the approach of these patients. One must keep in

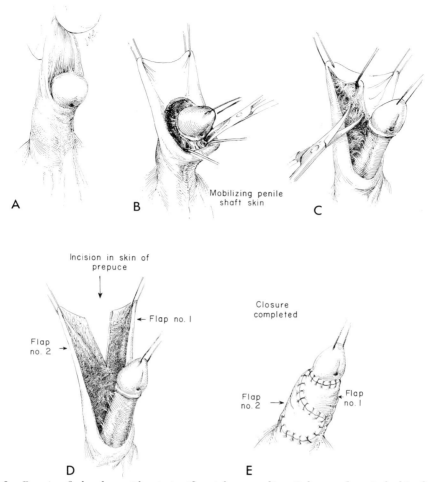

Figure 9–2. Repair of chordee without significant hypospadias. Release of ventral skin frees chordee virtually completely. The ventral skin defect created by the procedure is covered by transposed prepuce. (From Kelalis, P. P., King, L. R., and Belman, A. B.: Clinical Pediatric Urology, Vol. 1. Philadelphia, W. B. Saunders Co., 1976, p. 581.)

mind that when a more severe deformity is corrected by a single-stage technique, the risk of a complication (fistula) may be increased. This is certainly a justifiable risk since, under those circumstances, the second procedure is often quite minimal. Some of the currently popular single-stage procedures are illustrated in Figures 9–5 to 9–8. However, one must be aware that this is a highly individualized art and many other procedures of high quality are not listed.

Meatal Position

Functional positioning of the meatus requires only that it be placed at or distal to the coronal sulcus. More recently, surgical expectations have increased so that successful efforts to place the meatus toward or at the tip of the glans have been quite fruitful. Efforts by Horton and Devine in single-stage repairs (1973) and Smith (1973) in the planned two-staged approach have advanced the art considerably.

Temporary Urinary Diversion

During the acute healing period following urethral construction, most surgeons employ some means of diverting the urine from the newly constructed urethra. The simplest method is to use a form of urethral catheter or stent through the site of repair into the bladder. Many feel that this type of

Text continued on page 172

Step 1.

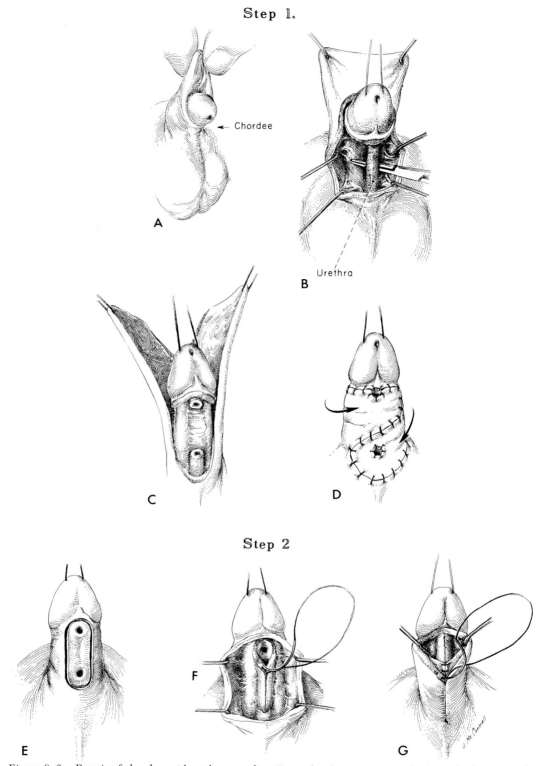

Figure 9–3.   Repair of chordee without hypospadias. Example of a situation in which urethral transection is necessary for complete straightening of the penis. Step 1: the ventral skin defect that results is closed with preputial flaps. Step 2: application of Johanson urethroplasty to close the urethral defect six months after straightening of the chordee. (From Kelalis, P. P., King, L. R., and Belman, A. B.: Clinical Pediatric Urology, Vol. 1. Philadelphia, W. B. Saunders Co., 1976, p. 580.)

1st stage

2nd stage

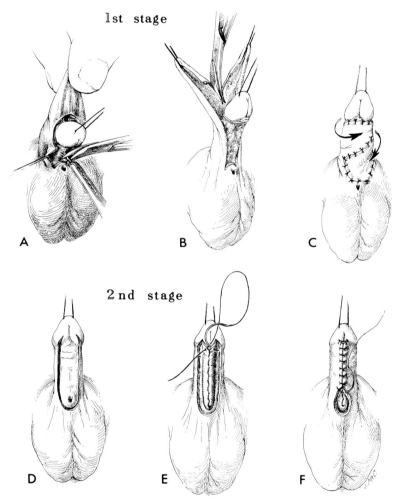

Figure 9–4. Two-stage repair of penoscrotal hypospadias (Byars modification). The ventral skin should be approximated as smoothly as possible to facilitate formation of the urethra at the second stage. After complete resolution of induration, the urethra is formed from the transposed skin. Multiple subcutaneous layers are closed over the new urethra to reduce the incidence of fistulae. (From Kelalis, P. P., King, L. R., and Belman, A. B.: Clinical Pediatric Urology, Vol. 1. Philadelphia, W. B. Saunders Co., 1976, p. 590.)

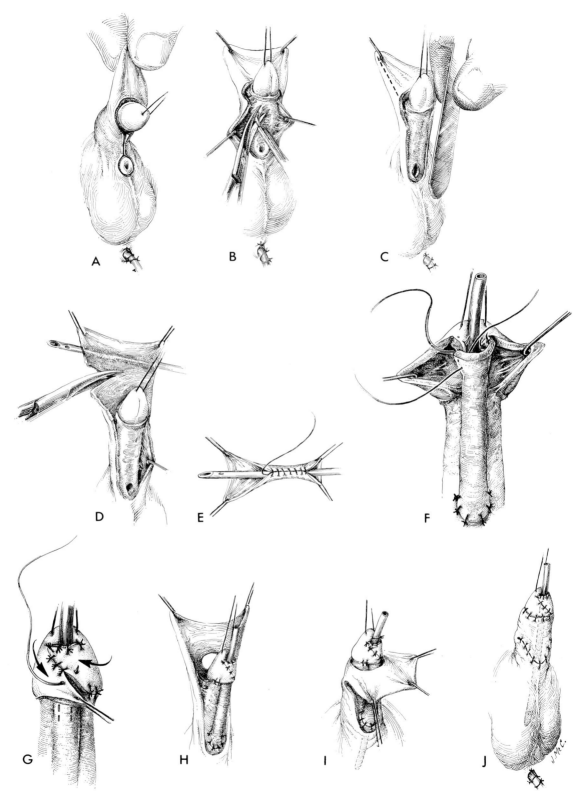

Figure 9–5. Devine and Horton hypospadias repair. Chordee is corrected by excising fibrous bands distal to the hypospadias urethral meatus. A free graft of preputial skin is then used to form the neourethra. Glanular dissection *(F)* allows distal placement of the meatus. The ventral skin defect is covered by transpositioning the remaining foreskin by the buttonhole technique. (From Kelalis, P. P., King, L. R., and Belman, A. B.: Clinical Pediatric Urology, Vol. 1. Philadelphia, W. B. Saunders Co., 1976, pp. 588–589.)

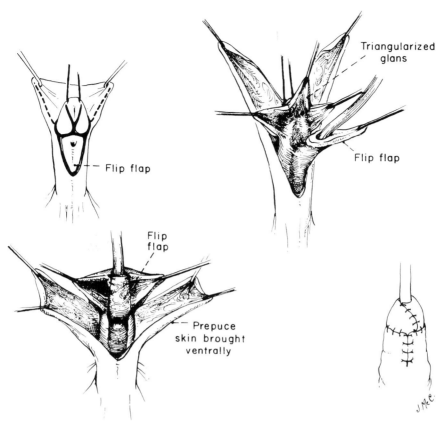

Figure 9–6. Single-stage repair for distal hypospadias resulting in a glanular meatus and straightening of any distal chordee that might exist. (from Harrison, J. H., Gittes, R. F., Perlmutter, A. D., et al.: Campbell's Urology, Vol. 2, 4th ed. Philadelphia, W. B. Saunders Co., 1979, p. 1587.)

Figure 9–7. A single-stage hypospadias repair using a rolled preputial pedicle graft. (From Harrison, J. H., Gittes, R. F., and Perlmutter, A. D., et al.: Campbell's Urology, Vol. 2, 4th ed. Philadelphia, W. B. Saunders Co., 1979, p. 1588.)

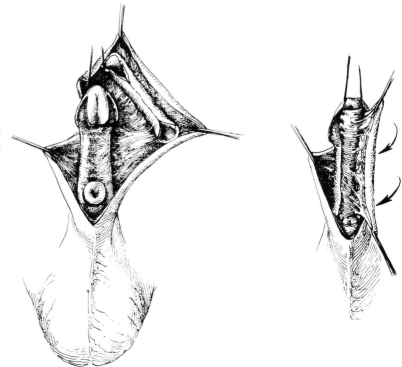

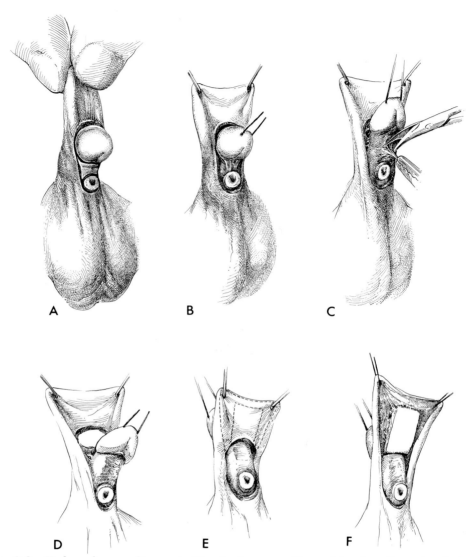

Figure 9–8. Hodgson hypospadias repair. Chordee is corrected by excising deep fibrous bands distal to the hypospadias meatus. Urethra is formed from deep preputial layer transposed ventrally. *E* outlines the lateral cutis, which is removed to isolate the island that is rolled into neourethra. *K* and *L* represent two methods of closing transposed foreskin. Lateral flaps are removed cautiously to avoid devascularization of the remaining prepuce. A subcuticular suture is then used to complete the semicircular closure. Alternatively, a wedge of redundant skin can be removed centrally, and a midline subcuticular closure can be used. (From Kelalis, P. P., King, L. R., and Belman, A. B.: Clinical Pediatric Urology, Vol. 1. Philadelphia, W. B. Saunders Co., 1976, pp. 586–587.)

Illustration continued on opposite page

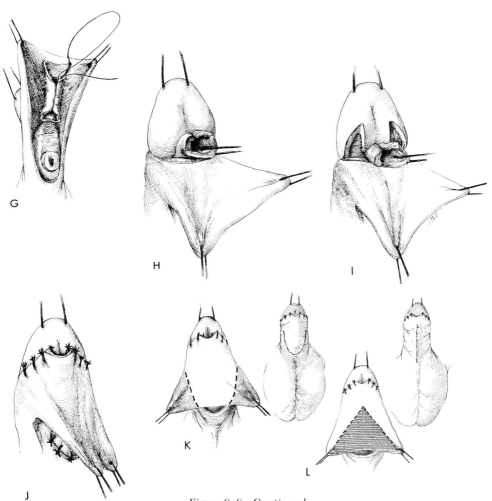

Figure 9–8 *Continued*

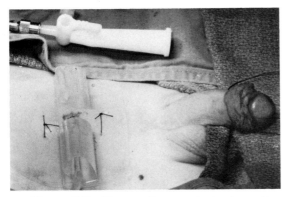

Figure 9–9. Hypospadias repair in immediate postoperative period. Note the plastic drainage tube in the background sutured to the abdomen. This is a form of percutaneous urinary drainage that is effective and easily inserted.

drainage is not adequate and prefer a higher form of diversion. Temporary suprapubic cystostomy is one choice done either formally through an abdominal incision or by insertion of a catheter percutaneously (Fig. 9–9). However, other surgeons prefer insertion of a temporary perineal urethrostomy — a catheter inserted through an opening made in the bulbous urethra which then enters the bladder. In either case, removal of these tubes results in prompt closure of the temporary surgical defect unless there is distal obstruction.

COMPLICATIONS OF HYPOSPADIAS REPAIR

The technical problems associated with hypospadias repair are legion. Occasionally hypospadias cripples result from a multiplicity of poorly planned, poorly executed procedures. However, even in the most experienced hands, the possibility exists for complications. The primary physician must be aware of this risk.

PERSISTENT CHORDEE

It is essential for the penis to be straight prior to urethral construction. The advent of the "artificial erection," produced by injecting sterile saline into the corpora after the application of a tourniquet to the base of the

penis (Fig. 9–10), has resulted in fewer errors in correction of chordee. Failure to correct chordee completely prior to definitive urethroplasty may then result in the necessity for more extensive surgery at a later date to include re-formation of the urethra.

FISTULA

All repairs that entail construction of a urethra are at risk for urethrocutaneous fistulae. The incidence of fistula formation varies from procedure to procedure and surgeon to surgeon. Fortunately, most fistulae are relatively small and require only simple closure (Fig. 9–11).

MEATAL STENOSIS AND URETHRAL STRICTURE

One must be ever aware that fistula formation may be secondary to distal obstruction. Meatal stenosis and urethral stricture formation must both be sought and corrected prior to attempt at fistula closure. Failure to recognize either limits the chances for fistula closure.

Other signs of stenosis or stricture include urinary tract infection, spraying and dribbling of the urinary stream, and severe hesitancy. Simple meatotomy may be the only step required for meatal stenosis, although this can result in some loss of

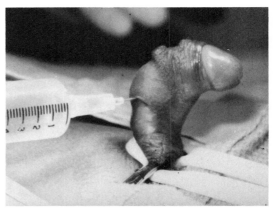

Figure 9–10. Artificial erection demonstrating chordee in a child without hypospadias.

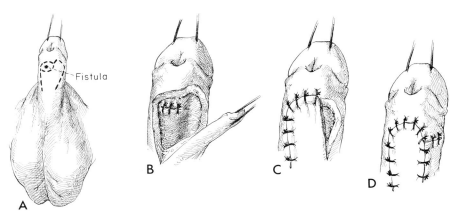

Figure 9–11. A method of closing a urethral fistula. Following closure of the fistula, a pedicle graft of penile skin completely covers the suture lines. This greatly lessens the chance of recurrence. (From Kelalis, P. P., King, L. R., and Belman, A. B.: Clinical Pediatric Urology, Vol. 1. Philadelphia, W. B. Saunders Co., 1976, p. 593.)

urethral length. Stricture formation may necessitate urethral reconstruction, often carried out in two stages but recent experience with transurethral direct vision urethrotomy suggests that the need for some of these secondary operations may be obviated.

URETHRAL DIVERTICULA

Rarely, an acquired diverticulum forms following urethral construction (Fig. 9–12). This is probably the result of infection following repair with formation of an epithelialized cavity in communication with the urethra. However, it might also follow a blowout proximal to distal obstruction (stricture). Excision of the diverticulum with primary urethral reconstruction is recommended.

OTHER URETHRAL ABNORMALITIES

EPISPADIAS

Although isolated epispadias is similar in terms of reparative approach to hypospadias, its pathologic embryologic origins are

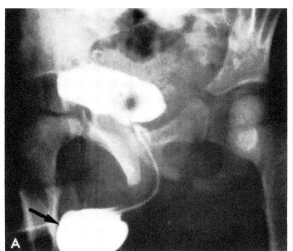
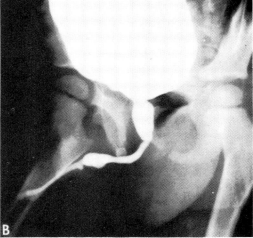

Figure 9–12. A, Large urethral diverticulum (arrow) at the site of the junction of hypospadiac meatus and neourethra. B, Postoperative urethrogram after excisison of diverticulum. (From Kelalis, P. P., King, L. R., and Belman, A. B.: Clinical Pediatric Urology, Vol. 1. Philadelphia, W. B. Saunders Co., 1976, p. 594.)

more closely related to the problem of bladder exstrophy, and it will be discussed in more detail in that section.

URETHRAL DUPLICATION AND ACCESSORY URETHRA

It is not uncommon to see a glanular urethral dimple in a child with hypospadias. In this instance, the true urethral meatus may be missed on examination if special effort is not made to look for it in a more ventral location (Fig. 9–13). Actual urethral duplication is uncommon; those completely extending from the bladder are very rare (Fig. 9–14). When present, urethral duplication may be part of an embryologic attempt at complete duplication of the lower genitourinary tract with a septate or double bladder and even penile duplication. Total urinary incontinence from one of these urethras may occur if it originates outside the normal sphincteric mechanism. Surgical excision of the more abnormal urethra may then be necessary. Voiding cystourethrography is the study best suited for evaluation of this abnormality, although it may be necessary to perform retrograde injections of contrast medium through each orifice to define the anatomy in detail.

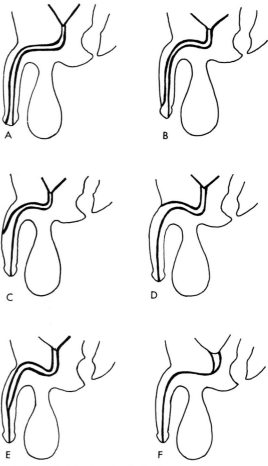

Figure 9–14. Urethral duplication arising from the bladder. *A* to *D* are complete forms. *E* and *F* are incomplete forms. This lesion may be associated with some form of urinary incontinence. (From Gray, S. W., and Skandalakis, J. E.: Embryology for Surgeons. Philadelphia, W. B. Saunders Co., 1972.)

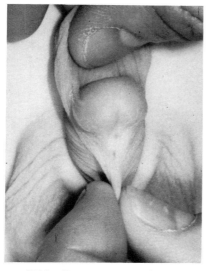

Figure 9–13. Demonstration of the hypospadiac urethral meatus by retraction of the ventral skin. This maneuver will open the meatus allowing its absolute identification, thus distinguishing it from a "dimple."

Most patients with an accessory urethra (Fig. 9–15) require no specific treatment as the finding is often an incidental one and unassociated with symptoms. Infection in a blind-ending tube, particularly in a sexually active male at risk for gonorrhea, is an indication for ablation of this structure. Finally, inability to direct the urinary stream may require excision of one of these tubes or consideration of division of the intervening septum if the urethras are closely apposed to one another. Less severe abnormalities often require only cosmetic repair. It is essential, however, that an unusual-looking but functional penis not be destroyed by an ill-conceived, poorly executed procedure.

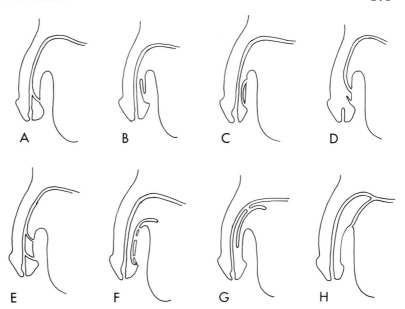

Figure 9–15. Accessory urethra. Urinary symptoms are rare. *G* is more representative of a form of urethral diverticulum than of actual incomplete duplication. (From Gray, S. W., and Skandalakis, J. E.: Embryology for Surgeons. Philadelphia, W. B. Saunders Co., 1972.)

PENILE TORSION

In our experience, congenital twisting of the penis occurs almost always to the patient's left (Fig. 9–16). There are no symptoms other than maldirection of the urinary stream. Although most commonly seen in association with hypospadias, this abnormality may occur independently. It may be associated with incomplete development of

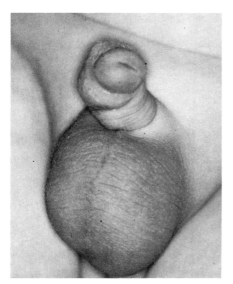

Figure 9–16. Penile torsion. The ventral foreskin is typically incomplete, and the penis twists to the left.

the ventral foreskin even if hypospadias is not involved.

Surgical correction, if necessary, is accomplished with ease by making an encircling subcoronal incision, denuding the penis of its skin to the base. Straightening results from reapproximating the skin in its normal relationship using the raphe as a midline guide. If a mild degree of hypospadias coexists, the tissue layers between the urethra and ventral skin are usually very thin. Unless extreme caution is exercised when performing the ventral dissection, a urethrocutaneous fistula may result.

MICROPHALLUS

Microphallus is often described as simply an abnormally small phallus with little reference to measured size. Hinman (1972) reviewed his clinical experience with 20 cases and stated that the mean penile (stretched?) length in the newborn with microphallus was 0.96 cm vs. 3.75 cm for the normal. For those seen at one year of age, the mean length of those with microphallus was 0.65 cm vs. 4.59 for the normal length. Feldman and Smith (1975) determined that the mean newborn penile length in the stretched state, measuring from the pubic ramus to the tip of the glans, was 3.5 cm with a shaft diameter of 1.1 cm. In their review, the third and 97th percentiles for length were 2.8 cm and 4.2 cm, respectively. It is apparent, then, that there is a great discrepancy in size between the normal phallus and the microphallus. This variance should be recognizable to any observer. Nevertheless, measurement is simple and should be carried out in the questionable situations.

The true microphallus (Fig. 9–17) must be differentiated from the concealed penis (Fig. 9–18) and those held in marked chordee. Palpation is the key to this differentiation, paying particular attention to the development of the paired corporal bodies.

Failure of adequate testosterone stimulation during late fetal development is one of the causes of microphallus. This may be primary in those with anorchia, assuming that fetal testosterone was produced earlier to evoke a male phenotype, or secondary in those with a pituitary-hypothalamic abnormality. Kallman's syndrome (hypogonadotropic hypogonadism and anosmia) is the best example of this.

The important clinical question is whether these children will have sufficient penile growth ultimately to allow sexual function as a male. In those both with and without hypospadias, the ability to respond to testosterone is essential for penile growth. Wilson and colleagues (1974) reviewed related types of familial hypogenitalism in which androgen production is normal but in which there is a genetic resistance to its action at the cellular level. These are variants of the testicular feminization syndrome. Although this class of abnormality is rare in the newborn period, it becomes essential to determine that the boy with a small phallus has the potential to respond to testosterone and that significant penile growth can be anticipated at puberty (Klugo and Cerny, 1978). Testosterone cream (2.5 to 5 per cent) applied locally to the penis two or three times daily should demonstrate within three weeks whether a response is forthcoming. Systemic depotestosterone has also been successfully employed (Burstein et al., 1979) and may be more reliable. Permanent side effects are not a threat with short-term treatment.

Potential penile growth is probably limited even in those children with an abnormally small penis that does respond to testosterone. Prepubertal treatment apparently borrows from future growth potential. Although it is highly desirable psychologically for the penis to be more normal in size in childhood, it is not known whether

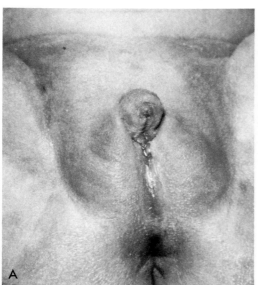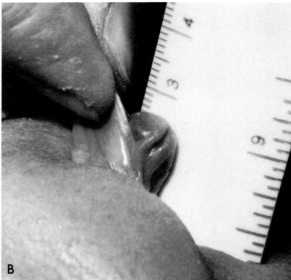

Figure 9–17. A, Genetic male born with ambiguous genitalia. B, The stretched length of the phallus measures less than 2.8 cm.

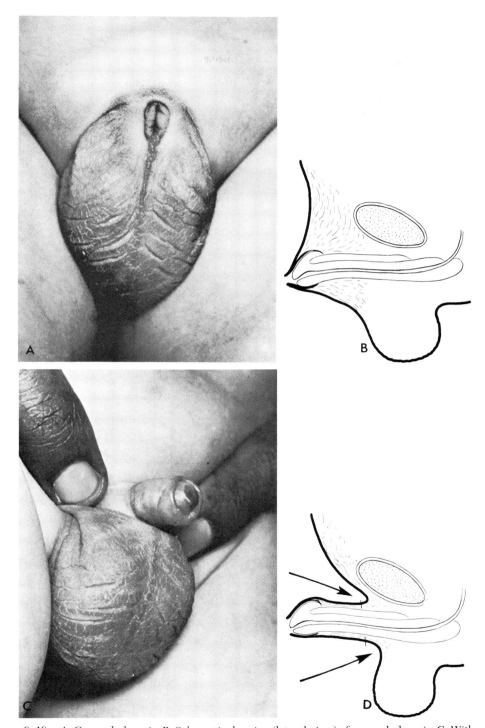

Figure 9–18. A, Concealed penis. B, Schematic drawing (lateral view) of concealed penis. C, With compression of the pubic fat pad and retraction of the foreskin, a normal penis is visualized. D, Schematic drawing of C. (From Eckstein, H. B., Hohenfellner, R., and Williams, D. I.: Surgical Pediatric Urology. Philadelphia, W. B. Saunders Co., 1977, p. 409.)

treatment affects the ultimate size at maturity. The underlying question, which may not be answerable in advance, is whether a particular child will ever have sexual functional capability.

Hinman (1972) elected to raise all his patients with microphallus as males. Our approach would be to determine first, on examination, if corpora are present. In the absence of significant corporal tissue, sex reassignment should be seriously considered. The approach to those who do have a growth response to testosterone is not clearcut, and each case must be carefully individualized. There is no single correct answer. If possible, this decision should be made before the child is sent home from the newborn nursery.

PENILE AGENESIS

Complete absence of the penis is a rare abnormality related undoubtedly to complete failure of development of the genital tubercle. The presence of a fully formed normal scrotum with or without descended testes suggests the separate embryogenesis of these structures (Fig. 9–19). The urethra may open into the perineum or the most distal part of the rectum, under which circumstance voiding occurs initially into the large bowel (Fig. 9–20). The importance of

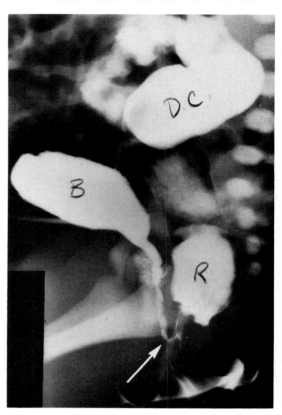

Figure 9–20. Urethrorectal communication (arrow) in the child with penile agenesis. Percutaneous cystogram demonstrates bladder (B), filling of urethra and rectum (R), and descending colon (D.C.). Note filling of the prostatic ducts just below the bladder neck.

early sex conversion to female with plans for formation of appropriate sexual structures in all these unfortunate babies (Fig. 9–21) cannot be overstressed.

DUPLICATION OF THE PENIS

Both penis and clitoris develop from the genital tubercle, which forms a mound in the midline between the cloacal plate and allantois. Actual sexual differentiation of this structure does not begin until about eight weeks of fetal life, and recognizable sexuality is not apparent until the third month.

Duplication of the penis may be complete or incomplete. Two forms exist, the less common being complete duplication of the phallus, in which paired corpora and

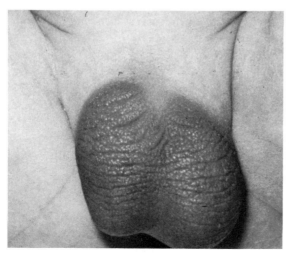

Figure 9–19. Complete penile agenesis in an otherwise normal male. The scrotum is fused, and the testes are normal and descended bilaterally.

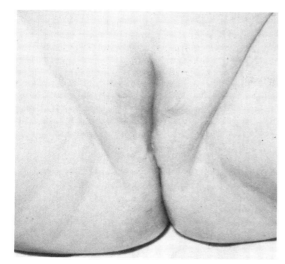

Figure 9–21. Results of genital reconstruction in the child in Figure 9–19 following castration and labial reconstruction.

separate glans exist entirely independently. Separate urethras lead to paired bladders, either or both of which may be functional (Fig. 9–22). These separate penes may be found in either a horizontal or vertical rela-

tionship and do not necessarily reside side by side. Since this is obviously an early developmental abnormality, multiple congenital anomalies are the rule, and complete evaluation of not only the urinary tract but also other organ systems is recommended.

More common but still extremely rare is the bifid penis. A spectrum of developmental pathologic processes exists in this problem, including an attempt at duplication of the glans in which a cleft may exist, duplication of the glans (Fig. 9–23), separation of the individual corpora, or completely separate single corporal bodies. The latter finding is the rule in both males and females with cloacal exstrophy (Fig. 9–24) and in girls with epispadias.

Treatment of penile duplication must be individualized and most often plays a less important role than management of the more life-threatening associated anomalies. However, early assignment of gender of rearing is paramount. In boys with cloacal exstrophy, for example, it is generally un-

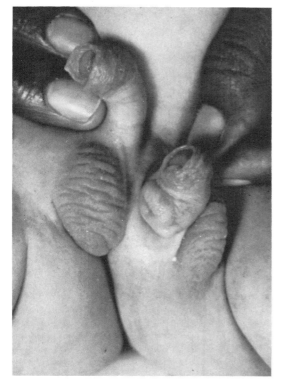

Figure 9–22. Complete diphallia. (Courtesy of Dr. Roy Witherington.) (From Kelalis, P. P., King, L. R., and Belman, A. B.: Clinical Pediatric Urology, Vol. 2. Philadelphia, W. B. Saunders Co., 1976, p. 641.)

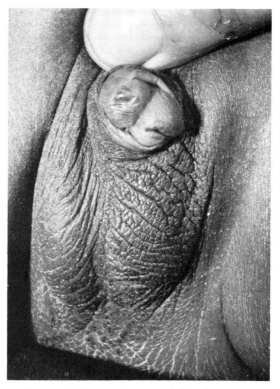

Figure 9–23. Duplication of the glans in a two-year-old boy. (From Kossow, J. H., and Morales, P. A.: Duplication of bladder and urethra and associated anomalies. Urology, *1*:71–73, 1973, by permission.)

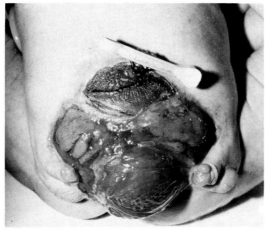

Figure 9–24. Cloacal exstrophy in a newborn boy. Note the lower midline colonic mucosa separating the two halves of the bladder mucosa (upper lateral aspect) and omphalocele. The bifid phallus and scrotum are far apart. (From Belman, A. B.: Imperforate anus and urogenital anomalies. *In* Glenn, J. F. (Ed.): Urologic Surgery, 2nd ed. New York, Harper and Row, 1975.)

reasonable to attempt penile reconstruction since normal sexual function is unlikely.

THE FORESKIN

The prepuce forms initially as a roll of epithelium at the coronal sulcus that fuses ventrally. The frenulum is the hallmark of this fusion. Failure of urethral development restricts foreskin formation; witness the absence of ventral foreskin in hypospadias and dorsal foreskin in epispadias.

Although the prepuce is formed distinctly separately from the glans, as it grows to cover the glans the two opposing epithelial surfaces fuse to separate gradually later. Almost no males have retractile foreskins at birth. Desquamated epithelial cells build up between the two layers in the intervening period and can be seen as accumulations of white pearls, often labeled as smegma. As the layers separate, these deposits are shed naturally (Fig. 9–25).

A point of confusion exists in terminology when one lumps the nonretractile foreskin and true phimosis into the same category. In Denmark, in a series of 9545 boys ages six to 17, Øster (1968) noted that one third of the total had some degree of failure of complete separation of the layers, whereas only 4 per cent had true phimosis. In those ages six to seven, 63 per cent had foreskins that were not entirely retractile. The foreskin in the newborn is not designed to retract. Not only is it fused to the glans but, in addition, the orifice of the foreskin has not gradually been stretched to fit over the glans. Forcible retraction, a practice common in this country, produces small tears. The inflammation that results when these are in contact with urine lead to scarring of this orifice.

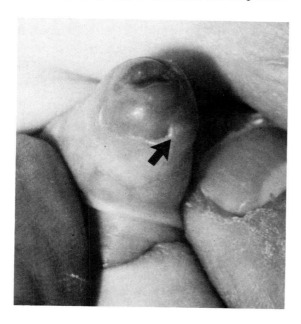

Figure 9–25. Accumulation of "pearls" under the foreskin of a normal uncircumcised European boy. Note that the foreskin remains adherent to the glans and cannot be completely retracted. This is a normal phenomenon and should not be categorized as phimosis.

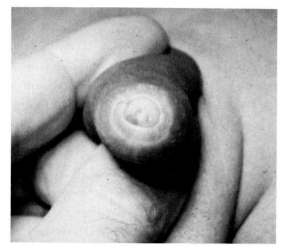

Figure 9–26. Phimotic scar in a boy in whom the foreskin has been forcibly retracted. Circumcision then becomes necessary.

PHIMOSIS

Phimosis is the inability to retract the foreskin because of an acquired circumferential cicatrix actually too small to admit the glans (Fig. 9–26). This is often the result of early forced retraction. The compulsion Americans have for the uncovered glans has provoked a self-fulfilling prophecy:

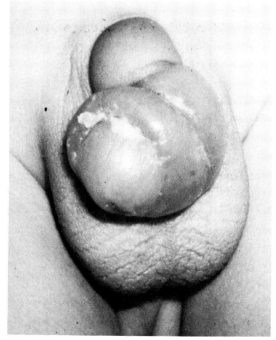

Figure 9–27. Paraphimosis of 24 hours' duration.

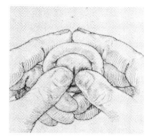

Figure 9–28. Manual decompression of paraphimosis by expressing the glans into the foreskin. (From Campbell, M. F.: Clinical Pediatric Urology. Philadelphia, W. B. Saunders Co., 1951.)

Those children who are not circumcised have their foreskins forcibly retracted, producing tears, leading to phimosis, requiring circumcision.

PARAPHIMOSIS

In paraphimosis, the same basic underlying pathologic process exists, but the phimotic ring has been brought proximal to the corona and cannot readily be returned to its normal position because of secondary distal edema (Fig. 9–27). Manual reduction of paraphimosis can be accomplished in essentially all patients seen within 24 hours. Persistent pressure must be applied to the glans for reduction (Fig. 9–28). This can be facilitated by the injection of local anesthetic (without epinephrine) at the penile base. If reduction is impossible, a dorsal slit interrupting the circumferential band, preferably under general anesthesia, is required (Fig. 9–29). In either case, circumcision is recommended when inflammation has resolved. Unfortunately, paraphimosis often follows a child's visit to his doctor.

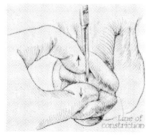

Figure 9–29. Dorsal slit — incision of the constricting phimotic band. (From Campbell, M. F.: Clinical Pediatric Urology. Philadelphia, W. B. Saunders Co., 1951.)

Forcible retraction of the foreskin with failure to return it to its normal position is a misguided cause for this problem.

CIRCUMCISION

The ritual of circumcision predates biblical history. One of its likely origins was the sanctification of the organ of reproduction to a deity. The Judaic custom dates to the time of the Patriarch Abraham over 4000 years ago. Other possibilities include the concept of a tribal mark or as a step toward marriage, particularly in those groups performing circumcision after puberty but prior to sexual activity (Hastings, 1911). The often referred to consideration of improved hygiene probably played no role in the initiation of this custom.

Circumcision today is carried out for a multitude of reasons not apparently related to its historical origins. The medical indications rest on the prevention of both carcinoma of the penis and phimosis. The incidence of carcinoma of the penis appears to be related to poor hygiene. Proper cleansing in the uncircumcised male requires retraction of the foreskin. As noted by Øster, in many boys retraction of the foreskin often is not possible, even as late as age 17.

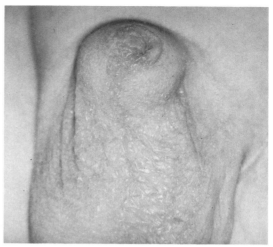

Figure 9–30. Complication of circumcision. The glans has retracted beneath the residual foreskin to which it has adhered.

This would seem to suggest that routine newborn circumcision should be strongly advocated. However, it is apparent from the low incidence of penile carcinoma in Western Europe, where forcible retraction of the foreskin is not advocated but where hygiene is stressed, that this delay is of little consequence. Objectivity appears to be lacking on the subject (Preston, 1970), and the indications are probably only cosmetic. For further discussion, the interested reader is referred to the monograph by Kaplan (1977b).

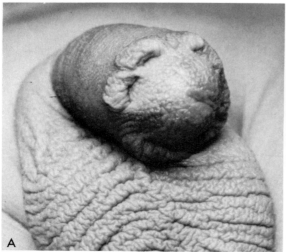 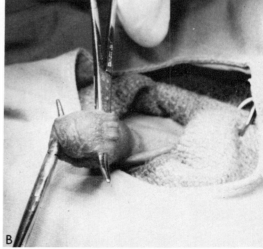

Figure 9–31. A, Adherent skin bands between residual foreskin and glans. B, Hemostat under the ridges of fibrous skin bands. These require incision to separate.

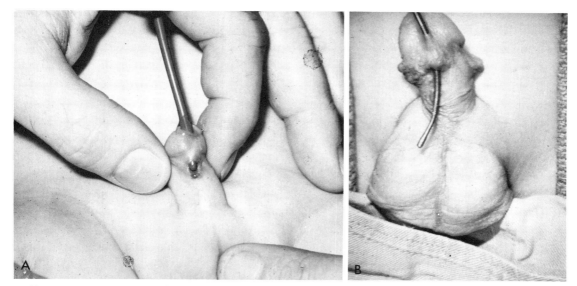

Figure 9–32. Two examples of urethrocutaneous fistulae secondary to circumcision. The meatus in *B* is slightly hypospadiac, suggesting that ventral foreskin was absent. Routine clamp circumcisions have a higher risk for fistula formation in this situation.

COMPLICATIONS OF CIRCUMCISION

In a review of 5882 neonatal circumcisions, the incidence of complications was 0.2 per cent (Gee and Ansell, 1976). None of these were major. Wound infection occurred more often in those using the Plastibell* device as compared to the Gomco clamp.

More serious complications requiring surgical repair do occur in spite of this report and are seen not infrequently at pediatric urologic centers. A common and most disconcerting complication is adherence of a sleeve of skin to the glans. The initial appearance suggests absence of the glans (Fig. 9–30). The underlying cause is inadequate removal of skin, which then rides over the glans as a sleeve. The subcutaneous tissue of this sleeve is adjacent to the glanular epithelium which has been made raw by forcible disruption of the normal adhering layers. Healing together of these two surfaces results in dense scarring, which, in its most extreme form, requires sharp dissection for separation, leaving a mutilated, pocked glans. Less severe degrees of the same problem are seen as individual dense fibrous bands between subcoronal skin and the glans itself (Fig. 9–31). These also require sharp dissection for separation.

An even more difficult complication therapeutically is a urethrocutaneous fistula secondary to removal of excessive ventral tissue. The fistula is generally found at the level of the coronal sulcus, where little flexible tissue is available for ease of repair (Fig. 9–32).

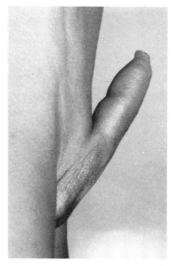

Figure 9–33. Priapism in a child with sickle cell disease.

*Hollister, Inc., Chicago, IL.

PRIAPISM

Persistent penile erection is uncommon in childhood. When it occurs, an underlying pathologic condition leading to an increased coagulative state is invariably present. The idiopathic variety of priapism frequently related to sexual excess or with no known cause is unusual in children.

PRIAPISM WITH SICKLE CELL ANEMIA

The most commonly noted underlying cause for priapism in boys is sickle cell disease. The child, usually five to 13 years of age, awakens with a persistant, painful erection and often is unable to void (Fig. 9–33). Contrary to expectations, few have active sickle cell crisis or intercurrent infection at the time of presentation.

Sludging of irreversibly sickled erythrocytes in the paired penile corpora is responsible, leading to a pernicious cycle, with sludging, less oxygenation, more sickling, and so on. The usual conservative treatment regimens of ice packs, anticoagulation, caudal anesthesia, hot enemas, intravenous ketamine, or irrigation are not directed at the underlying cause and so are not usually effective. Theoretically, ice packs may contribute to a decrease in blood flow and may exacerbate the condition.

Treatment of Priapism Secondary to Sickle Cell Disease

Often children with priapism associated with sickle cell disease will have spontaneous resolution of the problem. Many give a history of one or more episodes abating spontaneously prior to the sustained erection that prompted the seeking of medical care.

When the erection persists, an effective approach has been rapid hypertransfusion of normal red blood cells to reduce sludging (Seeler, 1973). Reports in the older literature discrediting this approach were proba-

bly the results of inadequate treatment using either whole blood or smaller volumes of red cells than required. The amount of blood to be given is the amount that will double the hemoglobin according to the formula below.

The transfusion is given over as short a period as can be tolerated without causing cardiovascular overload. The infused, more normal cells carry oxygen to the sequestered area, reducing sickling and sludging. When successful, discomfort disappears by 24 hours after the child's hemoglobin concentration has been doubled, and penile softening follows by three days. Since a clotting disorder is not the underlying problem, use of anticoagulants is not recommended. With no treatment, resolution of priapism can be expected in eight to 13 days (Sousa et al., 1962). Normal erectile ability can be anticipated in those in whom a surgical procedure was not deemed necessary.

Surgical Treatment

Shunting procedures using the saphenous veins were the first means of accomplishing alternate drainage (Grayhack et al., 1964). When it was recognized that the corpus spongiosum was not involved, side-to-side shunts between the spongiosum and paired penile corpora were found to be equally effective and less complicated (Garrett and Rhamy, 1966). Recently the same result has been found to be even more easily accomplished by the percutaneous removal of the fibrous interface between the corpora and the glans by means of a biopsy needle (Winter, 1976). The cutaneous defect produced in the glans is then sutured to control bleeding. Although we continue to recommend surgical intervention in the otherwise nonresponsive cases, our own success in these with sickle cell disease has been disappointing in the majority, although improvement if not resolution of the priapism, has been noted. When an invasive

$$\frac{\text{Volume of packed cells required (ml)}}{} = \frac{\text{Patient's hematocrit } (\%) \times \text{patient's blood volume (ml)}}{\text{Hematocrit } (\%) \text{ of packed cells}^*}$$

---

*Packed cell hematocrit is generally 75 to 85 per cent.

approach is elected, it should not be delayed beyond 24 hours. Permanent fibrosis of the erectile tissue may otherwise prevent the ability to have normal erections in the future.

PRIAPISM AND LEUKEMIA

Leukemia is an even less common cause of priapism in childhood. However, when it occurs, the chronic granulocytic type with its extremely high white blood cell count is to be anticipated. Sludging of large numbers of white cells in the penile venous outflow tract as well as in the corpora themselves is the most tenable explanation.

Treatment of Priapism Secondary to Leukemia

The obvious approach to this problem is to attack the primary underlying cause. Aggressive combined chemotherapy in association with local radiation therapy is recommended. Resolution of the priapism generally coincides with reduction of the leukocytosis. Neither surgical intervention nor anticoagulation is recommended since the risk of infection or bleeding in these patients is high.

TRAUMA

Trauma is the least frequently encountered cause of priapism in children. If a severe perineal straddle injury is associated with priapism, confirmation of urethral integrity by retrograde urethrography is mandatory prior to any therapeutic endeavors to resolve the priapism. After first exhausting conservative treatment, including simple insertion of an indwelling catheter, it may be necessary surgically to establish alternate means of venous drainage from the paired corpora.

OTHER CAUSES

Wilson and colleagues (1973) reported two patients with angiokeratoma corporis diffusum (Fabry's disease) and priapism. Fabry's disease is a glycosphingolipoid li-

posis caused by a defect of the enzyme ceramide trihexosidase. Patients with this defect are known to improve when a plasma transfusion temporarily replaces the missing enzyme. Plasma transfusion as an approach in the patient who has priapism and Fabry's disease may be a therapeutic consideration. Since lipoid infiltration is present in the kidneys, one should be suspicious of this rare abnormality in the patient with priapism and renal insufficiency.

TRANSPOSITION OF THE PENIS AND SCROTUM

Abnormal positioning of the genital tubercle in relationship to the scrotal folds is the likely embryologic explanation for penoscrotal transposition (Fig. 9–34). Phallic development is variable, and meatal position and formation of the urethra are not predictable. The complete variety of this abnormality (Fig. 9–35) is far less common than milder forms, which are frequently seen with hypospadias. In either situation, functional repair would depend upon the presence of corporal tissue and the ability to direct the penis to a position above the scrotum and in normal relationship to the symphysis pubis. Inadequate phallic size and inability to position the penis normally are the potential problems. In the more severe cases, sexual reassignment at birth is the best overall choice with emasculation and formation of a vagina at a later time.

The less severe forms can be corrected by circumferentially freeing the base of the penis and transposing it to a higher position. The dislocated scrotal skin is then used to cover the ventral defect created (Glenn and Anderson, 1973).

CONDYLOMA ACUMINATUM (VENEREAL WARTS)

Wart-like growths on the foreskin or in the area of the urethral meatus rarely occur in children (Fig. 9–36). Condyloma acuminatum is caused by a virus that is also respon-

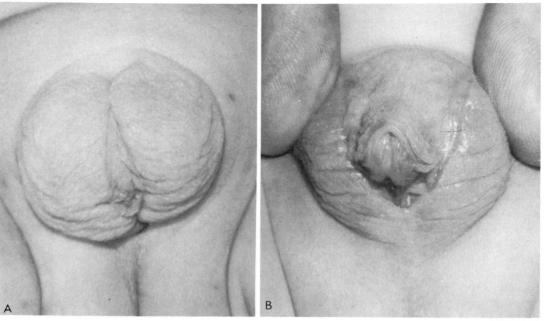

Figure 9–34. *A*, Moderately severe penoscrotal transposition in a boy with hypospadias *(B)*. (From Kelalis, P. P., King, L. R., and Belman, A. B.: Clinical Pediatric Urology, Vol. 2. Philadelphia, W. B. Saunders Co., 1976, p. 644.)

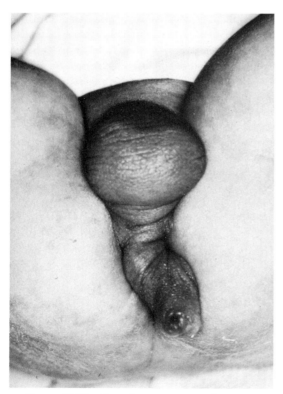

sible for verruca vulgaris and verruca plana (Bofverstedt, 1967). It prefers moist areas (meatus, foreskin). The mode of transmission in children is not known.

Treatment in children should probably be confined to circumcision or fulguration. Podophyllum and 5-fluorouracil have also been used in adults (Nickel and Plumb, 1979).

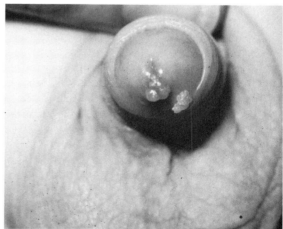

Figure 9–35. Complete penoscrotal transposition. This child has had severe bilateral renal dysplasia and did not survive.

Figure 9–36. Condyloma acuminatum of unknown etiology involving both the meatus and glanular surface.

ABNORMALITIES OF THE TESTES AND SCROTAL CONTENTS

Cryptorchidism

The term cryptorchidism derives from the Greek roots *crypto*, meaning hidden, and *orchio*, pertaining to the testis. This seems to be an appropriately general term since a variety of underlying pathologic states may exist when a testis is not found in its normal scrotal position (Fig. 9–37).

Retractility based on an active cremasteric reflex is probably the most common cause for initial inability to palpate a testis. This reflex is absent during the first few months of life; however, it becomes a normal phenomenon present until puberty requiring no specific treatment. Careful exam-

ination will aid in its recognition. With the patient supine, preferably in the frog-leg position or with the legs separated, the inguinal area should be gently ballotted with the palmar aspect of the fingers. The testis is felt as a mobile, rounded elevation. The testis is then trapped at this level by exerting pressure superior to the gonad. By working the examining fingers down toward the scrotum, the retractile testis can be coaxed into the scrotum and secured with the fingers of the other hand. Another trick is to have the child sit in the tailor position or cross-legged. Retractile testes often can be located or more easily manipulated into the scrotum in this position. If the testis can be manipulated well into the scrotum, there is no need for surgical fixation; it will come down and stay down at or before puberty. If a palpable gonad cannot be manipulated completely into the scrotum, this is then an ectopic testis. Occasionally even after the most thorough examination, a child will be noted to have a testis that can easily be manipulated into the scrotum after induction of anesthesia at the time of planned orchidopexy.

Ectopic testes are generally in the inguinal area but cannot be milked into the scrotum because there is an abnormal attachment of the gubernaculum. Most often this attachment is to the pubic tubercle with the testis being located between the fascia of the external oblique muscle and the fascia of the anterior abdominal wall. Other abnormal areas in which ectopic testes can be found include the perineum (Fig. 9–38), thigh, or, even more rarely, subcutaneously along the penile shaft. Ectopic testes have little chance of descending into their normal scrotal position in view of this abnormal fixation.

Undescended testes (intra-abdominal) are often not palpable or if they are felt along the inguinal canal, tend to readily slip back intraperitoneally. They cannot be manipulated into the scrotum. Although failure of descent may be due to mechanical obstruction along the pathway of descent, it is more likely of hormonal origin (Villee, 1969). Inadequate testosterone production as the result of an intrinsic testicular defect

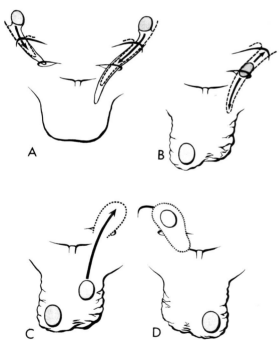

Figure 9–37. Failure of testicular descent. *A*, The intra-abdominal testis. The right side shows no descent; the left side depicts an elongation of the gubernaculum with a long patent processus vaginalis. In either case the testis may enter the canal. *B*, The canalicular, emergent testis with its range of movement. *C*, The high scrotal testis that easily retracts into the superficial inguinal pouch. *D*, The ectopic testis held in the closed superficial inguinal pouch. (From Harrison, J. H., Gittes, R. F., Perlmutter, A. D., et al.: Campbell's Urology, Vol. 2, 4th ed. Philadelphia, W. B. Saunders Co., 1979, p. 1554.)

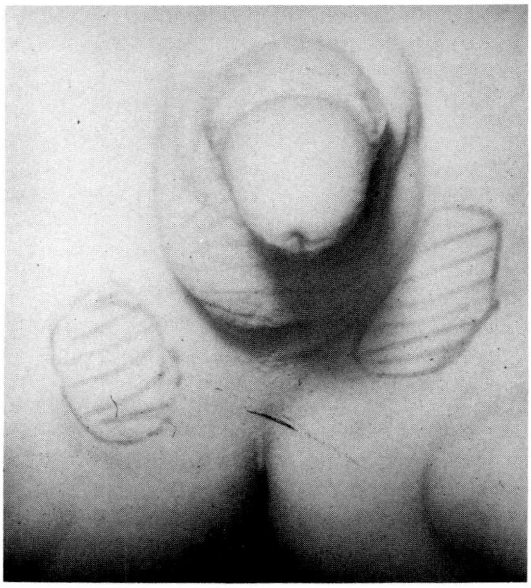

Figure 9–38. Two-and-one-half-year-old boy referred with nonpalpable undescended testis. On careful examination, the testes were evident lateral to the scrotum in a perineal location. Note the small scrotal size.

or as an expression of an extrinsic endocrine abnormality interfering with testicular stimulation (hypothalamic-pituitary-gonadal axis) may be responsible.

There is no question of the adverse effect on otherwise normal testes remaining in the extrascrotal position. The age at which these changes become permanent is controversial. Generally there is agreement that fibrosis as noted on light microscopy is evident after five years of age. More detailed histologic evaluation, including counting of spermatogonia and numbers of seminiferous tubules seen per microscopic field, suggests significant changes at age two (Hedinger, 1977). Electron microscopic evaluation demonstrates an increased collagen fiber zone at age two years (Hadziselimovic and Herzog, 1977), and basement membrane changes have been appreciated as early as six months (Minninberg, 1980).

Based on this knowledge, our clinical approach is to recommend orchidopexy at no later than two years of age in those who have ectopic testes (Hadziselimovic, et al., 1975). A trial of gonadotropin is attempted at the same age in those with nonpalpable or inguinal testes with surgical fixation of the testis in the scrotum in the nonresponders.

Retractile testes require no operative or hormonal therapy.

EXOGENOUS HORMONAL STIMULATION (GONADOTROPIN)

Frequently there is some difficulty in differentiating retractile testes from undescended testes. Exogenous hormonal stimulation in the form of human chorionic gonadotropin may be helpful in determining which testis will ultimately descend and which requires surgery. Additionally, those testes that have not descended because of failure of adequate maternal gonadotropin stimulation may benefit from hormonal stimulation. Human chorionic gonadotropin (HCG) stimulates testosterone secretion and has been noted to produce testicular descent effectively in 15 to 40 per cent of cases (Ehrlich et al., 1969). We use gonadotropin to differentiate the testis that has no chance of descending at puberty from that which is most likely to descend. A dose of 100 IU per lb per week divided into three separate injections (on Mondays, Wednesdays, and Fridays) is given for three weeks. As anticipated, the likelihood of a successful response to gonadotropins is increased in those with bilateral undescended testes (Bierich, 1977) and in those with a primary hypothalamic-pituitary pathologic condition (Prader-Willi syndrome).

The family and the older patient himself should be forewarned that since the response to gonadotropin stimulation is the production of endogenous testosterone, an increase in penile erections along with some minimal growth of the phallus and pubic hair should be anticipated. Masturbatory activity will also temporarily increase. These changes revert to normal upon cessation of hormonal stimulation, although there may be some residual pubic hair present. If shaved these will not generally grow back.

It is not our practice to operate on those patients whose testes descend following hormonal stimulation. Occasionally, however, these testes again retract following withdrawal of the hormone. If these cannot then be seen to spend a significant amount of time in the scrotum, consideration should be given to surgical fixation.

GENITOURINARY ABNORMALITIES ASSOCIATED WITH CRYPTORCHIDISM

One should not expect to find an increased incidence of urinary tract abnormalities in boys with undescended testes since failure of testicular descent is either mechanical or hormonal. Routine radiographic survey of the urinary tract, therefore, is not indicated (Donahue et al., 1973) except in those rare instances in which a vas deferens and epididymis are not found at the time of orchidopexy. The relationship between the wolffian duct and the ureteral bud suggests that failure of formation of the wolffian duct (the precursor of the vas deferens and ureteral bud) will lead to ipsilateral renal agenesis. There is a recognized association between hypospadias and undescended testes (probably on a hormonal basis), however.

TESTICULAR MALIGNANCY IN UNDESCENDED TESTES

The incidence of testis tumors in any segment of the population is small; however, men with a history of an undescended testis are about 35 times more likely to develop a testicular tumor than the remainder of the population. It is unclear as to whether malignant degeneration is a response to the increased environmental temperature alone or if the underlying defect is an intrinsic one. Martin (1979) and Altman and Malament (1967) suggest that early orchidopexy may reverse this tendency. Data to support this are not yet available. In any event, the scrotal position is preferable not only for psychological reasons and for its possible prevention of malignancy but also for the opportunity to periodically palpate the testis that is at increased risk for malignancy.

FERTILITY

The data regarding fertility in boys with undescended testes are very unsatisfactory. Unquestionably, those with bilateral intra-abdominal testes are infertile if uncorrect-ed. However, it is not known if early orchidopexy changes their chances or how a unilateral intra-abdominal undescended testis affects fertility.

Knorr and colleagues (1977) reported the fertility rates in boys with unilateral and bilateral undescended testes treated with gonadotropin alone and with gonadotropin plus surgery (Table 9–1). It is clear that sperm counts are reduced in all groups. However, none were treated before seven years of age. Lipschultz and coworkers (1978) have demonstrated decreased fertility in men with unilateral undescended testes even in the presence of prophylactic orchidopexy. Again, however, the results of early surgery are awaited.

Truly retractile testes, on the other hand, have no apparent negative effect upon fertility. Puri and Nixon (1977) reported on 164 boys with bilateral retractile testes. Fertility in those who were contacted was no different than the rate in the general population.

TESTICULAR ABSENCE VS. CRYPTORCHIDISM

It is common to either find a testis or evidence of a testis having been previously present (a small fibrotic remnant) in the child with a nonpalpable gonad. Primary testicular agenesis is rare. Theoretically, complete failure of development of the genital ridge and mesonephros results in ipsilateral gonadal and renal agenesis. This has led to the suggestion that when a testis is not palpable, an excretory urogram must be carried out. The conclusion that follows is that testicular exploration is not then necessary if the ipsilateral kidney is absent. It would seem that both unilateral renal agenesis (1:552) and unilateral testicular agenesis (1:2678) are common enough to expect to find each synchronously occasionally (Campbell, 1963). Therefore, renal absence and a nonpalpable testis does not justify the assumption of testicular agenesis in our minds.

Surgical exploration, including intra-peritoneal exposure, is required in all boys in whom a testis cannot be found along the

Table 9–1.   Sperm Counts in Normal, Unilateral Cryptorchidism Responsive to
Gonadotropin, and Those Requiring Surgery for Unilateral Undescended Testis (Top)
Vs. Those with Bilateral Undescended Testis (Bottom)

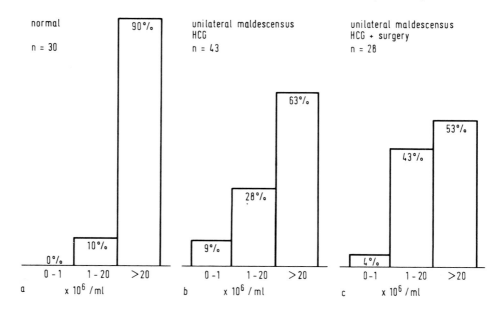

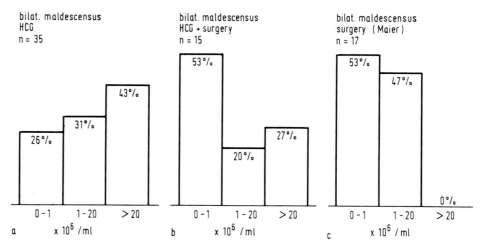

(From Bierich, J. R., Rager, K., and Ranke, M. B. (Eds.): Maldescensus Testis. Colloquium at Tübingen,
February 14, 1976. Baltimore, Urban and Schwarzenberg, 1977.)

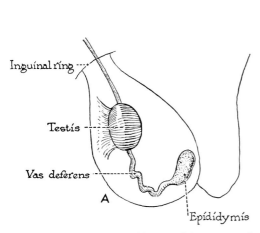
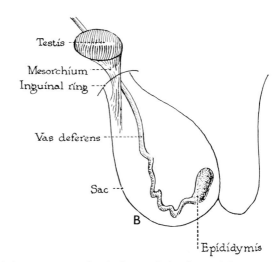

Figure 9–39.   Failure of fusion of the testis and epididymis. *A*, Completely descended right epididymis with incompletely descended testis. *B*, Completely descended right epididymis intra-abdominal testis. (From Badenoch, A. W.: Failure of the urogenital union. Surg. Gynecol. Obstet., 82:471-474, 1946.)

course of the inguinal canal. Prior to opening the abdominal cavity, the superficial inguinal area should be exposed. The presence of a small gonadal remnant or termination of the vas *and* gonadal vessels in fibrous tissue should be searched for, removed, and sent for histologic evaluation. However, since there can be complete separation of the testis from the epididymis and vas (Fig. 9–39), failure to identify the gonadal vessels at this juncture requires an adequate intraperitoneal search. In the event that an obviously dysgenetic testis is discovered, orchiectomy is advised provided the contralateral testis is normally descended. If both testes are dysgenetic, placement of at least one of these in the scrotum or, in the event that is impossible, in a subcutaneous position in the region of the external inguinal ring is probably best. Secondary removal of this testis after puberty may be considered to prevent the risk of malignancy. The alternative is removal of both gonads, necessitating lifetime extrinsic hormonal stimulation.

Recently, venography has been utilized as a means of testicular localization in those in whom testes are not palpable (Greenberg et al., 1979). Selective catheterization with injection of the spermatic veins allows identification of the pampiniform plexus and testicular location. However, we suggest

this study be reserved for exceptional cases.

BILATERAL TESTICULAR AGENESIS (ANORCHIA)

Failure to palpate any testicular tissue in the phenotypic male suggests the necessity for additional preoperative studies prior to surgical exploration. Chromosomal anomalies are occasionally present. In the neonatal nursery, the child with nonpalpable testes should have a buccal smear prior to hospital discharge to avoid missing the totally masculinized female with adrenal hyperplasia.

Recently, the gonadotropin stimulation test has proved efficacious in determining if testicular tissue is present. The absence of a significant (ten-fold) testosterone response to short-term gonadotropin stimulation (300 to 500 IU daily for three days) following determination of baseline levels obviates the need for exploration. In the unresponsive chromosomally normal male, one can assume testicular absence (Levitt et al., 1978). In the pubertal male, markedly elevated FSH and LH levels suggest an uncontrolled pituitary feedback system due to failure of testosterone production. Gonadotropin stimulation would then be redundant.

Table 9–2.   Differential Diagnosis of Testicular Torsion

	TESTICULAR TORSION	TORSION OF APPENDAGE	EPIDIDYMITIS	TUMOR
Pain	+	+	+	0
Pyuria	0	0	+	0
Fever	0	0	+	0
Testicular swelling	+	0	0	+
Epididymal swelling	+	0	+	0
Acute hydrocele	+	+	+	0
Increased testicular tenderness to palpation	+	±	0	0
Increased epididymal tenderness to palpation	+	±	+	0
Point tenderness to palpation	0	+	0	0

TESTICULAR TORSION

Exploration and orchiectomy should always be performed in the XO-XY male with gonadal dysgenesis in view of the high risk of gonadal malignancy. Agonadic boys require exogenous hormonal stimulation at puberty for masculinization and the capability for normal but infertile sexual activity.

TESTICULAR TORSION

There are few true emergency situations in pediatric urology. One of these is torsion of the testis. The diagnosis is suspected when a boy, usually an adolescent, presents with acute painful swelling of one testis. Fever and leukocytosis are not present in the first 24 hours. Owing to the abdominal origin and innervation of the testis, significant abdominal pain may coexist. Because of embarrassment peculiar to the age of the patient in question, he may be reluctant to point out that he has a swollen testis. Examination of the genitalia is imper-

ative in a boy with complaints of abdominal pain.

The entire scrotal contents are exquisitely sensitive to touch, and the testis is often elevated. A secondary hydrocele is present if several hours have elapsed since the onset. Delay must be avoided in determining the diagnosis; the differential diagnosis includes torsion of an appendage of the testis or epididymis, epididymitis, testis tumor, and trauma (Table 9–2).

There are two types of testis torsion. The least common is secondary to twisting of the spermatic cord and the entire tunica vaginalis (extravaginal torsion) and occurs in the prenatal or perinatal period. The defect is presumed to be inadequate fixation of the tunica vaginalis to the scrotum in the unborn or newborn male, allowing the entire intrascrotal contents to twist (Fig. 9–40A). The chances of early recognition in this group are poor, and the justification for surgery is questionable. Lately, however, we have been told of a few cases in which

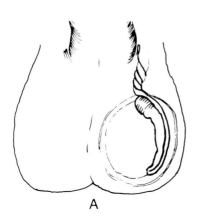

A

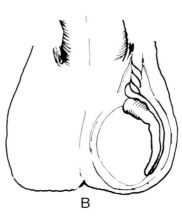

B

Figure 9–40. A, Extravaginal testicular torsion. Entire intrascrotal contents twist around the cord. This occurs almost exclusively in the prenatal or perinatal period. *B,* Intravaginal testicular torsion. The testis and epididymis turn on the spermatic cord within the tunica vaginalis. This is seen most commonly in adolescent males and is the result of a congenitally inadequate fixation of the testis to the tunic. (Courtesy of Dr. Arnold Willis.)

bilateral neonatal torsion has been recognized and testes have been thought to have been salvaged. This suggests that early surgical intervention may be advisable in selected cases. Failure to document this rare phenomenon probably accounts for atrophic testes noted in later years in some boys.

Torsion of the spermatic cord within the tunica vaginalis (intravaginal torsion) is seen far more commonly in postpubertal boys; however, it can occur at any age (Table 9–3). It is the result of inadequate posterior fixation of the tunica vaginalis to the testis and is referred to as the "bell and clapper" abnormality since the testis hangs freely within the tunica vaginalis (Fig. 9–40B). No known specific underlying activity is responsible for this phenomenon; however, a significant number of those affected awaken in the night or early morning with symptoms provoked by decreased vascular perfusion of the involved testis and epididymis. This suggests that physical activity is not the underlying cause.

To save the testis, immediate surgical detorsion of the cord is required. Fixation of the tunica albuginea to the tunica vaginalis and scrotum prevents its recurrence. Following completion of this simple procedure on the involved side, it is recommended that the contralateral side also be fixed since the predisposing abnormality may be bilateral. Detorsion should be carried out as quickly as possible. For those with a 360° twist, there is little likelihood of testis survival beyond six hours; however, those testes with intermittent or partial torsion may survive longer. Spontaneous untwisting occasionally occurs, and some boys give a history of previous episodes of pain and swelling. It is suggested that surgery be carried out in all patients in whom torsion is suspected, even if untwisting has occurred.

Unfortunately, it is often impossible to differentiate torsion of the testis (spermatic cord) from the other more benign intrascrotal conditions. Surgical exploration has classically been recommended in all boys with acute scrotal swelling since the ability to make an accurate preoperative diagnosis has been poor. The recent addition of isotope scanning provides a new dimension in determining the presence or absence of testicular arterial perfusion (Fig. 9–41). On

Table 9–3. Review of 159 Boys with Torsion*

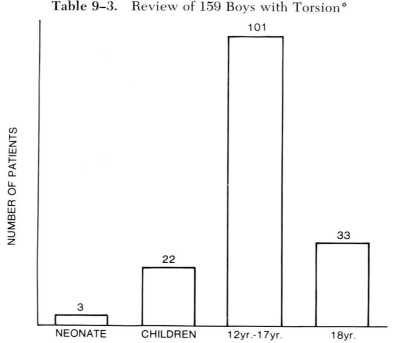

*The most common age of testis torsion is in adolescence. (Courtesy of Dr. Arnold Willis.)

the basis of this simple, minimally invasive (venipuncture) study, one can often rule out torsion of the entire cord by determining the presence of vascular perfusion. The differentiation can be made between appendiceal torsion and epididymitis, neither of which is a threat to the testis per se; these are then left to their individual clinical courses. However, the delay in exploration may not be justifiable. Additionally, interpreting this study is an art form. We, therefore, continue to recommend early surgical exploration in adolescent boys, a group in which torsion is highly likely.

Another simple means of evaluating testicular perfusion employs the pencil tip Doppler ultrasonic stethoscope (Levy, 1975). We have not been satisfied with the accuracy of this modality and cannot, for the moment, recommend its use (Nasrallah et al., 1977).

TORSION OF TESTICULAR OR EPIDIDYMAL APPENDAGES

Embryologic rests a few millimeters in size may be attached to the testis and epididymis. Those attached to the epididymis are of wolffian derivation, whereas those attached to the testis are of müllerian origin. All have the potential for torsion and, in spite of their small size, can cause an amazing degree of scrotal discomfort and swelling. Appendiceal torsion occurs most commonly in boys less than 14 years old (Puri and Boyd, 1976).

If the patient is seen early in the course of the illness, one may be able to identify a single point of tenderness, usually at the upper pole of the testis. The infarcted appendage may occasionally be seen as a blue dot underlying the scrotal skin in fair-skinned individuals (Dresner, 1973). A secondary hydrocele forms within hours of onset.

The natural history of torsion of an appendage includes a period of discomfort, which may last for several days in the unoperated patient. For this reason, as well as the necessity for making a definitive diagnosis, exploration and surgical excision have been advocated as a means of diminishing the period of morbidity. However, if the experienced examiner can make the diagnosis of appendiceal torsion with a great deal of confidence, exploration may not be necessary.

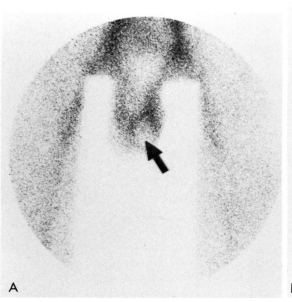 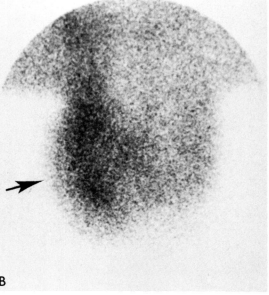

A   B

Figure 9–41.   *A,* Testicular torsion. The nonperfused testis (lucent area) is surrounded by increased perfusion due to scrotal reaction. *B,* Epididymitis. Increased perfusion (arrow) secondary to inflammation is present. (Courtesy of Dr. Massoud Majd.)

THE EPIDIDYMIS AND VAS DEFERENS

Developmental abnormalities of these structures independent of those associated with cryptorchidism are rare. Additionally, since an obstructive pathologic condition is generally manifested in problems related to fertility, its presentation in the pediatric population is uncommon. The only situation in which one might predict difficulties along these lines is the known association between cystic fibrosis and absence or atresia of the vas deferens (Klotz, 1973).

The incidental discovery of epididymal and vasal agenesis at the time of orchidopexy or herniorrhaphy suggests failure of development of the wolffian duct. Since this influences ureteral bud development and, therefore, kidney development, ipsilateral renal agenesis is to be anticipated. This can be verified by sonography.

ORCHITIS

Viral orchitis is either extremely rare or does not exist in prepubertal males. We have made this diagnosis only once in our urologic experience and that was in a pubertal 15-year-old boy. Scrotal swelling seen in a prepubertal male with parotitis should be regarded as an independent lesion, which should be evaluated and pursued on its own clinical merits.

HYDROCELE-HERNIA

A hydrocele is defined as fluid between the tunica vaginalis and tunica albuginea. The fluid surrounds the testis. If this fluid is transmitted from the peritoneal cavity through a patent processus vaginalis and is not a product of the tunica vaginalis itself, a defect must exist. This is potentially an indirect inguinal hernia. Hydroceles in children should be considered to be hernias since a patent processus vaginalis is almost always present. Based on this concept, operative correction is carried out by means of an inguinal incision with ligation of the neck of the sac. A transscrotal approach is applicable only in those patients who have had previous herniorrhaphy or in whom closure of the processus vaginalis has been proved by herniogram.

Many newborn males have hydroceles, often of large size, which may take a variable period of time to resolve. The general rule is that surgical repair should be delayed at least one year unless evidence of a hernia defect is present or the hydrocele is of giant proportions. Evidence of a hernia includes bulging along the course of the inguinal canal or significant changes in the amount of fluid present over relatively short periods of time (hours).

VARICOCELES

The finding of dilated veins in the scrotum (the pampiniform plexus) is virtually always confined to the left side. This is apparently the result of the relatively perpendicular course the left spermatic vein follows to the left renal vein. Stasis and backflow are the alleged causes of varicoceles.

Clinically, other than the unsightly bag-of-worms appearance, subfertility is the only recognized byproduct of this abnormality. Surgical ligation of the spermatic vein above the internal ring, where only two vessels are present, has been helpful in improving fertility in many. However, this procedure has not generally been advocated in adolescents, although varicoceles are not uncommon after 10 years of age (Øster, 1971).

Recently, Lipschultz and Corriere (1977) reported noting a significant decrease in size in the left testis of a group of men with varicoceles when compared to normal controls. Hotchkiss in 1944 suggested that prophylactic treatment of varicoceles was the key to prevention of progressive atrophy. This is not unlike orchidopexy.

We remain confused as to what to advise the patient and his parents when seeing an adolescent with a varicocele. If one could be sure that the changes leading to subfertility or infertility in those with varicoceles were progressive and more likely to

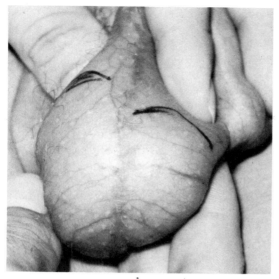

Figure 9-42. Hypoplastic left testis in a pubertal boy with a moderately large left varicocele. The left testis is measurably smaller than the right one.

reverse with early surgery, then this simple procedure should be advised in the otherwise healthy patient who is not a special anesthetic risk. As it now stands, our policy remains one of recommended ligation of the spermatic vein only in those with a demonstrable diminution in size of the ipsilateral testis when compared to its mate (Fig. 9-42).

ABNORMALITIES OF THE SCROTUM

BIFID SCROTUM

This abnormality is most commonly seen with hypospadias or as a part of the complex of penoscrotal transposition. It can occur independently but is not a significant abnormality. No therapy is necessary, although simple Z-plasty can be performed to normalize the scrotal appearance.

ACCESSORY SCROTUM

Dislocation of the scrotum from its normal location may be anticipated in boys born with cloacal exstrophy or duplication of the genitalia; however, occasionally ec-

topic scrotal tissue may be found in a child with otherwise normal genitalia (Lamm and Kaplan, 1977). A testis may or may not be associated with the ectopic scrotum, a factor that must be taken into consideration when planning treatment.

Simple excision of the extra scrotal tissue is reasonable only when adequate scrotum exists in the normal location or if transposition by a pedicle graft is not possible (Fig. 9-43). If a testis is located in an ectopic scrotal pouch, transposition to the normal location may be carried out either simultaneously with the scrotal correction or as a planned secondary procedure.

INFLAMMATORY CONDITIONS OF THE SCROTUM

The pediatrician is more familiar than the urologist with diaper rashes. It would be presumptuous for us to discuss this problem in this text.

Scrotal gangrene (Fournier's gangrene) is a rare condition occurring in adults but apparently was reported at least once in a child (Werner and Falk, 1964). Its origin is likely bacterial in nature, producing a rapidly progressive necrosis of a portion or all of the scrotum. The testes are spared, however.

Treatment requires rapid institution of broad-spectrum bactericidal antibiotics as

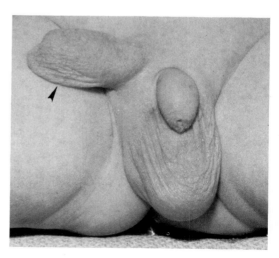

Figure 9-43. Ectopic scrotum containing undescended testis (arrow). (From Lamm, D. L., and Kaplan, G. W.: Accessory and ectopic scrota. Urology, 9:149, 1977.)

well as surgical debridement after demarcation of the necrotic areas has occurred. Complete destruction of the scrotum requires repositioning of the testes to the superficial inguinal area with secondary creation of a scrotum from skin swung from the thighs. Usually, however, some scrotal tissue remains, and regeneration can be anticipated, allowing ultimate replacement of the testes in their previous normal location.

Acute (idiopathic) scrotal edema is characterized by the sudden onset of unilateral swelling of the scrotal wall, although occasionally the involvement is bilateral. The process may extend into the inguinal area or the perineum.

The scrotal skin is erythematous and tender, although the tenderness is superficial. The testicles themselves are not involved — an important distinction since differentiation from testicular torsion is essential. To verify the normality of the intrascrotal contents, palpation should be carried out along the course of the spermatic cord. The testes may then be manipulated upward into the superficial inguinal area away from the edematous area for adequate examination.

There are no distinctive laboratory studies that corroborate the diagnosis of idiopathic scrotal edema and no specific recognized underlying cause. Allergy, insect bite, infection, trauma, and urinary extravasation have all been suggested but not corroborated as possibilities. The process is confined to the superficial scrotal layers, is self-limiting, and generally resolves in 12 to 24 hours without treatment (Kaplan, 1977a).

HENOCH-SCHÖNLEIN SYNDROME

Scrotal swelling not dissimilar to that of idiopathic scrotal edema has been noted in conjunction with Henoch-Schönlein purpura. The scrotal skin is usually hemorrhagic, however, and the typical rash present on other areas of the body suggests the diagnosis. Vasculitis is probably the underlying cause, and if testicular torsion can be ruled out, specific therapy is unnecessary. To confuse the issue, torsion has been reported in

association with Henoch-Schönlein purpura, and exploration may be necessary (Turkish et al., 1976). Scrotal isotope scanning has been successfully used to differentiate inflammation from torsion in this group (Naiman et al., 1978).

REFERENCES

Aarskog, D.: Clinical and cytogenetic studies in hypospadias. Acta Paediatr. Scand (Suppl.), *203*:1, 1970.

Aarskog, D.: Maternal progestins as a possible cause of hypospadias. N. Engl. J. Med., *300*:75, 1979.

Allen, T. D., and Spence, H. M.: The surgical treatment of coronal hypospadias and related problems. J. Urol., *100*:504, 1968.

Altman, B. L., and Malament, M.: Carcinoma of the testis following orchiopexy. J. Urol., *97*:498, 1967.

Bauer, S. B., Bull, M. J., and Retik, A. B.: Hypospadias: A familial study. J. Urol., *121*:474, 1979.

Bierich, J. R., Rager, K., and Ranke, M. B. (Eds.): Maldescensus Testis. Colloquium at Tübingen, February 14, 1976. Baltimore, Urban and Schwarzenberg, 1977.

Bofverstedt, B.: Condyloma acuminata. Acta Derm. Venereol., *47*:376, 1967.

Burstein, S., Grumbach, M. M., and Kaplan, S. L.: Early determination of androgen-responsiveness is important in the management of microphallus. Lancet, Nov. 10, 1979, p 983.

Campbell, M. F.: Urology, 2nd ed. Philadelphia, W. B. Saunders Co., 1963.

Donahue, R. E., Utley, W. L. F., and Maling, T. M.: Excretory urography in asymptomatic boys with cryptorchidism. J. Urol., *109*:912, 1973.

Dresner, M. L.: Torsed appendage: Diagnosis and management; blue dot sign. Urology, *1*:63, 1973.

Ehrlich, R. M., Dougherty, L. J., Tomashefsky, P., et al.: Effect of gonadotropin in cryptorchidism. J. Urol., *102*:793, 1969.

Fallon, B., Devine, C. J., and Horton, C. E.: Congenital anomalies associated with hypospadias. J. Urol., *116*:585, 1976.

Feldman, K. W., and Smith, D. W.: Fetal phallic growth and penile standards for newborn male infants. J. Pediatr., *86*:395, 1975.

Felton, L. M.: Should intravenous pyelography be a routine procedure for children with cryptorchidism or hypospadias? J. Urol., *81*:335, 1959.

Garrett, R. A., and Rhamy, D. E.: Priapism: Management with corpus-saphenous shunt. J. Urol., *95*:65, 1966.

Gee, W. F., and Ansell, J. S.: Neonatal circumcision: A ten year overview. Pediatrics, *5*:824, 1976.

Glenn, J. F., and Anderson, E. E.: Surgical correction of incomplete penoscrotal transposition. J. Urol., *110*:603, 1973.

Grayhack, J. T., McCullough, W., O'Conor, V. J., Jr., and Trippel, O.: Venous bypass operation to control priapism. Invest. Urol., *1*:509, 1964.

Greenberg, S. H., Ring, E. J., Oleaga, J., and Wein, A. J.: Gonadal venography for preoperative localization of nonpalpable testes in adults. Urology, *12*:453, 1979.

Hadziselimovic, F., and Herzog, B.: Development of normal and cryptorchid human testes. An ultrastructural study. *In* Bierich, J. R., Rager, K., and Ranke, M. B. (Eds.): Maldescensus Testis. Colloquium at Tübingen, February 14, 1976. Baltimore, Urban and Schwarzenberg, 1977.

Hadziselimovic, F., Herzog, B., and Seguchi, H.: Surgical correction of cryptorchism at 2 years: Electron microscopic and morphometric investigations. J. Pediatr. Surg., *10*:19, 1975.

Hastings, J.: Encyclopedia of Religion and Ethics. New York, Charles Scribner's Sons, 1911.

Hedinger, C.: The histopathology of the cryptorchid testis. *In* Bierich, J. R., Rager, K., and Ranke, M. B. (Eds.): Maldescensus Testis. Colloquium at Tübingen, February 14, 1976. Baltimore, Urban and Schwarzenberg, 1977.

Hinman, F., Jr.: Microphallus: Characteristics and choice of treatment from a study of 20 cases. J. Urol., *107*:499, 1972.

Horton, C. E., and Devine, C. J.: Developmental anomalies — hypospadias, one-stage repair — III. *In* Horton, C. E. (Ed.): Plastic and Reconstructive Surgery of the Genital Area. Boston, Little, Brown and Co., 1973.

Jones, H. W., Jr., and Scott, W. W.: Hermaphroditism, Genital Anomalies and Related Endocrine Disorders, 2nd ed. Baltimore, The Williams and Wilkins Co., 1971, pp. 376–405.

Kaplan, G. W.: Acute idiopathic scrotal edema. J. Pediatr. Surg., *12*:647, 1977a.

Kaplan, G. W.: Circumcision — An Overview. Current Problems in Pediatrics. Year Book Medical Publ., Inc., 1977b.

Klotz, P. G.: Congenital absence of vas deferens. J. Urol., *109*:662, 1973.

Klugo, R. C., and Cerny, J. C.: Response of micropenis to topical testosterone and gonadotropin. J. Urol., *119*:667, 1978.

Knorr, D., Proschold, U., and Richter, W.: Fertility after treatment of maldescensus testis. *In* Bierich, J. R., Rager, K., and Ranke, M. B. (Eds.): Maldescensus Testis. Colloquium at Tübingen, February 14, 1976. Baltimore, Urban and Schwarzenberg, 1977.

Lamm, D. L., and Kaplan, G. W.: Accessory and ectopic scrotum. Urology, *9*:149, 1977.

Levitt, S. B., Kogan, S. J., Engel, R. M., et al.: The impalpable testis: A rational approach to management. J. Urol., *120*:515, 1978.

Levy, B. J.: The diagnosis of torsion of the testicle using the Doppler ultrasonic stethoscope. J. Urol., *113*:63, 1975.

Lipschultz, L. I., Caminos-Torres, Jr., Greenspan, D., and Snyder, P. J.: Testicular function after unilateral orchiopexy. N. Engl. J. Med., *295*:15, 1978.

Lipschultz, L. I., and Corriere, J. N., Jr.: Progressive testicular atrophy in the varicocele patient. J. Urol., *117*:175, 1977.

McArdle, R., and Lebowitz, R.: Uncomplicated hypospadias and anomalies of the upper urinary tract: Need for screening? Urology, *5*:712, 1975.

Martin, D. C.: Germinal cell tumors of the testis after orchiopexy. J. Urol., *121*:422, 1979.

Minninberg, D.: Cryptorchidism: Observation on the ultrastructure of the undescended testis. 49th annual meeting, American Academy of Pediatrics, Detroit, Oct. 27, 1980.

Naiman, J. L., Harcke, T., Sebastianelli, J., and Stein, B. S.: Scrotal imaging in the Henoch-Schönlein syndrome. J. Pediatr., *92*:1021, 1978.

Nasrallah, P. F., Manzone, D., and King, L. R.: Falsely negative Doppler examinations in testicular torsion. J. Urol., *118*:194, 1977.

Neyman, M. A., and Schirmer, H. K. A.: Urinary tract evaluation in hypospadias. J. Urol., *94*:439, 1965.

Nickel, W. R., and Plumb, R. T.: Other infections and inflammations of the external genitalia. *In* Harrison, J. H., Gittes, R. F., Perlmutter, A. D., et al. (Eds.): Campbell's Urology, 4th ed. Philadelphia, W. B. Saunders Co., 1979.

Øster, J.: Further fate of the foreskin. Arch. Dis. Child., *43*:200, 1968.

Øster, J.: Varicocele in children and adolescents: An investigation of the incidence among Danish school children. Scand. J. Urol. Nephrol., *5*:27, 1971.

Page, L. A.: Inheritance of uncomplicated hypospadias. Pediatrics, *63*:788, 1979.

Preston, E. N.: Whither the foreskin? J.A.M.A., *213*:1853, 1970.

Puri, P., and Boyd, E.: Torsion of the appendix testis. Clin. Pediatr., *15*:949, 1976.

Puri, P., and Nixon, H. H.: Bilateral retractile testes — subsequent effects on fertility. J. Pediatr. Surg., *12*:563, 1977.

Ross, J. F., Farmer, A. W., and Lindsay, W. K.: Hypospadias: A review of 230 cases. Plast. Reconstr. Surg., *24*:357, 1959.

Section on Urology, American Academy of Pediatrics: The timing of elective surgery on the genitalia of male children with particular reference to undescended testes and hypospadias. Pediatrics, *56*:479, 1975.

Seeler, R. A.: Intensive transfusion therapy for priapism in boys with sickle cell anemia. J. Urol., *110*:360, 1973.

Smith, E. D.: A de-epithelialized overflap, flap technique in the repair of hypospadias. Br. J. Plast. Surg., *26*:106, 1973.

Sousa, C. M., Catoe, B. L., and Scott, R. B.: Studies in sickle cell anemia. XIX. Priapism as a complication in children. J. Pediatr., *60*:52, 1962.

Sweet, R. A., Schrott, H. G., Kurland, R., et al.: Study of the incidence of hypospadias in Rochester, Minn., 1940–1970 and a case control comparison of possible etiologic factors. Mayo Clin. Proc., 49–52, 1974.

Turkish, V. J., Traisman, H. S., Belman, A. B., et al.: Scrotal swelling in the Schönlein-Henoch syndrome. J. Urol., *115*:317, 1976.

Villee, D. B.: Development of endocrine function in the human placenta and fetus. N. Engl. J. Med., *281*:473, 533, 1969.

Wachtel, S. S.: H-Y antigen and the genetics of sex determination. Science, *198*:797, 1977.

Werner, H. J., and Falk, M.: Acute gangrene of the scrotum in an 8-year-old. J. Pediatr., *65*:133, 1964.

Wilson, J. D., Harrod, M. J., Goldstein, J. L., et al.: Familial incomplete male pseudo hermaphroditism, type 1: Evidence for androgen resistance and variable clinical manifestations in a family with the Reifenstein syndrome. N. Engl. J. Med., *290*:1097, 1974.

Wilson, S. K., Klionsky, B. L., and Rhamy, R. K.: A new etiology of priapism: Fabry's disease. J. Urol., *109*:646, 1973.

Winter, C. C.: Cure of idiopathic priapism. Urology, *4*:389, 1976.

Chapter Ten

GENITAL ABNORMALITIES IN THE FEMALE

Treatment of abnormalities of the female genital tract frequently falls to the pediatric urologist by default. Other disciplines often lack interest in nonsurgical problems that may involve these organs. Additionally, abnormalities of the female genitalia may be intimately involved in urinary tract problems. For these reasons, it seems appropriate to include a discussion of this area herein.

To best understand the congenital abnormalities of the female genital tract, one should first review its embryology (Gray and Skandalakis, 1972). The müllerian ducts, from which these structures eventually arise, appear during the first week of gestation as depressions in the urogenital ridges. These paired ducts grow caudally, crossing the wolffian ducts and coming to lie in apposition medial to the wolffian ducts. The müllerian ducts contact the posterior wall of the urogenital sinus at the müllerian tubercle. (In the male, this point eventually forms the seminal colliculus.) The müllerian ducts then fuse and canalize to form the uterovaginal canal, from which the fallopian tubes, uterus, and upper two thirds of the vagina eventually arise. (Fig. 10–1). The urorectal fold begins to divide the cloaca at five to six gestational weeks to form the anterior urogenital sinus and the posterior rectum. The lower vagina and

vestibule arise from the urogenital sinus. The bladder and urethra in the female correspond to the bladder and posterior urethra in the male.

VAGINAL AGENESIS

Vaginal agenesis (Fig. 10–2) occurs when the müllerian ducts do not canalize in their distal-most portion, presumably resulting in failure of development of the urogenital sinus (Jones and Scott, 1958). In reality, vaginal epithelium can usually be histologically identified in such cases so that it might be more appropriate to name this problem vaginal hypoplasia rather than vaginal agenesis. The uterus in these cases may be absent, extremely hypoplastic, or, in some cases, normal. The diagnosis of agenesis may be made at birth or during childhood but usually is not considered until puberty when the patient presents with amenorrhea or dysmenorrhea. Renal abnormalities have been reported in 29 to 51 per cent of girls with vaginal agenesis; unilateral renal agenesis and pelvic kidneys are the most common (Leduc et al., 1968). Vaginal agenesis should always be considered in the girl with a solitary pelvic kidney.

The vaginal opening may be absent or

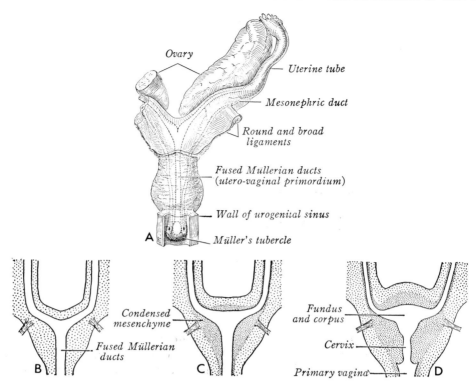

Figure 10–1. *A*, Genital tract of the human female, in ventral view at 10 weeks. *B*, *C*, and *D*, Diagrams illustrating the later history of the transverse limbs of the müllerian ducts within the genital cord. (From Arey, L. B.: Developmental Anatomy, 7th ed. Philadelphia, W. B. Saunders Co., 1974, pp. 326 and 327.)

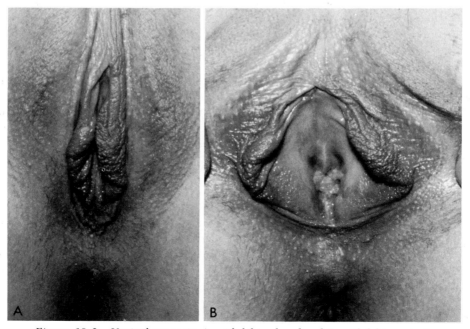

Figure 10–2. Vaginal agenesis. *A*, with labia closed and *B*, with labia spread.

may just be a shallow depression; the labia majora and minora, however, are completely normal. The age at which vaginal construction is performed depends on the presence or absence of the uterus. If the uterus is present, reconstruction should be performed when the patient is menarchal. However, if the uterus is absent, reconstruction is often delayed until the patient contemplates becoming sexually active. Prior to formation of a vagina, the status of the uterus must be determined; initial evaluation can be accomplished ultrasonographically with confirmation by either laparotomy or laparoscopy. If the uterus is present, then some connection to the external genitalia should be made.

There are multiple techniques available for vaginal reconstruction. One, applicable only to patients without a uterus, is nonoperative. Here pressure is applied against the perineum with dilators of gradually increasing depth and size until such time as a vaginal canal is firmly established (Huffman, 1968). A vagina can be surgically created by opening the area between the urethra and the rectum and lining this cavity with split thickness skin grafts (Ortiz-Monasterio et al., 1972), skin flaps developed from adjacent skin, or intestinal segments (Pratt, 1972). Both the nonoperative and surgical methods require that the newly constructed vagina be periodically dilated to prevent contraction. It is for this reason that vaginal reconstruction is often delayed until sexual activity is contemplated.

VAGINAL DUPLICATION

If the müllerian ducts fail to fuse, uterus didelphys (with two cervices and complete vaginal duplication) will result (Fig. 10–3). A partial failure of fusion would cause localized septa either in the uterus or the vagina (Fig. 10–4). These septa are usually oriented anteroposteriorly. Rarely, one side of a septate vagina may be blind, presenting the same propensity for ipsilateral renal agenesis as does complete vaginal agenesis (Milne, 1965).

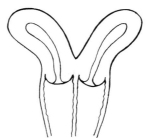

Figure 10–3. Uterus didelphys and vaginal duplication. (From Gray, S. W., and Skandalakis, J. E.: Embryology for Surgeons. Philadelphia, W. B. Saunders Co., 1972, p. 654.)

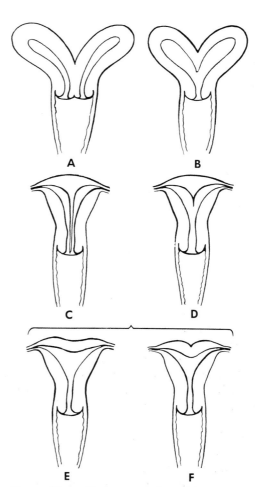

Figure 10–4. Fusion anomalies of the uterus. A, Uterus duplex bicollis. B, Uterus duplex unicollis. Both bicollis and unicollis forms are often lumped together as "bicornuate." C, Uterus septus. D, Uterus subseptus. E and F, Uterus arcuatus. The fundus is flattened or notched. (From Jarcho, J.: Malformations of the Uterus. Am. J. Surg., 71:106–166, 1946.)

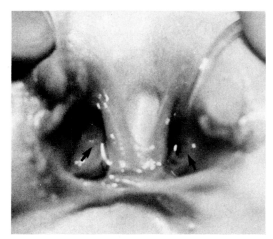

Figure 10–5. Vaginal and urethral duplication. Note catheters in the two urethras (arrows). The bladder itself was single, that is, it was not duplicated.

Other than vaginal agenesis with a uterus present, the lesions discussed are usually symptomless. The significance of vaginal and uterine septa lies in their adverse effect on fertility. Excision of the septa may improve the outlook for successful pregnancies in these patients (Strassmann, 1966). In rare instances complete vaginal and urethral duplication coexist (Fig. 10–5). In such instances the bladder is usually single (Boissonant, 1961).

IMPERFORATE HYMEN

Two relatively common abnormalities of variable severity are those caused either by an imperforate hymen or by a persistent transverse septum at the junction of the upper two thirds and lower one third of the vagina. Imperforate hymen may be detected at birth as a membrane that bulges between the labia (Fig. 10–6). There may be a mucocolpos behind an imperforate hymen caused by vaginal secretions that have been produced in response to maternal estrogens (Huffman, 1968). These secretions can result in a rather sizable abdominal mass (Fig. 10–7). Imperforate hymen may be familial and if so may be inherited as an autosomal recessive disorder.

A large hydrocolpos can obstruct the urethra and rectum and occasionally will

even occlude the venous return from the lower extremities. If hydrocolpos is present at birth and a bulging membrane is identified emerging between the labia majora, treatment consists of incision of this membrane and drainage of the fluid. Obstructive uropathy, if present, will usually promptly resolve (Fig. 10–8). One must be aware that a prolapsing ureterocele, also producing hydronephrosis, may present similarly (see Fig. 12–18). It is of interest (and also unexplained) that in some cases of imperforate hymen, there is no associated hydrocolpos. Where there is no hydrocolpos, presentation is delayed until puberty, at which time hematocolpos develops.

TRANSVERSE VAGINAL SEPTUM

Another form of vaginal obstruction is at a higher level and is caused by a high transverse vaginal septum (Brews, 1957). These girls may also present at birth with an abdominal mass and urinary and intestinal

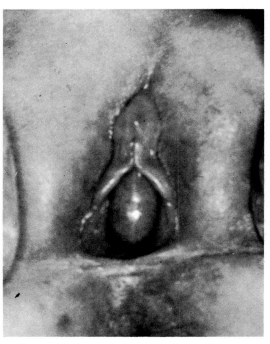

Figure 10–6. Imperforate hymen wih mucocolpos in a six-month-old infant. Approximately 75 cc. of mucoid material escaped when the hymen was incised. (From Huffman, J. W.: The Gynecology of Childhood and Adolescence. Philadelphia, W. B. Saunders Co., 1968, p. 183.)

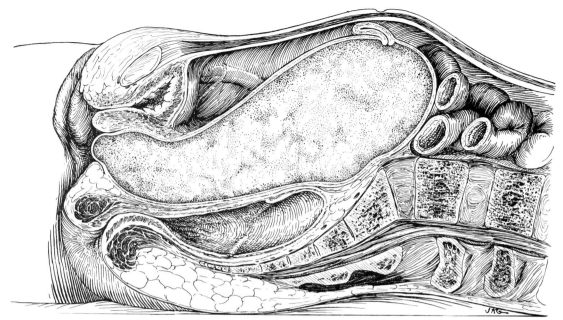

Figure 10–7. During infancy, mucoid material above an imperforate hymen may make a mass simulating a tumor. The tiny uterus sits atop the huge, fluid-filled cystlike vagina. (From Huffman, J. W.: The Gynecology of Childhood and Adolescence. Philadephia, W. B. Saunders Co., 1968, p. 184.)

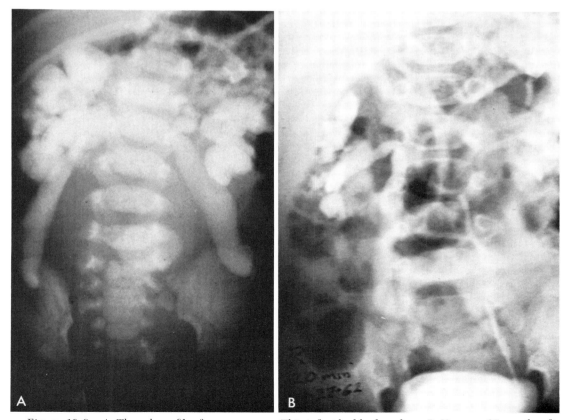

Figure 10–8. *A,* Three hour film from a urogram. This infant had hydrocolpos. *B,* Urogram 20 months after incision of the hymenal membrane.

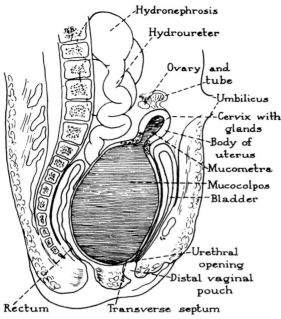

Figure 10–9. Hydrocolpos due to a transverse vaginal septum. (From McKusick, V. A., Bauer, R. L., Koop, C. E., and Scott, R. B.: Hydrometrocolpos as a simple inherited malformation. J.A.M.A., *189*:813–816, 1964. Copyright 1964; American Medical Association.)

obstruction (Fig. 10–9); however, the introitus will appear normal. Sometimes these masses are so large that they impinge on the diaphragm so that the infant may have respiratory distress. Rectal examination will reveal that the mass is located anterior to the rectum. If an excretory urogram is performed, the presence of a mass will be confirmed; usually bilateral hydrouretero-

nephrosis will be identified. Again, treatment consists of incision of the membrane or septum.

UROGENITAL SINUS ABNORMALITIES

Perhaps a more common cause of hydrocolpos than those discussed before is the anomaly best termed a persistent urogenital sinus (Fig. 10–10). Those anomalies discussed in the previous section are recognizable because there are two orifices present within the introitus: the vagina and urethra. In the persistent urogenital sinus, only one orifice is evident, representing the embryonic urogenital sinus from which the urethra and vagina emanate. Most of these children present with an abdominal mass, which usually causes moderate to severe hydronephrosis and can also be responsible for edema of the lower extremities (Reed and Griscom, 1973). The anatomy is often best defined by genitography and endoscopy. Treatment requires separation of the urinary tract from the vagina. This can often be accomplished as an abdominovaginal pull-through (Raffensperger and Ramenofsky, 1973) (Fig. 10–11) or perineally (Hendren, 1977). These children must be followed closely since poor bladder emptying is a frequent complication that may lead not only to urinary tract infection but also to hydronephrosis.

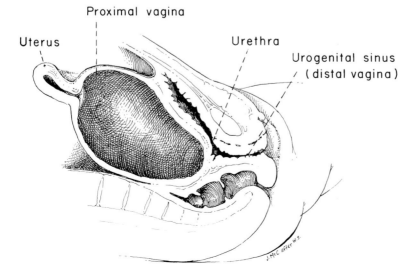

Figure 10–10. Diagram of hydrometrocolpos in a newborn infant, illustrating the urogenital sinus. (From Kelalis, P. P., King, L. R., and Belman, A. B.: Clinical Pediatric Urology, Vol. 2. Philadelphia, W. B. Saunders Co., 1976, p. 670.)

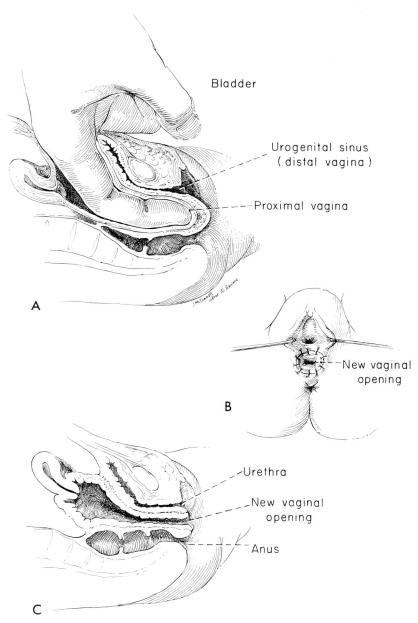

Figure 10–11.   The abdominovaginal pull-through operation. *A,* The huge vagina has been opened, and the posterior vaginal wall is being displaced downward by an assistant's finger. *B,* An inverted v incision is made on the perineum, and the vagina becomes visible. It is sutured to the perineal skin. *C,* Lateral diagram of completed operation. (From Kelalis, P. P., King, L. R., and Belman, A. B.: Clinical Pediatric Urology, Vol. 2. Philadelphia, W. B. Saunders Co., 1976, p. 672.)

PERSISTENT CLOACA

One of the more complex of all the anomalies one may encounter in a neonate is the persistent cloaca in the female (Raffensperger and Ramenofsky, 1973) (Fig. 10–12). This results from failure of the urorectal fold to reach the cloacal membrane so that the rectum, proximal urethra, and upper two thirds of the vagina all enter a common channel. This is the counterpart of the supralevator imperforate anus in the male and should be considered in every female child born with imperforate anus in whom no rectoperineal or low vaginal fistula can be identified. Approximately 30 per cent of the

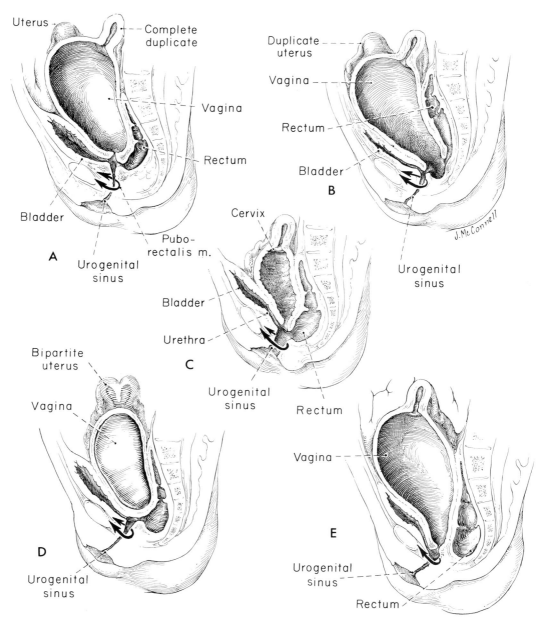

Figure 10-12. Varieties of cloacal anomalies. The double arrow indicates the position of the puborectalis muscle, which is essential to the development of fecal continence after operation. (From Kelalis, P. P., King, L. R., and Belman, A. B.: Clinical Pediatric Urology, Vol. 2. Philadelphia, W. B. Saunders Co., 1976, p. 673.)

girls with a persistent cloaca have hydrometrocolpos. There may often be vertebral anomalies and intestinal obstruction is always present. The urinary tract is also often obstructed, and in addition, roughly two thirds of these children have upper urinary tract abnormalities. Abnormalities also occur in other organ systems with increased frequency. Uterovaginal duplications occur in approximately 41 per cent of these patients.

It is essential that an accurate anatomic diagnosis be made as early as possible so that proper therapy can be employed. A "cloacogram," in which a small catheter is introduced into the common orifice on the perineum and contrast material is injected in a retrograde fashion, usually is the single most efficacious study for this purpose. If appropriate views are obtained, all three channels may be outlined. A transverse colostomy should be performed to proximally bypass the intestinal obstruction. If hydrometrocolpos is present, this may require some treatment in and of itself to relieve any resultant urinary tract obstruction. A vesicostomy may be necessary to relieve urinary obstruction. Once demonstrable obstructions have been relieved, it is usually best to delay definitive treatment until such time as the child has grown sufficiently that this can be accomplished with relative ease.

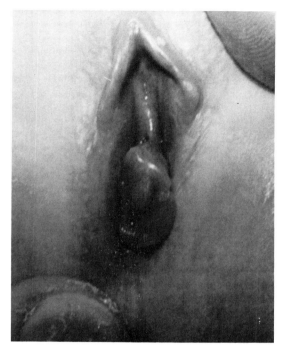

Figure 10–13. Vaginal inclusion cyst, presumably of Skene's duct origin, in a newborn girl.

Thorough excision of these cysts is difficult and usually unsatisfactory.

GENITAL PROLAPSE

Another lesion that does not have an embryologic basis is genital prolapse (Williams, 1968). This is quite rare and usually occurs during the first or second week of life in girls with a myelomeningocele or even more rarely in those who have undergone a difficult breech extraction. When genital prolapse occurs, it usually also causes bilateral ureteral obstruction. Treatment for that reason is mandatory for survival. The recommended treatment consists of manual reduction of the prolapse and catheter drainage of the bladder, after which the child's legs are bound together. If this position is maintained for one to two weeks, there is rarely recurrence of the prolapse.

Urethral prolapse is an entity occasionally seen in prepubertal girls, more often in blacks than whites (Klaus and Stein, 1973).

INTROITAL CYSTS

Other genital abnormalities that are infrequently noted at birth include cysts of either Gartner's duct or Skene's duct (Cohen et al., 1957) (Fig. 10–13). These often present as rather large masses that bulge out from the introitus. Although there is no need to differentiate them from each other, they must be differentiated from a prolapsed ectopic ureterocele. This is best accomplished by excretory urography. Once the lesion is shown to be a cyst, it can be observed for several months. Often these cysts will regress as the stimulus of maternal estrogens is withdrawn. If they do not regress, they are best marsupialized.

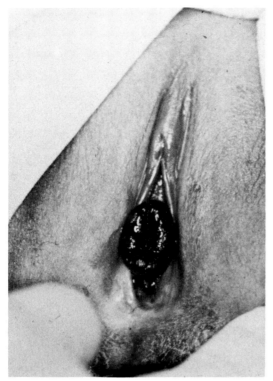

Figure 10–14.   Urethral prolapse in a seven-year-old girl.

The common mode of presentation is mild introital bleeding staining the underwear. Diagnosis is made by inspection (Fig. 10–14). The etiology is unknown. Excision of the prolapse usually suffices as therapy.

LABIAL ADHESIONS

A relatively frequent acquired problem is that of adhesions of the labia minora (Fig. 10–15). These are usually not present at birth and develop sometime during the first or second year of life. Presumably, these adhesions develop because maternal estrogen is withdrawn. Without estrogenic stimulation, the labia are thin and easily injured. If the labia are ulcerated by inflammation, the eroded surfaces then can adhere to one another. Even if no treatment is given for such labial adhesions, they will resolve spontaneously at adolescence, as estrogen stimulation causes thickening of the labial epithelium. Although the adhesions can be

separated manually or sharply in the office, this procedure is usually painful and is rarely successful since the inflamed areas in apposition are likely to readhere. For this reason, a preferred method of treatment is the daily application of an estrogen cream (Premarin) directly to the adhesions for approximately two weeks. This will usually cause spontaneous resolution of the problem. The mother must be cautioned that persistent use of estrogen creams can result in pubarche, and the child must be observed to prevent this complication. Occasionally manual lysis is required, in which case general anesthesia is recommended.

VAGINAL BLEEDING

The newborn female infant will often have a physiologic mucoid vaginal discharge. Occasionally, withdrawal bleeding occurs shortly after birth as a physiologic event because of the withdrawal of the maternal estrogenic stimulus. Withdrawal bleeding, should it occur, usually ceases within five to six days. Rarely, vaginoscopy may be necessary in some cases of unusually heavy bleeding to rule out the presence of a vaginal tumor (Huffman, 1968).

VULVOVAGINITIS

The most frequent pediatric gynecologic problem seen is unquestionably nonspecific vulvovaginitis (Gray and Ketcher, 1960). Nonspecific vulvovaginitis usually is a clinical problem in the two- to six-year-old age group. At this age, the vaginal and vulvar epithelia are quite thin and easily traumatized. These epithelia may be irritated by fecal contamination, by parasites (such as pinworms), by chemical irritants such as detergents (bubble bath), by the direct inoculation of upper respiratory tract pathogens (such as streptococcus), by fungal overgrowth after antibiotic therapy for other infections, and by foreign bodies.

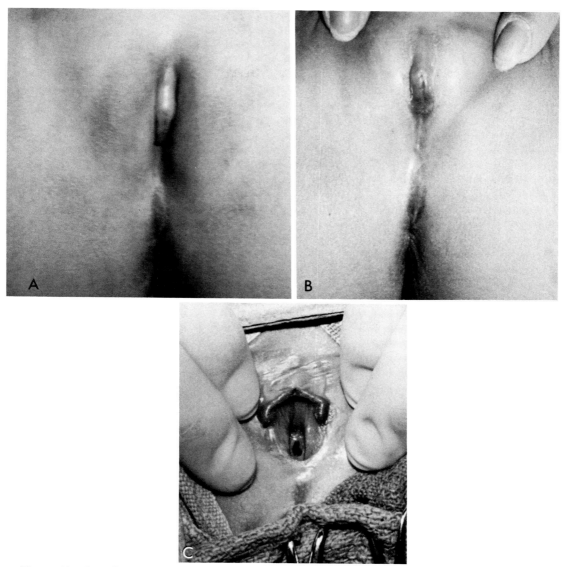

Figure 10–15.   Labial adhesions in a two-year-old girl *A*, before labia majora were spread, *B*, with labia majora spread, and *C*, after adhesions were lysed.

The symptoms of vulvovaginitis include a discharge that is usually yellowish and thin, erythema and irritation of the perineal skin, and, occasionally, marked dysuria. The dysuria may be severe enough to suggest urinary tract infection. The urinalysis, which is often contaminated by inflammatory cells from the vagina, tends to confuse the issue so that culture of a catheterized specimen may be required. Rectal examination will usually reveal most vaginal foreign bodies, although some will not be detected thereby.

One must be especially suspicious of the presence of a foreign body if the vaginal discharge is bloody or has a foul odor. Cultures should be obtained to rule out specific infections like gonococcal vulvovaginitis.

Most cases of nonspecific vulvovaginitis respond well to soothing sitz baths, like bicarbonate or oatmeal, and bland barrier ointments, such as Mycolog. Resistant cases may require a short course of estrogen cream therapy to produce resolution of any given episode. There is, unfortunately, a high incidence of recurrence of this problem, and the parents must be so advised.

REFERENCES

Boissonant, P.: Two cases of complete double functional urethra with a single bladder. Br. J. Urol., 33:453, 1961.

Brews, A.: Some clinical aspects of developmental anomalies of the female genitourinary tract. Proc. R. Soc. Med., 50:199, 1957.

Cohen, H. J., Klein, M. D., and Laver, M. R.: Cysts of the vagina in the newborn infant. Am. J. Dis. Child., 94:322, 1957.

Gray, L. A., and Ketcher, E.: Vulvovaginitis in childhood. Clin. Obstet. Gynecol., 3:165, 1960.

Gray, S. W., and Skandalakis, J. E.: The female reproductive tract. In Embryology for Surgeons. Philadelphia, W. B. Saunders Co., 1972, pp. 633–643.

Hendren, W. H.: Surgical management of urogenital sinus abnormalities. J. Pediatr. Surg., 12:339, 1977.

Huffman, J. W.: The Gynecology of Childhood and Adolescence. Philadelphia, W. B. Saunders Co., 1968, pp. 48, 183–186, 190–191.

Jones, H. W., and Scott, W. W.: Hermaphroditism, genital anomalies and related endocrine disorders. Baltimore, The Williams and Wilkins Co., 1958.

Klaus, H., and Stein, R. T.: Urethral prolapse in young girls. Pediatrics, 52:645, 1973.

Leduc, B., Campenhout, J., and Van Simard, R.: Congenital absence of the vagina. Am. J. Obstet. Gynecol., 100:512, 1968.

Milne, H. A.: Double uterus with unilateral haematocolpos and absence of ipsilateral kidney. Proc. R. Soc. Med., 58:238, 1965.

Ortiz-Monasterio, F., Serrano, A., and Barrera, G.: Congenital absence of the vagina. Plast. Reconstr. Surg., 49:165, 1972.

Pratt, J. H.: Vaginal atresia corrected by use of small and large bowel. Clin. Obstet. Gynecol., 15:639, 1972.

Raffensperger, J. G., and Ramenofsky, M. L.: The management of a cloaca. J. Pediatr. Surg., 8:647, 1973.

Reed, M. H., and Griscom, N. T.: Hydrometrocolpos in infancy. Am. J. Roentgenol. Radium Ther. Nucl. Med., 118:1, 1973.

Strassmann, E. D.: Fertility and unification of double uterus. Fertil. Steril., 17:165, 1966.

Williams, D. I.: Pediatric Urology. Kent, Butterworth & Co., 1968, p. 481, 1968.

Chapter Eleven

INTERSEX

Sexual ambiguity or one of the intersex states is a problem encountered relatively frequently in pediatric urologic practice. Often such patients pose difficult diagnostic and therapeutic challenges.

NORMAL EMBRYOGENESIS

Prior to attempting to unravel the mysteries of abnormal sexual differentiation, some discussion of normal differentiation seems pertinent (Fig. 11–1) (also see Chap. 9).

Normal sexual differentiation begins at the moment of fertilization, at which time one sex chromosome is provided by each parent. Inasmuch as the mother can provide only X chromosomes, the parent who actually determines the eventual sex of the child is the father, by providing either an X or Y chromosome. In early embryogenesis, it is impossible without a karyotype to determine the sex of the embryo, as there are no gross or microscopic distinguishing features.

In approximately the sixth week of intrauterine life, the gonad emerges from three primordia: primary germ cells, mesenchyme, and coelomic epithelium. The primary germ cells arise in the endoderm of the caudal portion of the yolk sac. These germ cells then migrate dorsally into the mesenchyme near the mesonephros at the root of the mesentery. The coelomic epithelium that overlies this area is the third element that eventually forms the gonad. These last two elements — the mesenchyme and its overlying coelomic epithelium — make up what is called the germinal ridge. In the seventh week, if a Y chromosome is present, a testis begins to develop from the medullary portion of this undifferentiated gonad. This appears to be mediated by an antigen from the Y chromosome labeled the H-Y antigen (Wachtel, 1975). If two X chromosomes are present, an ovary begins to form from the cortical portion of this undifferentiated gonad, but this event will not occur until the ninth gestational week. At the time the gonads differentiate, both müllerian and wolffian ducts are still present.

In a beautiful set of experiments, Jost (1960) demonstrated that early intrauterine castration in rabbits resulted in the development of internal and external female genitalia regardless of genetic sex. He further showed that in male embryos, early removal of one fetal testis would result in ipsilateral female genitalia and male internal genitalia contralateral to the site of castration. However, as long as one fetal testis remained, the external genitalia would be male (Fig. 11–2).

The explanation for these developments rests in the observation that the fetal

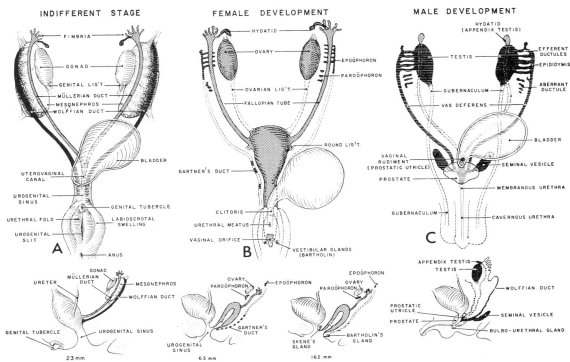

Figure 11–1. Embryonic differentiation of male and female genital ducts from wolffian and müllerian primordia. *A,* Indifferent stage showing large mesonephric body. *B,* Female ducts. Remnants of the mesonephros and wolffian ducts are now termed epoöphoron, paraoöphoron, and Gartner's duct. *C,* Male ducts before descent into scrotum. The only müllerian remnant is the testicular appendix. The prostatic utricle (vagina masculinis) is derived from the urogenital sinus. (From Williams, R. H.: Textbook of Endocrinology, 5th ed. Philadelphia, W. B. Saunders Co., 1974, p. 440.)

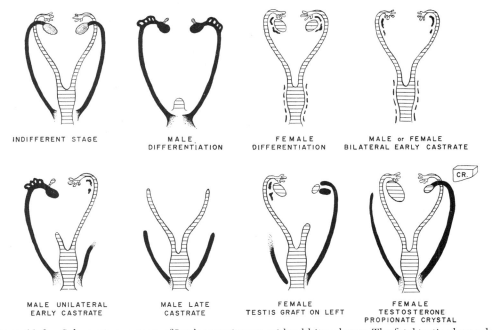

Figure 11–2. Schematic summary of Jost's experiments with rabbit embryos. The fetal testis plays a decisive role in determining the differentiation of genital ducts. Testosterone stimulates wolffian development but fails to effect involution of müllerian structures. (From Williams, R. H.: Textbook of Endocrinology, 5th ed. Philadelphia, W. B. Saunders Co., 1974, p. 440.)

testis secretes two hormones. One of these is a protein substance termed müllerian regression factor (müllerian inhibiting substance), which acts ipsilaterally to induce regression of the müllerian duct. The other substance is the androgenic steroid testosterone. This steroid causes the urogenital sinus to fuse posteriorly and the genital tubercle to enlarge. Additionally, fusion of the labioscrotal folds is prompted by the presence of this hormone. Fusion of the perineal part of the labioscrotal folds is completed in the human by the twelfth intrauterine week.

In the female, the müllerian ducts persist while the wolffian ducts regress because neither of the testicular substances is present. Additionally, the external genitalia remain female in appearance. During this period (the seventh to twelfth week of intrauterine life), other hormonal influences may come into play and may cause incomplete or excessive virilization. These factors are most prominent in the female and will be discussed more fully later.

CHROMOSOMAL DISORDERS

GONADAL DYSGENESIS

With the preceding information as background, we can now discuss the disorders of abnormal sexual differentiation. For any one of several reasons, there may be an alteration in an individual's chromosomal composition. These disordered karyotypes result in recognizable disorders. A classic example of such a disorder is Turner's syndrome (Fig. 11–3) first described in 1938. This phenotype is usually associated with a 45 XO karyotype, but mosaic forms may occur.

The clinical incidence of this disorder is estimated to be one in 2700 women. However, many aborted fetuses have this karyotype, and it has been estimated that the incidence of this abnormality at conception may be as high as one in 100 (Carr, 1971). If one performs buccal smears for cytologic examination, Barr bodies will not usually be seen.

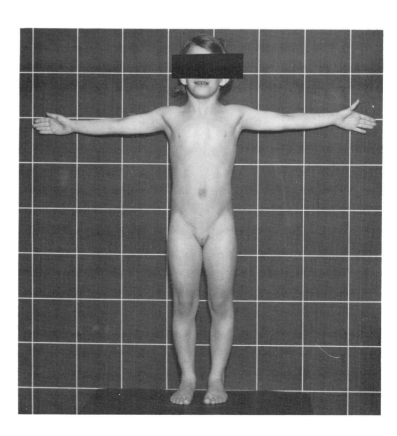

Figure 11–3. Patient with gonadal dysgenesis. (From Kelalis, P. P., King, L. R., and Belman, A. B.: Clinical Pediatric Urology, Vol. 2. Philadelphia, W. B. Saunders Co., 1976, p. 1006.)

The phenotype of a patient with Turner's syndrome is characteristic. Short stature is common; the eventual adult height is 50 to 60 inches. At birth, these patients have a low birth weight and decreased birth height. Their faces are also characteristic and include micrognathia, epicanthal folds, ptosis, and low-set ears. The palate is high and narrow; strabismus is common. One of the more consistent features is a short, broad neck with webbing and a low-set hairline that often looks like an inverted "M" (Fig. 11–4). During infancy, such webbing is present in 50 per cent of these children. Additionally, the neck is thrown into loose folds posteriorly. The chest is shield-shaped because the nipples are laterally placed. Lymphedema is often present at birth. The nails are hypoplastic. Cubitus valgus is present in 60 per cent of those with Turner's syndrome. Fifty to 85 per cent of these patients have renal abnormalities (Persky and Cowens, 1971). Horseshoe kidneys are the most common, but hydronephrosis occurs with some regularity. Congenital heart disease is similarly a frequent finding. Coarctation of the aorta

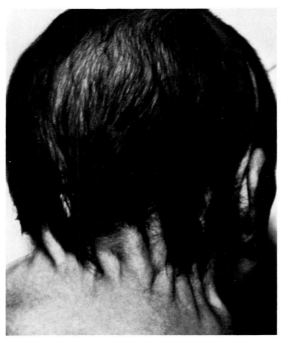

Figure 11–4. Webbed neck and low-set hairline in a patient with Turner's syndrome.

is one of the more common lesions seen. Aortic stenosis and aortic valve abnormalities also occur in some patients. Additionally, cystic medial necrosis of aortic aneurysms, as well as unexplained hypertension, have been reported. Additional abnormalities that have been reported in Turner's syndrome include multiple pigmented nevi, a tendency to keloid formation, mild mental retardation, and a shortened fourth metacarpal.

The external genitalia of these patients are normal. At puberty, the pubic hair is sparse, and other secondary sex characteristics are absent. The gonads themselves are merely fibrous streaks. The vagina, uterus, and fallopian tubes are normal. These patients are usually sterile, but pregnancy has been reported rarely in patients with Turner's syndrome (Nakashima and Robinson, 1971). If XY mosaicism is present, gonadectomy is advisable as there is a high incidence of gonadal malignancy in such patients (Schellhas, 1974).

Two variations of Turner's syndrome should be mentioned — Ullrich's syndrome (Ullrich, 1949) and Noonan's syndrome (Noonan, 1968). Ullrich's syndrome can occur in either males or females. These patients have the somatic abnormalities of Turner's syndrome but are normally fertile and are of normal stature. Congenital heart disease, especially pulmonic stenosis, is rather frequent in such patients, as are arthrogryposis, muscle agenesis, and neurologic abnormalities. The karyotype is normal in both Ullrich's and Noonan's syndrome. Patients with Noonan's syndrome are males with the somatic abnormalities of Turner's syndrome. Usually these boys are short, and, in addition, they have undescended testes with or without hypospadias and infertility.

KLINEFELTER'S SYNDROME

Another example of an abnormality determined by the patient's karyotype is Klinefelter's syndrome. As originally described, these are males with azoospermia, gynecomastia, small testes, eunuchoidism, elevated gonadotropins, and, upon testicular biopsy, hyalinized spermatic tubules (Klinefelter et al., 1942). Somewhat later, it was discovered that many of these patients have a chromatin-positive buccal smear. It was found still later that many had an XXY karyotype (Jacobs and Strong, 1959). The diagnosis of Klinefelter's syndrome is rarely made before puberty. However, it is possible to do so if one maintains a high index of suspicion when presented with a patient with small testes. After puberty, patients with Klinefelter's syndrome are taller than the average patient and have unusually long legs (Fig. 11–5). Approximately half the patients with Klinefelter's syndrome have gynecomastia; some also have signs of androgen deficiency. The phallus is usually small. Approximately two thirds of those who are chromatin-positive have a 47 XXY karyotype, and most of the rest have 46 XY/47XXY mosaicism. The estimated incidence of Klinefelter's syndrome in the general population is thought to be as high as one in every 400 males.

There is a variant of Klinefelter's syndrome that has a very characteristic appearance and therefore can be recognized clinically. These are patients with a 49 XXXXY karyotype (Cunningham and Ragsdale, 1972). These boys are usually quite retarded, have large ears, a short neck, hypertelorism, strabismus, and mandibular prognathism. The testes and penis are both small. Additionally, skeletal abnormalities such as radioulnar synostosis are present.

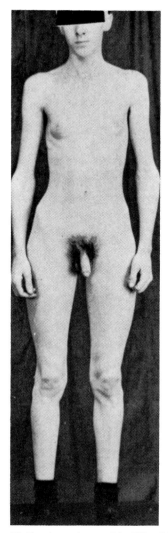

Figure 11–5. A patient with Klinefelter's syndrome. (Courtesy of Dr. Harry F. Klinefelter.) (From Harrison, J. H., Gittes, R. F., Perlmutter, A. D., et al.: Campbell's Urology, Vol. 2, 4th ed. Philadelphia, W. B. Saunders Co., 1979, p. 1493.)

TRUE HERMAPHRODITISM

True hermaphroditism is relatively rare. Approximately 400 cases have been reported to date. To qualify for this diagnosis, recognizable ovarian and testicular tissue must both be present. Patients with true hermaphroditism have been classified into three types (Jones and Scott, 1971). In the lateral form (34 per cent of the total), there is a testis on one side and an ovary on the other. Interestingly, the ovary is usually on the left side and the testis is on the right. In the bilateral form (20 per cent of the total),

there is an ovotestis on each side. The third form is the unilateral, which is the most frequent (46 per cent of the total), in which an ovotestis is found on one side and either an ovary or a testis on the other.

True hermaphrodites usually present at birth with ambiguous genitalia. The internal genitalia of these patients tend to mimic the external genitalia. For example, if the external genitalia tend to be masculine, then the internal genitalia are usually more masculine and vice versa. Approximately three quarters of true hermaphrodites are raised as males. However, if the sex of rearing is related to the appearance of the external genitalia, about 80 per cent of those with feminized external genitalia were raised as females, whereas more than 90 per cent of those with masculinized external genitalia were raised as males. About 70 per cent of the true hermaphrodites so studied have been chromatin-positive (Cloutier and Hayles, 1976). Upon karyotype, about half are XX, 20 per cent are XY, and the remainder are mosaics, usually XO/XY. Testicular tissue, when present, may not have any germ cells; occasionally, one will find testicular tissue without a Y chromosome. In some instances, true hermaphroditism is thought to be caused by a recessive gene.

MIXED GONADAL DYSGENESIS

In the syndrome of mixed gonadal dysgenesis, there is a unilateral testis with a streak gonad and müllerian structures on the contralateral side (Davidoff and Federman, 1973). These patients are usually XO/XY in karyotype and may have ambiguous genitalia. They are usually masculinized. All patients with mixed gonadal dysgenesis reported to date have had a uterus, in contradistinction to true hermaphrodites, in whom a uterus may not be present. Fallopian tubes are present bilaterally in most patients with mixed gonadal dysgenesis. Most of the patients with mixed gonadal dysgenesis should be raised as females as they are usually of short stature and have a small phallus. Those raised as females may masculinize at puberty; gonadal tumors are frequent in this syndrome. For both these reasons, it has been suggested that gonadectomy is routinely desirable in these patients.

PURE GONADAL DYSGENESIS

Individuals with pure gonadal dysgenesis are usually female in appearance, are of normal or above average height, and remain sexually immature (Sohval, 1965). They do not have a Turner's phenotype. Most have an XX karyotype, although a few have an XY

karyotype, which tends to be familial. Both external and internal genitalia are normal, but such patients have bilateral streak gonads and generally require hormone replacement as sexual development may be insufficient. Neoplasms are rare in those with XX gonadal dysgenesis as compared to those with XY karyotype, in whom gonadectomy is advisable.

CHROMOSOME INVERSIONS

Chromosome inversions have been reported. There are phenotypically male patients who have a 46 XX karyotype. Such patients have a Klinefelter's phenotype; the testis on biopsy has an appearance like that of Del Castillo's syndrome (germinal cell aplasia). The H-Y antigen has been found in some of these patients (Wachtel, 1975). The incidence of this problem has been estimated to be one in 45,000 males.

MALE PSEUDOHERMAPHRODITISM

Testicular Feminization. Sexual development can also be affected by intrauterine endocrinologic malfunction. We will first discuss disorders of the fetal testis. Such problems are often classified as male pseudohermaphroditism. The classic example of this problem, in which the karyotype is 46 XY, is the testicular feminization syndrome (Morris, 1953). At birth these children have a completely normal female phenotype. However, no female internal genitalia are present. The uterus is absent, and the vagina is shallow. Testes are present and are usually intra-abdominal, although occasionally they may be in the inguinal canal. As they grow, these "girls" are often of above average height. Between one half and two thirds present with inguinal hernias as the testes descend; the diagnosis will be detected at that time in these patients. The remainder will then usually present because of primary amenorrhea. At puberty they all have normal breast development, although the nipples may be slightly hypoplastic and underpigmented. Sexual hair will be present but scanty. Histologically, no spermatogenesis is present in adults; some testes contain Sertoli cell adenomata.

If the testes are retained intra-abdominally, there is a high incidence of dysgerminoma, and for this reason the testes should be removed. However, it is generally felt that the testes should be retained through puberty. Failure of the pituitary feedback system results in an abnormally high circulating testosterone level. Excellent feminization is a byproduct.

The underlying cause for testicular feminization is a failure in end-organ response to testosterone due to a defect in the protein binding of dihydrotestosterone, thereby interfering with its intracellular transport (Keenan et al., 1974). Testicular feminization is inherited as an X-linked recessive disorder. There are incomplete forms of testicular feminization in which there is more virilization (Wilson et al., 1974). Patients with the incomplete forms also have less breast development than those with the complete form and may present at birth with ambiguous genitalia. They also usually have more sexual hair than is seen in patients with the complete form of this disorder.

5-Alpha Reductase Deficiency Syndrome. Another problem in which there may be an intrauterine endocrine malfunction is pseudovaginal-perineoscrotal hypospadias (Simpson et al., 1971). These patients have a moderate-sized phallus, a perineal urethral meatus, and a blind perineal opening resembling a vagina. Occasionally, it may be possible to feel testes in the groin. The internal genital ducts are all male, and at puberty the phallus enlarges impressively. Hence, theoretically, if these patients were recognized at birth, it might be possible to raise them as males with the potential for fertility. Familial forms exist, one of which is inherited as an autosomal recessive trait. The basic defect in this problem has been shown to be an absence of 5-alpha reductase, the enzyme that converts testosterone to dihydrotestosterone. Dihydrotestosterone is responsible for external male genital stimulation in the fetus.

Hernia Uteri Inguinale. Hernia uteri inguinale is the result of persistence of müllerian structures despite an XY geno-type and a male phenotype (Brook et al., 1973). These patients present with a hernia containing a uterus and fallopian tube and cryptorchidism. This disorder is thought to represent an intrauterine deficiency of müllerian regression factor. It may be inherited as a recessive gene. Fewer than 100 such cases have been reported.

Other examples of male pseudohermaphroditism include Lubs' syndrome, Gilbert-Dreyfus syndrome, and the Reifenstein syndrome. Lubs' syndrome is one in which the patients have a small phallus, bifid labioscrotal folds, and a single urogenital orifice; at puberty these children are eunuchoid. The Gilbert-Dreyfus patients have ambiguous genitalia and a male karyotype. Patients with the Reifenstein syndrome are males with hypospadias and cryptorchidism; this syndrome has a familial pattern.

FEMALE PSEUDOHERMAPHRODITISM AND THE ADRENOGENITAL SYNDROME

Female pseudohermaphroditism may result from abnormalities in either exogenous or endogenous hormones. If the mother receives exogenous androgenic hormones such as progesterone to prevent abortion, the fetus might become virilized. Additionally, if the mother has a virilizing ovarian or adrenal tumor during pregnancy, the fetus might be virilized. These are relatively rare but should be recognized at birth in light of the mother's history.

A more common and more difficult problem that usually produces ambiguous genitalia is that of congenital adrenal hyperplasia. This occurs as the result of a block in the synthesis of cortisol. Cortisol, aldosterone, and testosterone all have common pathways of metabolism arising from cholesterol. If an enzyme deficiency exists resulting in a decreased production of cortisol, the pituitary will respond by increasing the production of ACTH. This will cause the adrenal cortex in turn to be stimulated to produce whatever hormones it can, usually some form of androgen. There are now five recognizable deficiencies in this metabolic pathway (Fig. 11–6).

The first is a deficiency in desmolase (Prader and Anders, 1976). This enzyme converts cholesterol to pregnenolone. When a desmolase deficiency is present, there is incomplete virilization of the male fetus. Patients with a desmolase deficiency are salt losers and have a virtual absence of circulating steroids. There have to date been no long-term survivors with desmolase deficiency. At autopsy, there is a large amount of cholesterol in the adrenal cortex; for this reason, this disorder has also been called lipoid hyperplasia. Females born with a desmolase deficiency basically have normal external genitalia.

Another enzyme deficiency that causes congenital adrenal hyperplasia is 3-β-hydroxysteroid dehydrogenase deficiency (Bongiovanni, 1961). This enzyme converts pregnenolone to progesterone; it is also involved in the conversion of dehydroepiandrosterone to androstenedione. If this enzyme is deficient, there will be decreased virilization of the males because the androgens produced are weak. Affected girls usually have a normal female phenotype or may have slight clitoral enlargement with labioscrotal fusion caused by the previously

mentioned weak androgen production. Most of these patients are salt losers as there is a decreased production of glucocorticoids and aldosterone.

A third enzyme is 17-α-hydroxylase (Alvarez et al., 1973); this enzyme converts progesterone to 17-hydroxyprogesterone and pregnenolone to 17-hydroxypregnenolone. If this enzyme is deficient, the production of both cortisol and androgens is decreased while the production of corticosterone is increased. Males with this deficiency have ambiguous genitalia; females will have normal genitalia and will present with primary amenorrhea and delayed pubarche. These children usually have mild hypertension due to hypervolemia. Laboratory abnormalities include hypokalemic acidosis, elevated serum ACTH, decreased circulating renin, and decreased urinary 17-ketosteroids. If glucocorticoids are given, the blood pressure will fall to normal.

A fourth enzyme is 21-hydroxylase, which, when deficient, results in decreased levels of 11-deoxycortisol (compound S) and cortisol and elevated levels of 17-hydroxyprogesterone (Marks and Fink, 1969). About one third of these patients lose

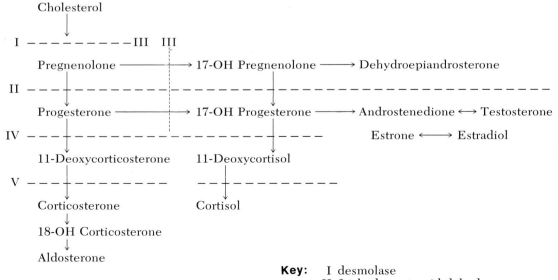

Key: I desmolase
       II 3β-hydroxysteroid dehydrogenase
      III 17α-hydroxylase
       IV 21-hydroxylase
        V 11β-hydroxylase

Figure 11–6. Pathways of steroidogenesis and blocks in congenital adrenal hyperplasia. (From Kelalis, P. P., King, L. R., and Belman A. B.: Clinical Pediatric Urology, Vol. 2. Philadelphia, W. B. Saunders Co., 1976, p. 1014.)

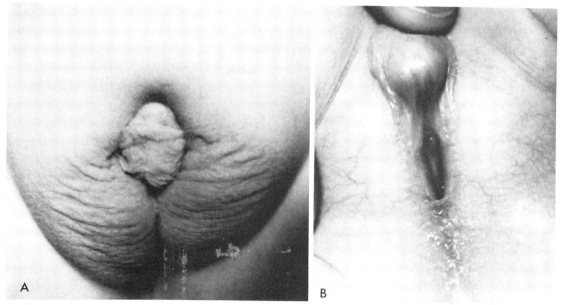

Figure 11–7. A and B, Newborn girl with the adrenogenital syndrome; there is mild clitoromegaly.

salt. This is the commonest form of congenital adrenal hyperplasia. The main metabolite of 17-hydroxyprogesterone is pregnanetriol, which is found in elevated levels in the urine of patients with a 21-hydroxylase deficiency.

The fifth enzyme is 11-β-hydroxylase, which converts compound S into cortisol and deoxycortisone into corticosterone (Gandy et al., 1960). 11-β-hydroxylase deficiency is rare. These patients present with virilization and hypertension; the latter is caused by elevated levels of DOC. Females with this deficiency are virilized at birth, and affected boys will virilize if they are not treated. If glucocorticoids are given, blood pressure will fall to normal levels.

Testosterone is the cause of virilization in all the patients with congenital adrenal hyperplasia; presumably the testosterone is produced by elevated circulating levels of androstenedione. Additionally, testosterone causes an increased growth rate and an advanced bone age, but its excess results in premature closure of the epiphyses with consequent short stature. Why some patients with congenital adrenal hyperplasia lose salt and others do not is incompletely understood. There may be a "salt-losing hormone" that has not yet been detected, or

it may be that this relates more to the severity of the deficit.

It is thought by some that cortisol is necessary for aldosterone function. In severe cases of congenital adrenal hyperplasia, there is little if any cortisol produced. Aldosterone production is decreased in salt-losing patients even if they are deprived of salt. This tendency to lose salt lessens with age; consequently, some salt-losing patients may not need treatment for salt-losing after age four or five years.

Girls with congenital adrenal hyperplasia usually have abnormal genitalia at birth. The genital abnormalities can vary from a normal vulva and introitus with mild clitoral enlargement (Fig. 11–7) to complete masculinization with a fully formed phallus and completely fused labioscrotal folds (Fig. 11–8). The most severely masculinized females tend to be the result of adrenal hyperplasia since hormonal stimulation occurs throughout fetal development. The ovaries, uterus, and fallopian tube are normal regardless of the degree of masculinization. If untreated, affected girls progressively virilize and will not enter pubarche.

In affected males, except those patients with 3-β-hydroxysteroid hydrogenase or desmolase deficiency, the genitalia are

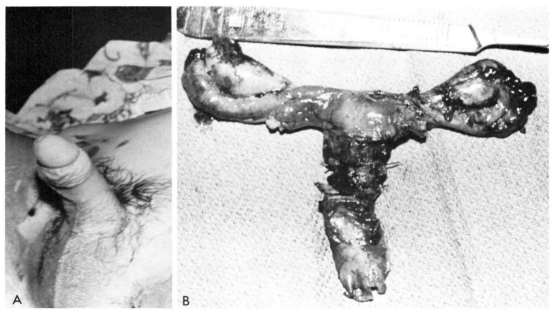

Figure 11–8. A seven-year-old 46XX who has been fully masculinized by the adrenogenital syndrome. *A,* External genitalia. *B,* Internal genitalia and gonads.

usually normal at birth. Virilization usually starts at about six months to two years of age if it occurs. The penis enlarges, but the testes remain small. In both boys and girls, growth rate is increased, and the epiphyses close prematurely so that the patient is ultimately short. In boys muscular development is accelerated and the voice deepens. The genitalia are often hyperpigmented in both sexes, more noticeably so in males and salt-losers.

Salt-losing patients do not manifest their salt loss at birth but usually do so between the second and fifth weeks of life. This is heralded by the sudden onset of irritability, failure to thrive, vomiting, and occasionally diarrhea. Dehydration and decreased circulating plasma volume develop as a result of the salt loss, and this may progress to circulatory collapse within 48 hours. If serum electrolytes are measured during a crisis or its prodrome, sodium levels are low and potassium levels are high.

Congenital adrenal hyperplasia is inherited as an autosomal recessive trait. The various types of hyperplasia tend to "run through" in families. When suspected in girls, a buccal smear can be obtained, which

will usually demonstrate Barr bodies. Because the risk of circulatory collapse is so serious, *one should entertain this diagnosis in all neonates when no testes can be palpated.* A buccal smear should be done in all neonates with male phenotype in whom testes cannot be palpated at birth. 17-Ketosteroid levels can be measured in the urine and are elevated in those affected; however, urinary 17-ketosteroid levels may normally be high during the first two weeks of life. If an elevated level is obtained, it should be subsequently measured again to ascertain that it is not a physiologic elevation. To further characterize which of the five enzyme deficiencies is responsible in any given patient, the abnormal steroid metabolites must be identified. Urethroscopy and genitography are often helpful in establishing a diagnosis of congenital adrenal hyperplasia (Fig. 11–9).

The object of hormonal treatment in patients with congenital adrenal hyperplasia is to prevent abnormal virilization and to obtain normal growth. Glucocorticoids will elevate serum cortisol levels and will decrease ACTH production, thereby decreasing androgen stimulus and normalizing urinary 17-ketosteroid excretion. Both cortisone acetate and hydrocortisone are effective for this purpose. Girls with this syndrome are fertile despite steroid therapy. Normal pregnancies and deliveries have been reported in patients with congenital adrenal hyperplasia; normal infants can result from such pregnancies.

Emergency treatment of patients who are salt-losers and who present in cardiovascular collapse consists of administration of intravenous saline and intramuscular deoxycorticosterone acetate. In addition, hydrocortisone can be given intramuscularly or intravenously. When the patient is able to tolerate oral medications, salt can be added to the diet. For maintenance therapy, deoxycorticosterone acetate can be administered either as subcutaneous pellets or depot injections. 9-α-Fluorocortisol (Fluorinef) can be given by mouth as an alternative. Maintenance hydrocortisone can be given orally instead of intramuscularly.

EVALUATION OF THE CHILD WITH AMBIGUOUS GENITALIA

The preceding discussion of intersex has followed an etiologic classification based on either chromosomal or hormonal abnormalities. The latter were then divided into exogenous and endogenous hormonal abnormalities. Another way to approach the intersex problem is to divide patients into those who present with ambiguous genitalia and those who do not. Those with ambiguous genitalia include the 49 XXXXY Klinefelter's syndrome, the true hermaphrodite, mixed gonadal dysgenesis, 5-alpha reductase deficiency, Lubs' syndrome, the Gilbert-Dreyfus syndrome, congenital adrenal hyperplasia, and girls masculinized by abnormal maternal androgen production or ingestion. The remainder of patients with intersex states do not present with ambiguous genitalia at birth, hence, their inclusion in any scheme for differential diagnosis of intersex is only confusing.

If a patient presents with ambiguous genitalia at birth, it is important to establish a diagnosis rapidly (Fig. 11–10). One can use either chromatin examination of a buccal smear or karyotype initially to separate patients into those with XX and those with XY karyotypes. Let us first consider those patients who are chromatin-positive, i.e., XX. Excessive maternal androgens can usually be detected by a history of either ingestion of progestational agents by the mother during pregnancy or the presence of a maternal virilizing tumor. If no such history is present, one can then measure urinary

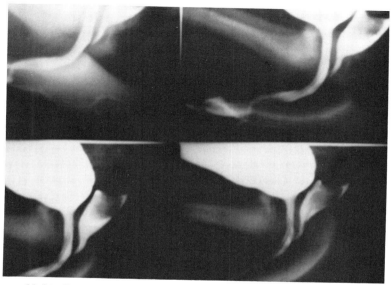

Figure 11–9. Genitogram of an infant with the virilizing adrenogenital syndrome.

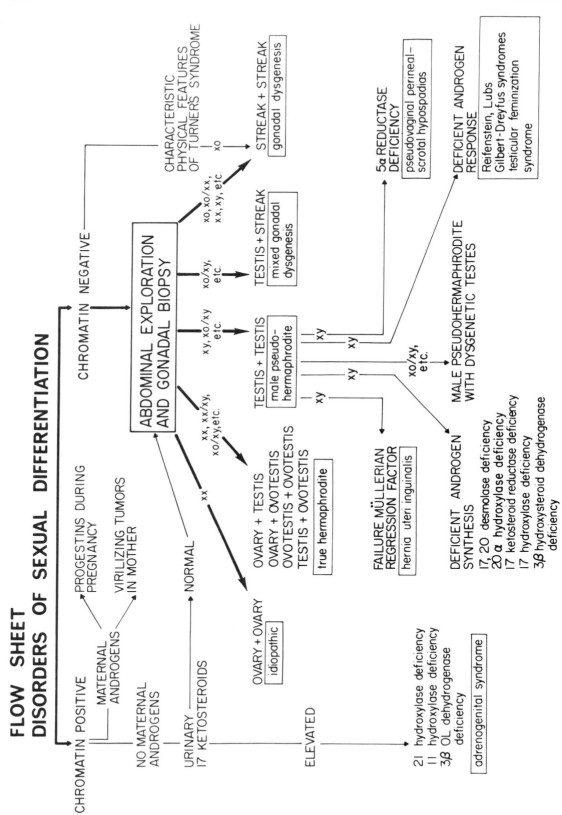

Figure 11–10. Disorders of sexual differentiation. (From Allen, T. D.: Disorders of sexual differentiation.

17-ketosteroids to identify the adrenogenital syndromes. Genitography is often of use at this point, for this may demonstrate the presence of internal müllerian structures in an infant who externally has predominantly masculine genitalia. If a diagnosis of adrenal hyperplasia is not established, it is then likely that one is dealing with either true hermaphroditism or mixed gonadal dysgenesis. These latter conditions require laparoscopy or abdominal exploration with gonadal biopsy for establishment of a firm diagnosis. If the patient's buccal smear is chromatin-negative or if the karyotype is XY, one may be dealing with a severe form of hypospadias, the 49 XY variant of Klinefelter's syndrome, true hermaphroditism, or mixed gonadal dysgenesis. Here again, abdominal exploration (or laparoscopy) and gonadal biopsy may be indicated.

Regardless of the underlying diagnosis, there are certain overriding principles of management of both the psyche and the genitalia. The most important factor in sexuality is probably the sex of rearing; this must immediately be established. If the patient is initially seen after 18 to 24 months of age, the sex of rearing cannot readily be reassigned; sex assignment should be changed after a few months of age in only the most unusual of circumstances. Consequently, in patients with ambiguous genitalia, it is very important to establish the sex of rearing conclusively prior to hospital discharge. The elements that enter into such a decision include (1) the patient's potential for fertility, (2) the potential that the gonads that are present will produce normal endogenous hormones so that exogenous hormones need not be administered, and (3) the potential for adequate sexual function in whichever sexual role is chosen. Specifically, in the male an adequate phallus is required for potency. The phallic adequacy of a neonate with ambiguous genitalia is a decision best made by a surgeon with experience in genital reconstruction and should not be made arbitrarily by someone with little appreciation of the surgical possibilities (Chap. 9). Such decisions are best made by a team that includes, at a minimum, a pediatric endocrinologist and a pediatric urologist. Unilateral decisions of this type are often fraught with hazard.

REFERENCES

Alvarez, M. N., Cloutier, M. D., and Hayles, A. B.: Male pseudohermaphroditism due to 17-α hydroxylase deficiency in two siblings. Pediatr. Res., 7:325, 1973.

Bongiovanni, A. M.: Unusual steroid pattern in congenital adrenal hyperplasia. J. Clin. Endocrinol. Metab., 21:860, 1961.

Brook, C. G. D., Wagner, H., and Zachman, M.: Familial occurrence of persistent Müllerian structures in otherwise normal males. Br. Med. J., 1:771, 1973.

Carr, D. H.: Cytogenetic aspects of induced and spontaneous abortions. Clin. Obstet. Gynecol., 15:203, 1972.

Cloutier, M. D., and Hayles, A. B.: Intersex and related disorders. In Kelalis, P. P., King, L. R., and Belman, A. B.: Clinical Pediatric Urology. Philadelphia, W. B. Saunders Co., 1976.

Cunningham, M. D., and Ragsdale, J. L.: Genital anomalies of an XXXXY male subject. J. Urol., 107:872, 1972.

Davidoff, F., and Federman, D. D.: Mixed gonadal dysgenesis. Pediatrics, 52:725, 1973.

Gandy, N. M., Keutmann, E. H., and Izzo, A. J.: Characterization of urinary steroids in adrenal hyperplasia. J. Clin. Invest., 39:364, 1960.

Jacobs, P. A., and Strong, J. A.: A case of human intersexuality having a possible XXY sex-determinant mechanism. Nature, 183:302, 1959.

Jones, H. W., Jr., and Scott, W. W.: Hermaphroditism, Genital Anomalies and Related Endocrine Disorders, 2nd ed. Baltimore, Williams and Wilkins, 1971.

Jost, A.: The role of fetal hormones in prenatal development. Harvey Lect., 55:201, 1960.

Keenan, B. S., Meyer, W. J., Hadjian, M. J., Jones, H. W., and Migeon, C. J.: Syndrome of androgen insensitivity in man. J. Clin. Endocrinol. Metab., 38:1143, 1974.

Klinefelter, H. F., Jr., Reifenstein, E. C., Jr., and Albright, F.: Syndrome characterized by gynecomastia, aspermatogenesis without A-Leydigism and increased excretion of follicle-stimulating hormone. J. Clin. Endocrinol., 2:615, 1942.

Marks, J. F., and Fink, C. W.: Incidence of salt losing form of congenital adrenal hyperplasia. Pediatrics, 43:636, 1969.

Morris, J. M.: The syndrome of testicular feminization in male pseudohermaphrodites. Am. J. Obstet. Gynecol., 65:1192, 1953.

Nakashima, T., and Robinson, A.: Fertility in a 45X female. Pediatrics, 47:770, 1971.

Noonan, J. A.: Hypertelorism with Turner phenotype: A new syndrome with associated congenital heart disease. Am. J. Dis. Child., 116:373, 1968.

Persky, L., and Cowens, R.: Genitourinary tract abnormalities in Turner's syndrome (gonadal dysgenesis). J. Urol., 105:309, 1971.

Prader, A., and Anders, G.: Quoted by Allen, T. D.: Disorders of sexual differentiation. Urology (Suppl.), 7:1, 1976.

Schellhas, H. F.: Malignant potential of the dysgenetic gonad. Obstet. Gynecol., *44*:455, 1974.

Simpson, J. L., New, M., Peterson, R. E., and German, J.: Pseudovaginal perineoscrotal hypospadias in sibs. Birth Defects, *7*:140, 1971.

Sohval, A. R.: The syndrome of pure gonadal dysgenesis. Am. J. Med., *38*:615, 1965.

Turner, H. H.: A syndrome of infantilism, congenital webbed neck, and cubitus valgus. Endocrinology, *23*:566, 1938.

Ullrich, D.: Turner's syndrome and status Bonnevie-Ullrich. Am. J. Hum. Genet., *1*:179, 1949.

Wachtel, S. S.: H-Y antigen and the genetics of sex determination. Science, *198*:797, 1975.

Wilson, J. D., Harrod, M. J., Goldstein, J. L., et al.: Familial incomplete male pseudohermaphroditism, type 1: Evidence for the androgen resistance and variable clinical manifestations in a family with the Reifenstein syndrome. N. Engl. J. Med., *290*:1097, 1974.

Chapter Twelve

DEVELOPMENTAL ABNORMALITIES OF THE KIDNEY AND URINARY COLLECTING SYSTEM

BILATERAL RENAL AGENESIS

Urinary output during fetal life plays an important role in fetal development. The infant born with bilateral renal agenesis not only has the characteristic facial appearance of a flattened nose, receding chin, wide interpupillary space, and large, low-set ears (Fig. 12–1) described by Potter (1946) but also may have pulmonary hypoplasia. Other abnormalities relating to the genitourinary tract, lower spine, and lower intestinal tract are often concurrently present. Obviously, total renal agenesis is incompatible with life.

Causes of renal agenesis include failure of formation of the urogenital ridge (a most rare occurrence also resulting in failure of ipsilateral internal genital formation), failure of budding of the ureter, absence of the nephrogenic blastema, and failure of renal vascularization. In the latter two circumstances, some degree of distal ureteral formation may be evident.

Absence of any urinary output during the first 24 hours of life is more commonly caused by poor fluid intake, acute tubular necrosis secondary to a period of neonatal hypotension, or severe obstruction. In chil-dren with urinary tract obstruction, one would expect to note a palpable mass, either the bladder in a boy with posterior urethral valves or one or both kidneys in the child with distal ureteral or ureteropelvic junction obstruction.

The diagnosis of renal agenesis is best established by angiography through an um-

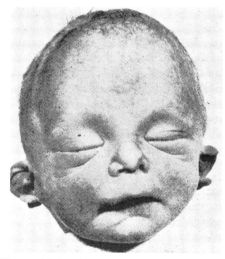

Figure 12–1.   Characteristic appearance of infants with bilateral renal agenesis (the Potter facies). (From Potter, E. L.: Facial characteristics of infants with bilateral renal agenesis. Am. J. Obstet. Gynecol., 51:885–888, 1946.)

225

bilical artery catheter. Renal arteries will not be present. Excretory urograms and isotope renal scans are not diagnostic in this situation since failure of function of existing kidneys can also produce complete non-visualization. Ultrasonography in the neonate may be worthwhile for delineating masses but may not offer sufficiently sensitive resolution in the tiny baby to exclude absolutely the presence of very small kidneys.

Survival in these infants can be distressingly prolonged. Unless death occurs from failure of some other organ system, they may survive for several days. The high incidence of other associated urinary tract anomalies and the extremely poor results of transplantation or dialysis in this age group obviate serious consideration for these procedures.

UNILATERAL RENAL AGENESIS

Unless associated with some other abnormality or condition leading to urologic evaluation, the diagnosis of unilateral renal agenesis is not likely to be made in the neonate since it is unassociated with symptoms. Its incidence is in the general range of 1:500 to 1000 (Longo and Thompson, 1952). Although a single kidney is adequate for a normal life span, congenital absence of one renal unit may suggest a higher incidence of disease in the remaining kidney. Emanuel and colleagues (1974) reviewed a series of 74 children with known unilateral agenesis. Five died within the neonatal period, and one third required surgical procedures on the remaining solitary unit. However, this series was gleaned from hospital records and is therefore biased.

Nonurologic abnormalities are frequently associated with unilateral renal agenesis. It is the commonest nonskeletal anomaly seen in children with supralevator imperforate anus (Belman and King, 1972) and is often associated with congenital scoliosis.

If suspected, screening can be carried out most safely with ultrasonography. Confirmation can be obtained by isotope renal scan to rule out ectopia.

The solitary kidney becomes stimulat-ed to hypertrophy, after birth. When one notes an apparently solitary kidney that is not hypertrophied in an older child (beyond six months of age), one should suspect that the contralateral kidney, rather than being absent, is acutely injured and nonfunctioning.

One of the questions frequently asked of the physician caring for a child with a solitary kidney refers to the need for limitation of physical activity, such as athletics. There are no conclusive data to support any absolute position; however, our rule of thumb is to allow these children to lead normal lives; however, we discourage their participation in contact sports.

SUPERNUMERARY KIDNEYS

Many people confuse duplication of the urinary collecting system, a common abnormality (p. 230), with the presence of an additional or supernumerary kidney. The presence of a third, separate kidney is one of the rarest urologic anomalies. The ureter from a supernumerary kidney may join the ureter of the normal ipsilateral kidney or separately may pass directly into the urinary bladder. The presence of a supernumerary kidney would be picked up as an incidental finding unless it was palpated as a mass. Its significance would depend upon any associated pathologic condition.

MALROTATION

Renal malrotation is in actuality renal nonrotation. The malrotated kidney, although normally positioned in the flank, maintains its fetal orientation with the pelvis directed anteriorly. This has no clinical significance unless aberrant vessels or bands interfere with normal urinary drainage.

RENAL FUSION

The most common form of renal fusion is the horseshoe kidney, in which the lower poles are fused in the midline. However, a variety of forms of horseshoe kidney exist

(Fig. 12–2). The horseshoe kidney deformity does not generally cause symptoms, although it may come to clinical attention as a midline abdominal mass that transmits the aortic pulse.

Owing to their location and subsequent intimate relationship with the bony spine, fused kidneys are more susceptible to trauma. Additionally, ureteropelvic junction obstruction secondary to abnormally located renal vessels is not uncommon.

RENAL ECTOPIA

The presence of a kidney in an abnormal position often presents itself as an abdominal mass. In older children, minimal

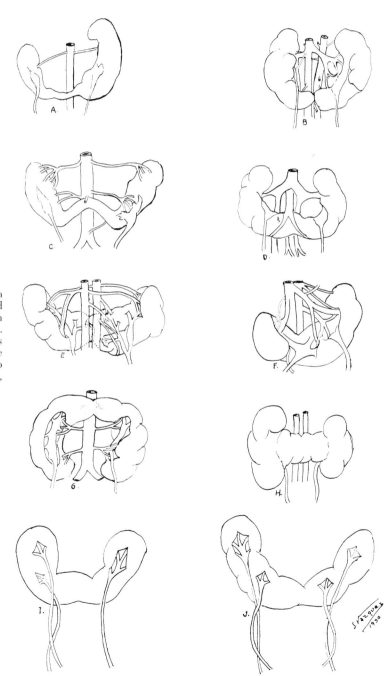

Figure 12–2. Variations in the shape of horseshoe kidneys and the number of their ureters. (From Benjamin, J. A., and Schullian, D. M.: Observations on fused kidneys with horseshoe configuration: The contribution of Leonardo Botallo (1564). J. Hist. Med., 5:315–326, 1950.)

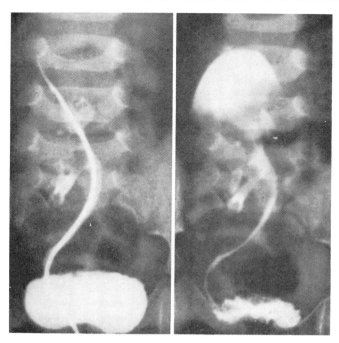

Figure 12–3. Retrograde pyeloureterograms, showing catheter penetration of unsuspected right ectopic pelvic kidney (left) and extensive subcapsular collection of contrast medium (right). The position of this ectopic kidney directly over the spinal column makes it highly susceptible to trauma. (Bellevue Hospital.) (From Kelalis, P. P., King, L. R., and Belman, A. B.: Clinical Pediatric Urology, Vol. 2. Philadelphia, W. B. Saunders Co., 1976, p. 1040.)

trauma may lead to hematuria (Fig. 12–3). Additionally, vesicoureteral reflux and ureteropelvic junction obstruction are frequently found in this group (Fig. 12–4).

The most common site of renal ectopia is in the true bony pelvis. Oftentimes it is radiographically difficult to appreciate the presence of a kidney in this location since adjacent bones and the urinary bladder obscure visualization. The isotope renal scan is extremely useful in making this determination (Fig. 12–5).

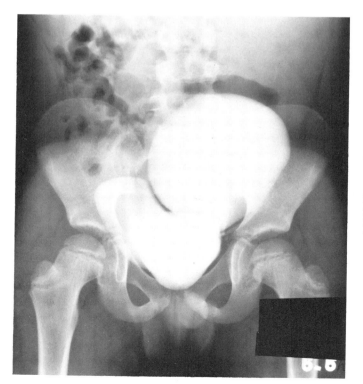

Figure 12–4. Pelvic kidney with hydronephrosis secondary to high insertion of ureter into pelvis. (From Kelalis, P. P., King, L. R., and Belman, A. B.: Clinical Pediatric Urology, Vol. 1. Philadelphia, W. B. Saunders Co., 1976, p. 484.)

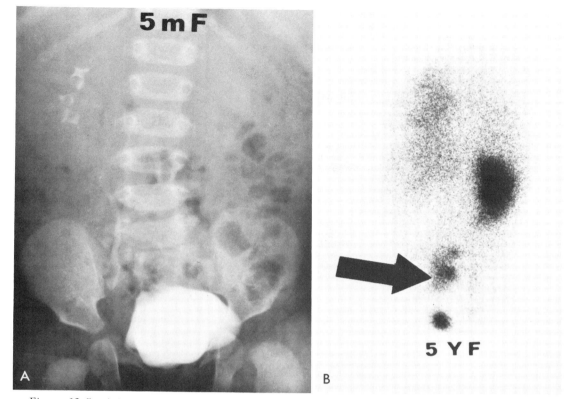

Figure 12–5. *A*, Excretory urogram in a five-month-old girl. Interpretation: solitary kidney. *B*, Posterior view renal scan in the same child at five years of age following discovery of a lower abdominal mass. The pelvic kidney is obvious (arrow), and, retrospectively, calices can be seen in the true pelvis in *A*.

In girls, a consistent relationship has been found between the solitary pelvic kidney and other anomalies. This has been referred to as the MURCS association (Duncan et al., 1979). The association includes müllerian duct aplasia, consisting clinically of vaginal and uterine agenesis, renal ectopia, and cervicothoracic vertebral anomalies.

Another form of ectopia is the crossed fused ectopic kidney (Fig. 12–6). The parenchyma of the two kidneys are confluent; however, the collecting systems remain separate. The crossed kidney is generally lower than the one normally situated.

There is no specific treatment for renal ectopy; however, recognition of abnormally placed kidneys carries with it the responsibility for determining that no additional pathologic condition exists. Patients and families should be forewarned regarding the increased risk of obstruction and renal trauma, and appropriate treatment must be provided if either should occur.

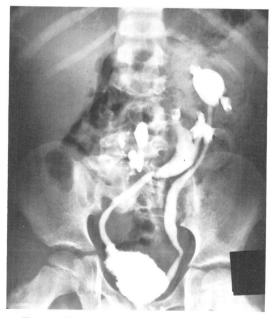

Figure 12–6. Crossed renal ectopy with fusion. The contrast medium in the midline is from a previous myelogram. (From Kelalis, P. P., King, L. R., and Belman, A. B.: Clinical Pediatric Urology, Vol. 1. Philadelphia, W. B. Saunders Co., 1976, p. 488.)

DUPLICATION OF THE URINARY COLLECTING SYSTEM

When two separate ureteral buds arise from the wolffian duct, complete duplication of the urinary collecting system results (Fig. 12–7). This is one of the most common genitourinary developmental aberrations. Complete duplication exists in about 1 in 500 persons (Campbell, 1951). Somewhere

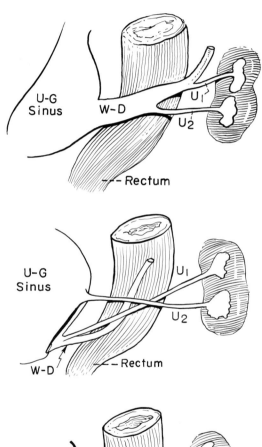

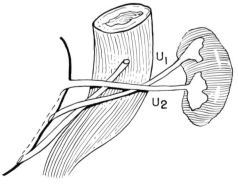

Figure 12–7.   Development of duplicated collecting system; two ureters (U₁ and U₂) are seen to bud from the wolffian duct (W-D). (From Kelalis, P. P., King, L. R., and Belman, A. B.: Clinical Pediatric Urology, Vol. 1. Philadelphia, W. B. Saunders Co., 1976, p. 510.)

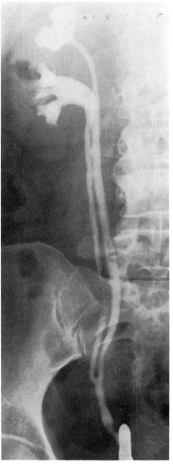

Figure 12–8.   Bulb pyeloureterogram. The junction of incompletely duplicated ureters is well shown to be just above the bladder. (From Witten, D. M., Myers, G. H., and Utz, D. C.: Emmett's Clnical Urography, Vol. 2, 4th ed. Philaelphia, W. B. Saunders Co., 1977, p. 648.)

between one fourth to one third of the duplications are bilateral. There appears to be a greater incidence of duplication in females than in males, and a familial propensity for duplication apparently exists (Whitaker and Danks, 1966).

Incomplete duplication of the collecting system results when the ureter bifurcates after its original budding. The extent of incomplete duplication can range from paired ureters that join just extravesically (Fig. 12–8) to a bifid renal collecting system (Fig. 12–9).

Duplication of the collecting system, either complete or incomplete, does not intrinsically suggest a uropathologic condition. Of itself, duplication is not responsible

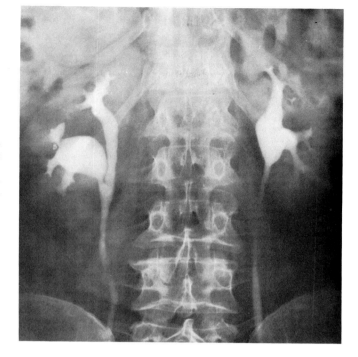

Figure 12–9. Excretory urogram. Y-type duplication of right ureter. There is dilatation of both forks above the stem. (From Witten, D. M., Myers, G. H., and Utz, D. C.: Emmett's Clinical Urography, Vol. 2, 4th ed. Philadelphia, W. B. Saunders Co., 1977, p. 653.)

URETER DUPLICATION
reflux and ectopy

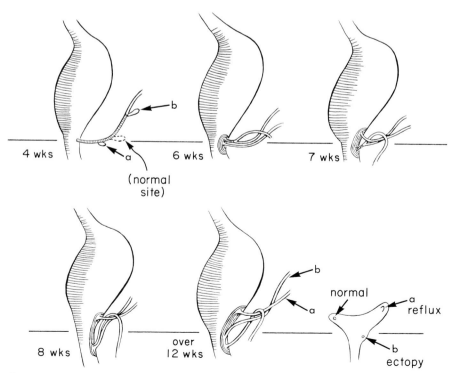

Figure 12–10. Simplified drawing of ectopic orifice position associated with abnormal budding of the ureter. When the takeoff of the ureteral bud (a) is more medial than normal, the ultimate position of the orifice is more lateral and more likely to reflux. (From Harrison, J. H., Gittes, R. F., Perlmutter, A. D., et al.: Campbell's Urology, Vol. 2, 4th ed. Philadelphia, W. B. Saunders Co., 1979, p. 1357.)

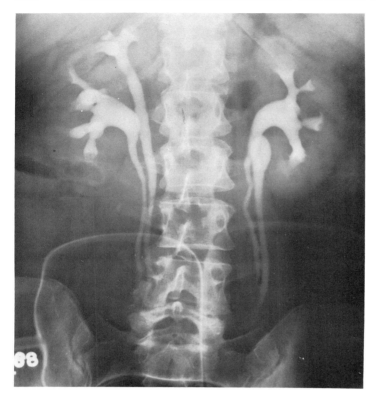

Figure 12–11. Excretory urogram. Retrograde peristalsis up blind-ending duplicated left ureter. Junction of ureters is at left of transverse process of L5. the blind-ending segment has been filled by retrograde flow of urine. (From Witten, D. M., Myers, G. H., and Utz, D. C.: Emmett's Clinical Urography, Vol. 2, 4th ed. Phiĺadephia, W. B. Saunders Co., 1977, p. 649.)

Figure 12–12. Surgical treatment of ureteroureteral reflux (yo-yo peristalsis). (From Kelalis, P. P., King, L. R., and Belman, A. B.: Clinical Pediatric Urology, Vol. 1. Philadelphia, W. B. Saunders Co., 1976, p. 507.)

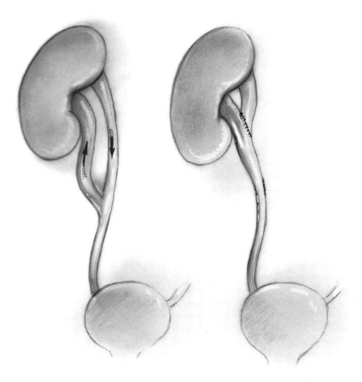

for urinary tract infection. However, certain pathologic situations are predictably associated with duplication. These are explainable embryologically.

Following ureteral budding from the wolffian (mesonephric) duct, both the distal duct and the distal ureter become incorporated into the bladder base. In the presence of complete ureteral duplication, the two ureters must by necessity become crossed. The result is a reversed relationship between the renal poles and their respective ureteral orifices: The upper pole ureteral orifice is lower on the bladder base than the orifice to the lower pole ureter (Fig. 12–10). This is referred to as the Weigert-Meyer law. The result is that vesicoureteral reflux tends to occur more commonly into the lower renal pole (see Fig. 4–10), although reflux may be present into both ureters of a duplicated system; when obstruction exists, it almost always affects the upper renal segment.

PARTIAL DUPLICATION OF THE COLLECTING SYSTEM

Incomplete duplication is rarely of clinical significance. Occasionally, stasis secondary to yo-yo peristalsis, that is, the to-and-fro flow of urine up and down the ureteral limbs, results in urinary tract infection (Fig. 12–11). Excision of the redundant ureter with a high ureteroureterostomy or ureteropyelostomy is the treatment of choice (Fig. 12–12).

BLIND-ENDING URETERAL DUPLICATION

Rarely, one limb of a duplicated system does not have any associated renal parenchyma, ending blindly (Fig. 12–13). Stasis may then result, and if it is associated with urinary tract infection, it may assume clinical significance. However, confirmation of the presence of bacteria in the ipsilateral

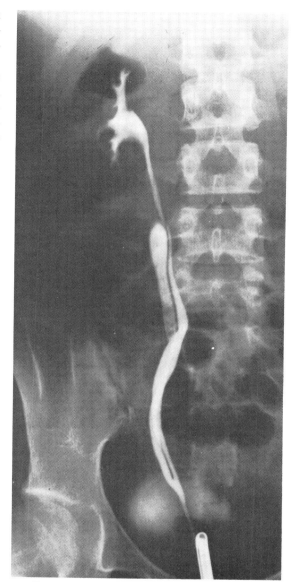

Figure 12–13. Retrograde pyelogram. Blind-ending duplication in an 18-year-old girl noted in evaluation of transitory hematuria. Only the distal portion of this blind-ending duplication had been visualized on IVP. (From Harrison, J. H., Gittes, R. F., Perlmutter, A. D., et al.: Campbells's Urology, Vol. 2, 4th ed. Philadelphia, W. B. Saunders Co., 1979, p. 1364.)

upper urinary tract by culturing urine collected from that system by ureteral catheterization is mandatory prior to surgical excision. Stasis in a blind-ending duplicated ureter or, for that matter, any portion of a dilated renal collecting system is not an explanation for bacteriuria confined to the bladder.

SUPERNUMERARY URETERS

Triplication of the ureter is very rare. When associated with obstruction or reflux, its management is similar to that of duplication.

VESICOURETERAL REFLUX AND DUPLICATION OF THE COLLECTING SYSTEM

The problem of reflux and duplication differs little from reflux into a single system. The reader is referred to Chapter 4 for a discussion of reflux.

The management of reflux in the duplicated system varies only in that the likelihood for the reflux to resolve spontaneously is apparently markedly reduced. Our clinical approach to the problem remains the same; that is, the decision to operate is made on the radiographic and endoscopic findings as well as the ability to prevent urinary tract infections. More often than is the case with single systems, however, the orifice to the refluxing lower renal pole ureter is more laterally located and has a significantly shortened submucosal tunnel.

Technically, the actual surgical procedure differs only in that the refluxing lower ureter as well as its ipsilateral mate, which shares a common vascular sheath, are by necessity implanted together. An alternative maneuver is to excise the refluxing ureter and to perform a high ureteroureterostomy to allow drainage entirely through the nonrefluxing upper renal segment ureter.

URETERAL ECTOPIA

When a ureter terminates anywhere other than at its anticipated trigonal position, it is considered to be ectopic. Ureteral ectopia is most frequently found in association with duplication of the collecting system and, corresponding to the Weigert-Meyer law, the upper renal segment ureter is inevitably the ectopic system (Fig. 12–10). The termination of the ectopic orifice may be anywhere in the genitourinary system in girls (Fig. 12–14); however, it is never found distal to the urogenital diaphragm in boys (Fig. 12–15).

Ectopia beyond the bladder neck may result in ureteral obstruction, urinary incontinence, or both. Obstruction is generally brought to clinical attention when a child with a urinary tract infection is radiographically evaluated. A peculiar type of incontinence occurs in girls who have an ectopic ureter outside the urinary tract, that is, at the introitus or in the vagina. Because the ureter is outside the bladder, these girls tend to be moist all the time, yet give a history of normal voiding habits. This is

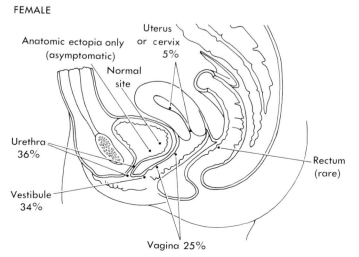

Figure 12–14. Sites of ureteral ectopia and their incidence in females. (From Gray, S. W., and Skandalakis, J. E.: Embryology for Surgeons. Philadelphia, W. B. Saunders Co., 1972, p. 536.)

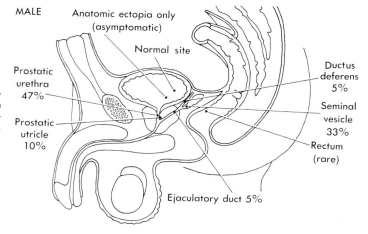

Figure 12–15. Sites of ureteral ectopia and their incidence in males. (From Gray, S. W., and Skandalakis, J. E.: Embryology for Surgeons. Philadelphia, W. B. Saunders Co., 1972, p. 536.)

termed paradoxical incontinence (Fig. 12–16).

Single system ureteral ectopia is rare. It produces varying degrees of hydroureteronephrosis and may or may not be associated with enuresis. When bilateral single ureteral ectopia occurs, the bladder develops poorly, lacking the in utero stimulus of filling.

URETEROCELES

Ureteroceles are cystic dilatations of the distal ureter within the bladder, urethra,

or both (Fig. 12–17). Two types exist; the simple type is infrequently seen in children and is usually nonobstructive. Simple ureteroceles usually affect single, not duplicated, systems, and morbidity is most often related to stone formation within the ureterocele. Treatment in the absence of a specific documented secondary pathologic condition is not required.

The more complex ectopic ureteroceles affect the ureter to the upper renal pole of a

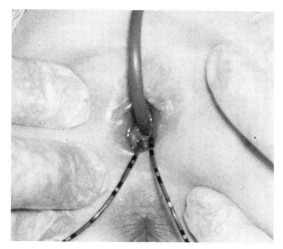

Figure 12–16. Ureteral catheters (seen coming inferiorly) entering ectopic orifices outside the urethra (Foley catheter identifies urethra). (From Kelalis, P. P., King, L. R., and Belman, A. B.: Clinical Pediatric Urology, Vol. 1. Philadelphia, W. B. Saunders Co., 1976, p. 519.)

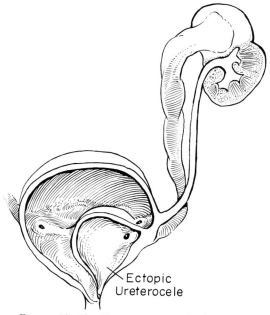

Figure 12–17. Ectopic ureterocele. (From Malek, R. S., Kelalis, P. P., Burke, E. C., et al.: Simple and ectopic ureterocele in infancy and childhood. Surg. Gynecol. Obstet., *134*:611–616, 1972. By permission of Surgery, Gynecology and Obstetrics.)

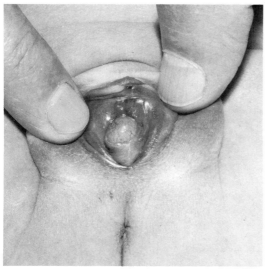

Figure 12–18. Prolapsing ureterocele. (From Kelalis, P. P., King, L. R., and Belman A. B.: Clinical Pediatric Urology, Vol. 1. Philadelphia, W. B. Saunders Co., 1976, p. 526.)

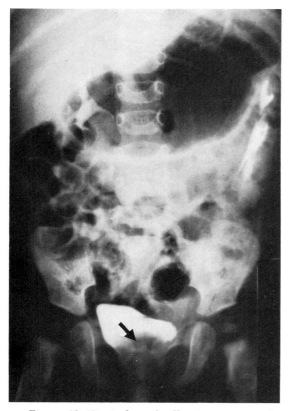

Figure 12–19. Left renal collecting system markedly distorted and laterally deviated. This picture is typical of neuroblastoma. However, note filling defect (arrow) in bladder. Child had duplication of left collecting system with obstructed upper segment secondary to a ureterocele. Massive dilatation of upper renal segment is responsible for distortion of visualized segment.

duplicated system. Just as in other ectopic ureters, ectopic ureteroceles tend to be obstructive and are recognized when a child is evaluated for urinary tract infection. Occasionally, girls present with prolapse of a ureterocele through the urethra (Fig. 12–18). This may totally obstruct the bladder outlet and cause bilateral hydroureteronephrosis. Theoretically, one might confuse a prolapsed ureterocele with either urethral prolapse or prolapsed sarcoma botryoides, although each has its own peculiar appearance. Urinary incontinence is rarely associated with a ureterocele.

The diagnosis of ureterocele can generally be made by excretory urography alone. The nonvisualizing obstructed upper renal segment pushes the normally functioning lower segment inferolaterally. This picture might be confused with the radiographic appearance of a suprarenal neuroblastoma if the filling defect of the intravesical ureterocele is not appreciated (Fig. 12–19). Additionally, most of these children have urinary tract infections, a presenting complaint uncommonly seen with neuroblastoma.

Excision of the upper renal segment and its involved ureter is the treatment of choice. The associated renal segment is often dysplastic. An argument exists as to whether the ureterocele itself must be excised (Hendren and Monfort, 1971) or whether it can be left intact following drainage of its contents (Belman et al, 1974). All agree, however, that total nephrectomy with sacrifice of the lower renal segment, which is often normal or affected only by mild reflux, is inappropriate. Additionally, transurethral incision or resection of the ureterocele without attention being paid to the upper system replaces obstruction with massive reflux. This mode of therapy must be applied only in the most unusual circumstance since it creates the necessity for further surgical treatment in the future.

REFERENCES

Belman, A. B., Filmer, R. B., and King, L. R.: Surgical management of duplication of the collecting system. J. Urol., 112:316, 1974.

Belman, A. B., and King, L. R.: Urinary abnormalities associated with imperforate anus. J. Urol., *108*:832, 1972.

Campbell, M. F.: Embryology and anomalies of the urogenital tract. *In* Clinical Pediatric Urology, Philadelphia, W. B. Saunders Co., 1951.

Duncan, P. A., Shapiro, L. R., Stangel, J. J., et al.: The MURCS association: Müllerian duct aplasia, renal aplasia, and cervicothoracic somite dysplasia. J. Pediatr., *95*:399, 1979.

Emanuel, B., Nachman, R., Aronson, N., et al.: Congenital solitary kidney: A review of 74 cases. Am. J. Dis. Child., *127*:17, 1974.

Hendren, W. H., and Monfort, G. J.: Surgical correction of ureteroceles in childhood. J. Pediatr. Surg., *6*:235, 1971.

Longo, V. J., and Thompson, G. J.: Congenital solitary kidney. J. Urol., *68*:63, 1952.

Potter, E. L.: Facial characteristics of infants with bilateral renal agenesis. Am. J. Obstet. Gynecol., *51*:885, 1946.

Whitaker, J., and Danks, D. M.: A study of the inheritance of duplication of the kidneys and ureters. J. Urol., *95*:176, 1966.

Chapter Thirteen

BLADDER EXSTROPHY, CLOACAL EXSTROPHY, AND IMPERFORATE ANUS

Bladder Exstrophy

Exstrophy of the bladder is one of the most catastrophic of congenital urinary tract abnormalities because it presents formidable anatomic and psychosocial problems for which there are only limited solutions. Children afflicted with exstrophy and left untreated are plagued by a lifetime of incontinence, discomfort, and social ostracism; despite this, exstrophy itself is compatible with life (MacFarland et al., 1979). Exstrophy is really a spectrum of abnormalities in which there may be defects in the abdominal wall, umbilicus, pubis, bladder, genitalia, and intestines. The incidence of exstrophy in the general population varies from one affected individual per 10,000 to 50,000 live births (Jeffs, 1979). Males are affected twice as frequently as females. The abnormality does not seem genetically determined, although a few familial instances have been reported.

EMBRYOLOGY

Exstrophy is embryologically unusual in that it is not the result of an arrest of normal development as are most congenital abnormalities (Figs. 13–1 and 13–2). There is no stage of normal embryogenesis that resembles the exstrophic condition. Patton and Barry have theorized that exstrophy occurs because the primordium of the genital tubercle arises more caudally than normally and, in addition, fails to migrate ventrally. The genital tubercle then fuses in this position and prevents the cloacal membrane from regressing. The cloacal membrane remains on the lower abdominal wall, interfering with the normal invasion of mesoderm. When the cloacal membrane ruptures, it then leaves a defect in the lower abdominal wall. Muecke (1964) has proposed instead that the cause of exstrophy lies in the cloacal membrane itself. If the cloacal membrane arises too far ventrally, it prevents mesodermal invasion with the same end result as previously described. He has experimentally produced this deficit in chick embryos by placing a millipore filter in the midline of the lower abdominal wall. When the chicks hatched, the resulting lesion was identical to that seen in cloacal exstrophy. Johnston and Kogan (1974) have postulated that exstrophy arises merely as a result of a delay of mesodermal invasion.

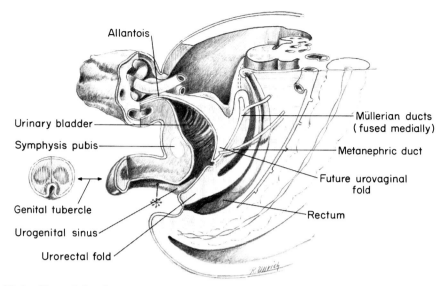

Figure 13–1. Normal development of the embryo at the eighth gestational week. The urethral groove (*) is ventrally placed. Note that the genital tubercle and phallus are dorsal to the urogenital sinus. The allantois has begun to obliterate at its umbilical end. (From Kelalis, P. P., King, L. R., and Belman, A. B.: Clinical Pediatric Urology, Vol. 1. Philadelphia, W. B. Saunders Co., 1976, p. 544.)

RENAL CHANGES ASSOCIATED WITH EXSTROPHY

In exstrophy patients, concomitant renal abnormalities per se are unusual. The most common of the kidney abnormalities seen in association with exstrophy are unilateral renal agenesis and horseshoe kidneys (Engel, 1973). Hydronephrosis is not usually present at birth in patients with exstrophy but does occur with some frequency thereafter, either spontaneously or

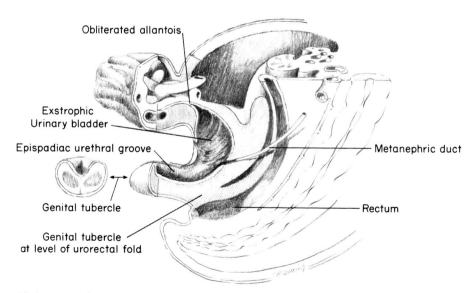

Figure 13–2. Sagittal section of an embryo with exstrophy during the eighth week of gestation. The anterior bladder wall is exstrophic, and the urethral groove is epispadiac. The genital tubercle is ventral and posterior to the urethral groove. (From Kelalis, P. P., King, L. R., and Belman, A. B.: Clinical Pediatric Urology, Vol. 1. Philadelphia, W. B. Saunders Co., 1976, p. 545.)

as a result of treatment (Williams, 1969). There is a mistaken notion in modern urologic literature that untreated exstrophy patients do not succumb to renal failure and that all hydronephrotic changes seen are complications of treatment. However, if one refers to the older urologic literature, one notes that approximately 50 per cent of patients with exstrophy had died by age 10, while two thirds had died by age 20 —mostly untreated patients (Hinman, 1935). If hydronephrosis occurs in untreated children, it is usually secondary to urinary tract infection or to local problems at the ureteral orifices, presumably due to inflammation or obstruction brought about by bladder irritation. After treatment, it could be due to infection, vesicoureteral reflux, or urinary outflow obstruction.

After functional closure of an exstrophic bladder, reflux occurs in approximately 85 per cent of patients unless specific measures for its prevention are employed. The ureter enters the exstrophic bladder at an abnormal angle such that reflux easily

occurs should the bladder actually store any urine (Chap. 4). Even without hydronephrosis present, the lower ureter of the exstrophy patient is frequently dilated in a characteristic manner (Fig. 13–3). This dilatation, however, is thought to be of no functional significance (Lattimer and Smith, 1966).

BLADDER CHANGES

The exstrophic bladder, in addition to being exteriorized, is abnormal in other ways. Both acute and chronic inflammatory changes are seen in the mucosa. Seventy-five per cent of patients with exstrophy develop squamous metaplasia, which can be present as early as two weeks after birth. Cystitis cystica or cystitis glandularis occurs in two thirds of these patients. These changes in the vesical mucosa may persist after closure so that exteriorization itself is presumably not the only cause (Culp, 1964). However, whether this is due to an intrinsic abnormality of the bladder mucosa or is a response to chronic irritation is not well documented. It is estimated that patients with exstrophy are 200 times more likely to develop a tumor of the bladder than are normal patients; adenocarcinomas are the histopathologic type most commonly seen (Engel and Wilkinson, 1970). Such tumors usually arise after the third decade of life in patients who have not had their bladders closed and are quite uncommon in those exstrophic bladders that are functionally closed. Two patients, each with adenocarcinoma and rhabdomyosarcoma of closed bladders, have been reported (Johnston and Kogan, 1974).

Just as the mucosa of the exstrophic bladder is abnormal, so is its muscle, which is often fibrotic and disorganized. The musculature of the pelvic floor is also abnormal. Because the pubic symphysis is absent and the pelvis is incomplete, these muscles are arranged in a semicircular rather than circular fashion. Consequently, the muscles insert in the approximate area of the laterally displaced pubic tubercles rather than in the midline.

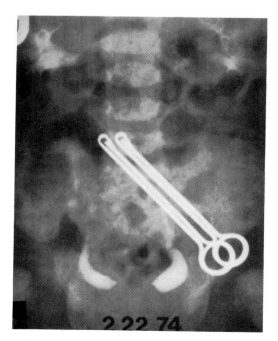

Figure 13–3. Excretory urogram of an untreated male infant with exstrophy. Note the widely separated pubes and the characteristic distal ureteral configuration. (From Kelalis, P. P., King, L. R., and Belman, A. B.: Clinical Pediatric Urology, Vol. 1. Philadelphia, W. B. Saunders Co., 1976, p. 547.)

GENITAL ABNORMALITIES

The external genitalia in both males and females are usually abnormal (Figs. 13–4 and 13–5). Epispadias is almost always a significant component of bladder exstrophy. In the male, the penis as well as the scrotum may be bifid or even duplicate. The scrotum is almost always anteriorly placed and quite broad and small, but after puberty it becomes more normally dependent. The prostate, although open ventrally, is itself normal; the verumontanum (utriculus masculinus) is intact, and ejaculation will occur, unless this structure is damaged consequent to surgical repair. The testes in most patients are intrinsically normal, although 40 per cent do have undescended testes.

In the female, the clitoris is usually bifid, and there is a dorsal separation of the labia majora and minora. In about two thirds of patients, the vaginal orifice is stenotic and may for this reason require revision. Rarely vaginal agenesis will occur. Vaginal duplications have also been reported. Fertility is possible in females with exstrophy, but at the time of delivery, there may be

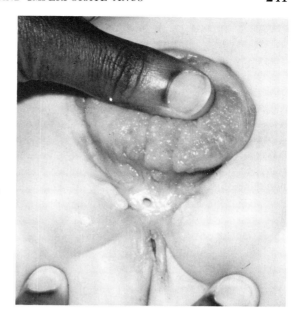

Figure 13–5. Female infant with exstrophy.

problems with genital prolapse, presumably because of the abnormal pelvic musculature.

In the male, the penile shaft is broad and tends to hug the anterior abdominal wall. The epispadiac urethra is dorsally rather than ventrally placed. The corpus spongiosum is absent. The ventral portion of the prepuce is present; however, its dorsal component is absent. Erections occur, but intromission in the untreated patient may be difficult because of the foreshortening and severe dorsal angulation of the penis.

OTHER ASSOCIATED ABNORMALITIES

The anus and rectum are abnormal in that they occupy a more ventral location than usual. Because the rectum passes through the pelvic floor musculature more anteriorly than normal, rectal prolapse is seen much more frequently in exstrophy patients than normal. This is especially true in girls.

Because the pubes are widely separat-

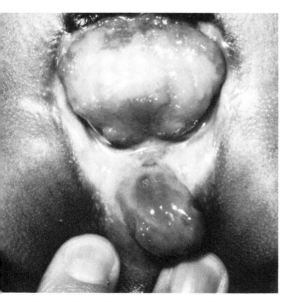

Figure 13–4. Newborn male with exstrophy. (From Kelalis, P. P., King, L. R., and Belman, A. B.: Clinical Pediatric Urology, Vol. 1. Philadelphia, W. B. Saunders Co., 1976, p. 547.)

ed, these children often have a waddling appearance to their gait. It has been suggested by some authors that this requires orthopedic correction in and of itself for normal ambulation. This is now known to be fallacious. We have studied several such patients using a computerized gait analysis and find their only deficit to be a degree of external rotation of no functional significance (Kaplan et al., 1980). Additionally, the appearance of the gait tends to improve with age.

Because the pubic symphysis is absent, the insertion of the rectus abdominus muscles tends to diverge laterally, leaving a midline defect that complicates attempts at bladder closure. In addition, inguinal hernias are much more common in patients with exstrophy than in the normal population. Because the rectus abdominus is abnormal, the repair of such hernias is dif-

ferent and often challenging. The umbilicus itself also tends to be low-set.

EXSTROPHY VARIANTS

In addition to the classic pictures of exstrophy and epispadias, there are some variants of this complex worthy of mention (Ignatoff et al., 1971). One has been termed pseudoexstrophy, in which the pubic symphysis is absent and the umbilicus is low-set (Fig. 13–6). Epispadias is not present in these children, but the scrotum tends to be broad and flat. Additionally, the scrotum and anus are both anteriorly placed. Another minor variation has been termed superior vesical fissure or fistula (Fig. 13–7). In this particular abnormality, there is a fistulous

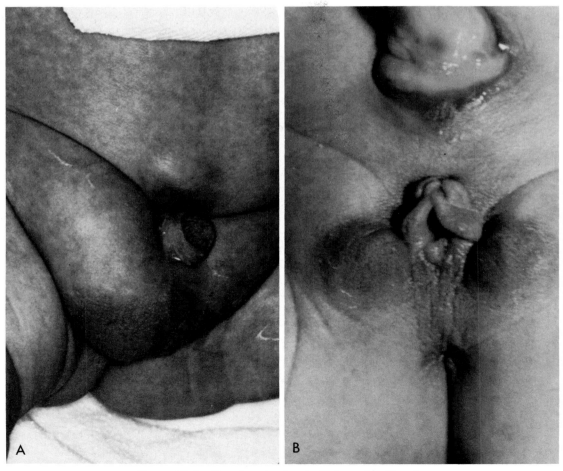

Figure 13–6. Pseudoexstrophy. A, Male, and B, Female.

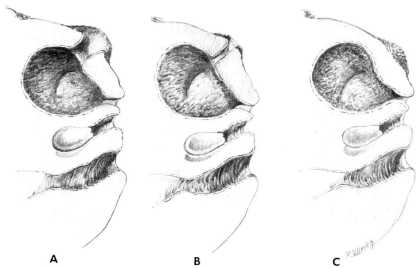

A   **B**   **C**

Figure 13–7. Exstrophy variants. *A,* Type A. Superior vesical fissure — a large opening between bladder and anterior abdominal wall. *B,* Type B. Superior vesical fistula — a small communication to the abdominal wall. *C,* Type C. Duplicate exstrophy — a mucosal disk having no communication with a completely closed and intra-abdominal bladder. (From Kelalis, P. P., King, L. R., and Belman, A. B.: Clinical Pediatric Urology, Vol. 1. Philadelphia, W. B. Saunders Co., 1976, p. 550.)

communication between the bladder and the anterior abdominal wall. The symphysis is usually split, and the rectus abdominus muscles tend to diverge. However, the pelvic floor is intact, and continence is usually present. The only treatment these children usually need is closure of the fistula or fissure. Since the bladder neck is intact, they will be rendered continent by such closure alone.

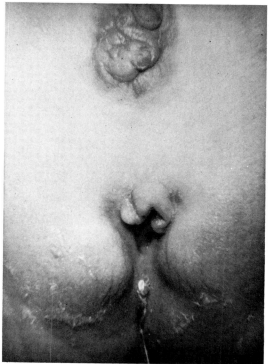

Figure 13–8. A girl with duplicate exstrophy. (From Kelalis, P. P., King, L. R., and Belman, A. B.: Clinical Pediatric Urology, Vol. 1. Philadelphia, W. B. Saunders Co., 1976, p. 550.)

Another minor variation that is important to recognize is duplicate exstrophy, in which the bladder itself is actually closed but there is a patch of bladder mucosa on the skin of the lower abdominal wall (Fig. 13–8). This abnormality is treated by simply excising this ectopic patch of mucosa. It is our opinion that this particular abnormality would best be termed ectopic vesical mucosa to distinguish it from its more serious cogeners.

TREATMENT

Primary Closure

In patients with the full-blown picture of exstrophy, there are several therapeutic options. These include no treatment, functional closure, or urinary diversion. Although no means of treatment is completely satisfactory, it is difficult to believe anyone in modern society would leave these children untreated, as their existence would then be miserable. The exstrophic bladder does cause discomfort, and, in addition, such patients are social outcasts. The concept of functional closure of the bladder is one that is quite attractive and is becoming increasingly more successful. In selected patients, recent reports have suggested success rates of just over 50 per cent (Jeffs, 1979).

Closure seems to be more satisfactory in females than in males. Early closure decreases the inflammatory changes in the bladder and may limit the degree of perimuscular fibrosis. The use of bilateral iliac osteotomies is an important adjunctive step, as it allows easier closure of the abdominal wall defect by enabling the pubes to be brought together. In the newborn the pelvic girdle is more malleable than it is in the older infant and approximation of the pubes can sometimes be achieved without osteotomy. It is for this reason that closure within 48 hours of birth has been recommended by some (Ansell, 1975).

At the time of initial closure, most modern authors do not feel that any attempt should be made to achieve continence.

Operations such as the Leadbetter modification of the Young-Dees operation that are designed to provide continence by lengthening the urethra in the region of the bladder outlet should be reserved for a later date at which time the results of such endeavors seem better. It is of interest that some patients who have had functional closure and initially are not continent will, at or about the time of puberty, become continent. The explanation for this observation is completely obscure, but one might speculate, at least in the male, that it relates to prostatic growth. In those children with untreated or unsuccessfully treated exstrophy, there is a high incidence of psychiatric problems, especially during the pubertal years. The incidence of suicide among boys with exstrophy who still have penile abnormalities is rather formidable.

Ureterosigmoidostomy

Because of the limited success rates of functional closure, particularly by those surgeons with less experience, many continue to prefer primary urinary diversion as treatment for this problem. Ureterosigmoidostomy is an operation that has been used for such purpose intermittently for the last 75 years (Chap. 8). Several long-term studies demonstrate conclusively that 50 per cent of patients with exstrophy so treated (by ureterosigmoidostomy) have survived, are continent, and have a normal upper urinary tract (Spence et al., 1975). It is for this reason that ureterosigmoidostomy still has many very vocal proponents. Lattimer has recently observed, however, that many "continent" ureterosigmoidostomy patients soil themselves to some degree (MacFarland et al., 1979). This operation certainly has the advantage of not requiring any external collecting devices.

Unfortunately, it has also become apparent with passing years that there is a propensity for tumor to arise at the site of ureteral implantation into the colon. The reasons for the problem are obscure, but it does require the mixture of urine and feces (Crissey et al., 1980). This propensity to oncogenesis continues even if urine is subsequently diverted away from this implantation site in the conversion of ureterosigmoidostomy to an ileal conduit. Whether tumors would still develop if the ureter were removed from the colon in toto when patients needed to abandon ureterosigmoid urinary diversion for some other procedure is moot. Nonetheless, patients with intact ureterosigmoidostomy should have frequent (perhaps annual) urography, for one of the earliest signs of such tumors is ureteral obstruction. Patients with abandoned ureterosigmoidostomy in whom portions of the ureter remain in the colonic wall probably should have yearly proctoscopy or colonoscopy. In both groups, rectal bleeding must be aggressively investigated.

A variation of ureterosigmoidostomy currently employed by Hendren (1976) is a two-stage approach. A colon conduit is constructed at a relatively young age, and the abdominal wall is repaired at that time. At a later date, when it can be proved that the child has anal continence, the colon conduit is converted surgically to a ureterosigmoidostomy. The advantage to this approach lies in the relatively early age at which "dryness" can be achieved. The disadvantage is the necessity for two operations.

A definite contraindication to ureterosigmoidostomy would seem to be hydronephrosis. It has been demonstrated time and again that the hydronephrotic upper urinary tract does not tolerate diversion into the intact intestinal tract. The long-term complications of ureterosigmoidostomy include pyelonephritis and hyperchloremic acidosis. Both of these problems are seen with some regularity in patients with hydronephrosis who have undergone ureterosigmoidostomy. It may unfortunately be necessary to abandon a well-functioning ureterosigmoidostomy because of either uncontrolled urinary tract infection and renal parenchymal loss or difficulties with hyperchloremic acidosis that cannot be controlled with bicarbonate management. Inasmuch as it is well known that acidosis is poorly tolerated by the growing child and interferes with somatic growth, it is of interest that there are no longitudinal studies available that document the growth of patients after ureterosigmoidostomy. It is a clinical impression, however, that these children do not grow as well as their nondiverted peers.

CUTANEOUS URINARY DIVERSION

Because ureterosigmoidostomy was associated with the problems just mentioned, many authors abandoned the procedure in favor of the ileal conduit urinary diversion. Unfortunately, long-term studies of patients after ileal conduit diversion have demonstrated that this operation, too, is not a panacea, for as many as 50 per cent of patients will show signs of renal deterioration within 10 years following ileal conduit diversion (Chap. 8). Consequently, many are now recommending the use of nonrefluxing colonic conduits in hopes that such anastomoses can prevent such upper tract deterioration from occurring. Whether or not such will prove to be the case is unknown at present.

Even if diversion is elected, one must still deal with the exstrophic bladder. Some have recommended total cystectomy, but this then leaves an abdominal wall defect that is difficult to close. Closure can be accomplished by rotating flaps of anterior rectus sheath across the midline, which thereby obliterates this defect somewhat. Another approach is to strip the mucosa from the exstrophic bladder and leave the muscle in situ to bolster this defect. It is important in the male to leave the bladder neck intact so that fertility is not impaired.

EPISPADIAS

Regardless of how the upper urinary tract is managed, one is left with the problem in the male of penile repair. Because the penis is short and broad and is tethered to the anterior abdominal wall, some attempt must be made to achieve length in addition to merely closing the epispadiac urethra. Multiple procedures have been described, but the simplest and most satisfactory seems that described by Johnston (1975) in which a V-Y-plasty of the urethral mucosa is accomplished after the corpora

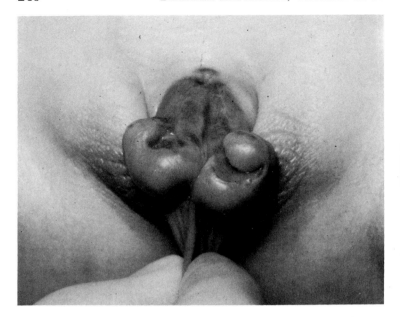

Figure 13–9. Complete epispadias without exstrophy. Note the duplicated glans penis. This child has associated urinary incontinence.

are partially detached from the ischia. This effectively lengthens the penis much as a wishbone would advance if its wings were brought together. At another stage, the urethra may then be closed and brought to the tip of the glans. In the female, the clitoris can be reapproximated, and, in addition, the mons can be reconstructed by rotating flaps of skin from the lateral pubic area ultimately to achieve a more normal pubic hair distribution and overall appearance.

Epispadias as an isolated defect occurs approximately once in 95,000 live births and has a 4:1 male to female preponderance (Fig. 13–9). In patients with epispadias alone, incontinence is not invariably present. Granted, the more severe the epispadias, the more likely the patient is to be incontinent. The surgical approach to the creation of a urethra for epispadias is not too dissimilar from the correction of hypospadias. However, even in those boys with isolated epispadias, there is separation of the pubes, and the penile angle can be improved upon to some degree by release of the corpora from their ischial attachments. Additionally, dissection of the dorsal shaft skin allows further straightening of the penis. By transferring the ventral prepuce (the prepuce in epispadias is present on the ventral surface; in hypospadias it is present

dorsally) to the denuded dorsal surface, the stage is set for creation of the urethra, generally accomplished as a second procedure 6 to 12 months later. Some surgeons prefer completing the repair in a single stage using a free graft of skin taken from the prepuce for the urethra.

In females, epispadias, if present, is more likely to be complete. Hence, over 90 per cent of girls with epispadias are incontinent. In those children with severe epispadias involving the bladder neck area, continence is provided using the urethral lengthening technique mentioned previously in the section on primary closure of the exstrophic bladder. Unfortunately, the success in any of these procedures is limited.

Interestingly, vesicoureteral reflux occurs in about 90 per cent of patients with epispadias, so that one presumes a similar abnormality of the ureterovesical junction to that seen in patients with exstrophy. Correction of the reflux can be carried out simultaneously with formation of the urethra or modification of the bladder neck.

REFERENCES

Ansell, J. S.: Vesical exstrophy. *In* Glenn, J. F.: Urologic Surgery, 2nd ed. New York, Harper and Row, 1975.

Crissey, M. M., Steele, G., and Gittes, R. F.: Rat model for carcinogenesis in ureterosigmoidostomy. Science, 207:1079, 1980.

Culp, D. A.: The histology of the exstrophied bladder. J. Urol., 91:538, 1964.

Engel, R. M.: Bladder exstrophy. Urology, 2:20, 1973.

Engel, R. M., and Wilkinson, H. A.: Bladder exstrophy. J. Urol., 104:699, 1970.

Hendren, W. H.: Exstrophy of the bladder — An alternative method of management. J. Urol., 115:195, 1976.

Hinman, F.: The Principles and Practice of Urology. Philadelphia, W. B. Saunders Co., 1935, p. 423.

Ignatoff, J. M., Kaplan, G. W., and Swenson, D.: Incomplete exstrophy of the bladder. J. Urol., 105:579, 1971.

Jeffs, R. D.: Exstrophy. In Harrison, J. H., Gittes, R. F., Perlmutter, A. P., et al.: Campbell's Urology, 4th ed. Philadelphia, W. B. Saunders Co., 1979, pp. 1691–1692.

Johnston, J. H.: The genital aspects of exstrophy. J. Urol., 113:701, 1975.

Johnston, J. H., and Kogan, S. J.: The exstrophied anomalies and their surgical reconstruction. Curr. Probl. Surg. 1–39, Aug., 1974.

Kaplan, G. W., Sutherland, D., and Brock, W. A.: Computerized gait analysis in patients with exstrophy. In preparation.

Lattimer, J. K., and Smith, M. J. V.: Exstrophy closure. J. Urol., 95:356, 1966.

MacFarland, M. T., Lattimer, J. K., and Hensle, T. W.: Improved life expectancy for children with exstrophy of the bladder. J.A.M.A., 242:442, 1979.

Muecke, E. C.: The role of the cloacal membrane in exstrophy. J. Urol., 92:659, 1964.

Patten, B. M., and Barry, A.: The genesis of exstrophy of the bladder and epispadias. Am. J. Anat., 90:35–37, 1952.

Spence, H. M., Hoffman, W. W., and Pate, V. A.: Exstrophy of the bladder. J. Urol., 114:133, 1975.

Williams, D. I.: Epispadias and exstrophy. Proc. R. Soc. Med., 62:1079, 1969.

Cloacal Exstrophy

The baby born with a large defect of the lower abdominal wall combining both bowel and bladder mucosa is frightening to both the physician and the family. The anatomy of cloacal exstrophy (vesicointestinal fissure) is predictable and consists of a central strip of cecum flanked by two halves of bladder, each with its own ureteral orifice (Fig. 13–10); additionally, the phallus is usually bifid. An opening at the upper portion of the exstrophic cecal component represents the ileocecal junction through which small intestine frequently prolapses.

The orifices of one or more vermiform appendices may be found adjacent to this cloacal junction. Finally, an opening to a variable length of blind-ending large bowel is found at the lower-most aspect of the exstrophic cecal segment. The large bowel is rarely completely formed.

An exomphalos is found superior to the intestinal and bladder defect and may be quite large. In addition, severe spinal abnormalities, including meningomyelocele (Fig. 13–11), and upper urinary tract anomalies are common in this group of pa-

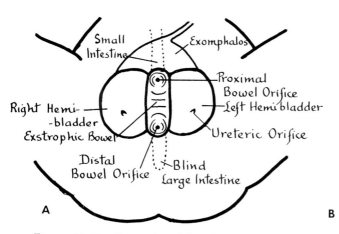

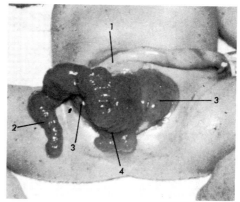

Figure 13–10. Exstrophy of the cloaca. *A,* Diagram of the external anatomy. *B,* Photograph of a patient showing exomphalos (1), prolapsed ileum (2), hemibladders lying on either side of exstrophic bowel (3), distal bowel orifice (4), and absence of anus and external genitalia. (From Johnson, J. H., and Penn, I. A.: Exstrophy of the cloaca. Br. J. Urol., 38:302–307, 1966.)

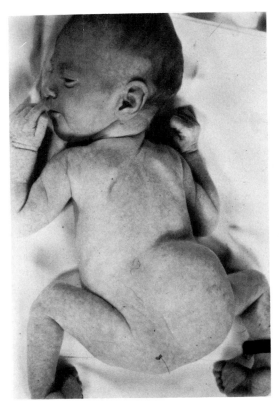

Figure 13–11. Child with cloacal exstrophy and associated abnormalities of the musculoskeletal system. Talipes equinovarus and large lumbosacral defect are obvious. (From Kelalis, P. P., King, L. R., and Belman, A. B.: Clinical Pediatric Urology, Vol. 2. Philadelphia, W. B. Saunders Co., 1976, p. 612.)

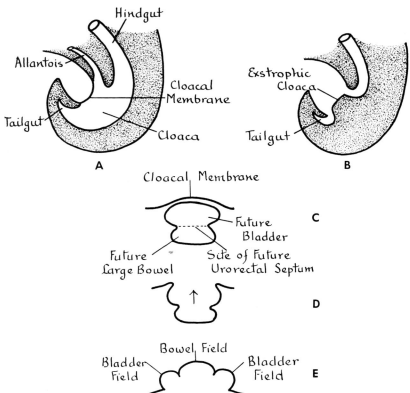

Figure 13–12. Presumed genesis of cloacal exstrophy. *A,* Normal condition of the embryo at 4 mm stage. *B,* Rupture of the cloacal membrane, perhaps from failure of local mesodermal development, leads to exstrophy. *C,* Transverse section through normal cloaca. *D, E,* Rupture of the cloacal membrane and resulting exstrophy. (From Johnson, J. H., and Penn, I. A.: Exstrophy of the cloaca. Br. J. Urol., 38:302–307, 1966.)

tients. This is a rare anomaly presenting once in every 200,000 to 250,000 live births.

EMBRYOLOGY

Cloacal exstrophy represents a type of embryologic defect similar to bladder exstrophy. However, its origins are probably at an earlier fetal date prior to completion of formation of the urorectal septum (Fig. 13–12) (Johnson and Penn, 1966).

CLINICAL COURSE

The congenital defects in these children are severe; however, most have the potential for survival. Although great strides have been made recently in bladder reconstruction, fecal continence cannot be anticipated. Assuming the absence of an anomaly incompatible with survival, reconstruction of the abdominal defect may be staged with turning in of the exstrophic colonic segment and creation of an end colostomy as the first step. Ileostomy alone often results in severe diarrhea and secondary fluid and electrolyte abnormalities. Use of whatever blind colon may be present as part of the functional intestinal tract requires extensive reconstruction but often prevents this difficulty. Ultimately, closure of the lower abdominal defect with some form of cutaneous urinary diversion will probably be necessary. Recent success in joining the bladder halves with an attempt at creating a functional urinary bladder or one that may be used as a reservoir for intermittent catheterization at a later date broaden the horizons in the care of these children (Tank, 1979).

Because most of these patients, regardless of genetic sex, have a bifid phallus separated by the abdominal defect (see Fig. 9–24), the likelihood of creating a functional penis in the male is slim. On this basis, it is advisable to assign all these children to the female gender at birth. Castration and union of the phallic portions to serve as a clitoris can be made a part of one of the many future reconstructive procedures.

The prognosis for these children has changed quite markedly in the past few years. Spectacular advances in neonatal care as well as daring and imaginative reconstructive surgery have given some of these children a chance for a functional future. Nevertheless, the responsibility imposed upon the families of these children is awesome and requires extensive support from all medical and paramedical facilities available.

REFERENCES

Gray, S. W., and Skandalakis, J. E.: The anterior abdominal wall. *In* Embryology for Surgeons. Philadelphia, W. B. Saunders Co., 1972.

Johnson, J. H., and Penn, I. A.: Exstrophy of the cloaca. Br. J. Urol., 38:302, 1966.

Tank, E. S.: The urologic complications of imperforate anus and cloacal dysgenesis. *In* Harrison, J. H., Gittes, R. F., Perlmutter, A. D., et al.: Campbell's Urology, 4th ed. Philadelphia, W. B. Saunders Co., 1979.

Imperforate Anus

Imperforate anus presents itself either as a misplaced anal opening located somewhere anterior to its anticipated position or as complete absence of a visible anus. Rarely, the anus itself is normal, but an atretic segment of distal colon obstructs the passage of stool. The relationship of imperforate anus and the urinary tract resides not only in physical proximity but also in common embryologic origins and developmental timing. It is, therefore, not surprising that children born with imperforate anus may be anticipated to have a high incidence of associated urinary tract abnormalities.

URINARY ANOMALIES ASSOCIATED WITH IMPERFORATE ANUS

Children born with supralevator imperforate anus, one in which the rectum ends blindly above the puborectalis sling of the levator ani muscle (type III of Ladd and Gross (Fig. 13–13), are most likely to have associated urologic and lower spinal abnormalities. Supralevator imperforate anus is the result of a fetal injury in the first six weeks of gestation. The most extreme variant of this abnormality is the human sirenomelus. These monsters have fusion of their lower extremities, severe sacral abnormalities, imperforate anus, and absence of the entire genitourinary tract except gonads (Fig. 13–14). Duhamel (1961) labeled this entity the "syndrome of caudal regression," relating the constellation to a single, early anatomic injury. Less severe forms compatible with survival demonstrate the close association between the formation of the distal intestinal tract, lower spine, and urinary tract. About half of those children born with supralevator imperforate anus have associated urinary tract abnormalities, and slightly more have lower spine anomalies.

Classification of imperforate anus has been slightly confusing. However, four major types have been defined (Ladd and Gross, 1934). Types I and II conform to the infralevator lesions, whereas type III represents the supralevator lesion (Fig. 13–13).

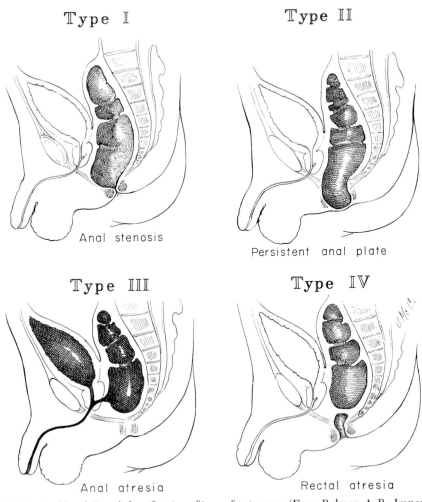

Type I — Anal stenosis

Type II — Persistent anal plate

Type III — Anal atresia

Type IV — Rectal atresia

Figure 13–13. Ladd and Gross' classification of imperforate anus. (From Belman, A. B.: Imperforate anus and urogenital anomalies. *In* Glenn, J. F.: Urologic Surgery, 2nd ed. New York, Harper and Row, 1975.)

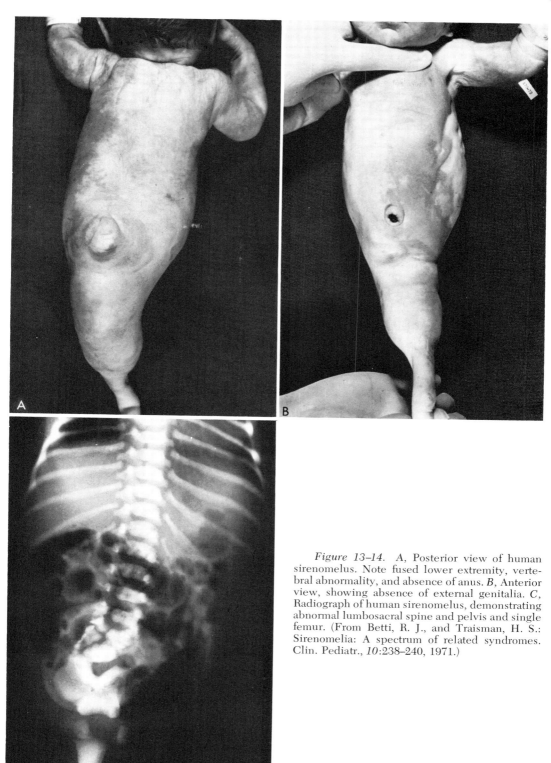

Figure 13–14. A, Posterior view of human sirenomelus. Note fused lower extremity, vertebral abnormality, and absence of anus. B, Anterior view, showing absence of external genitalia. C, Radiograph of human sirenomelus, demonstrating abnormal lumbosacral spine and pelvis and single femur. (From Betti, R. J., and Traisman, H. S.: Sirenomelia: A spectrum of related syndromes. Clin. Pediatr., *10*:238–240, 1971.)

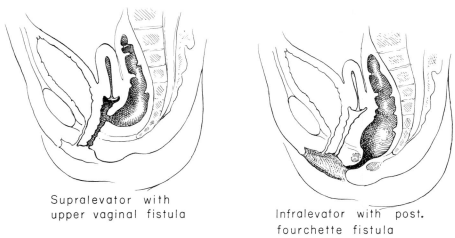

Supralevator with
upper vaginal fistula

Infralevator with post.
fourchette fistula

Figure 13–15.   *A,* Rare supralevator lesion in the female with a high vaginal fistula. *B,* More common infralevator abnormality in the female with rectocutaneous fistula at the posterior fourchette. (From Belman, A. B.: Imperforate anus and urogenital anomalies. *In* Glenn, J. F.: Urologic Surgery, 2nd ed. New York, Harper and Row, 1975.)

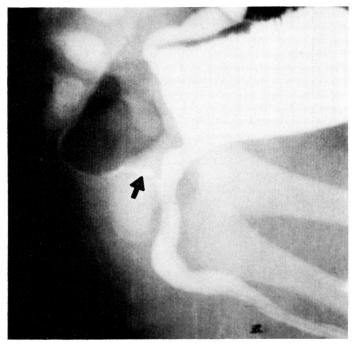

Figure 13–16.   Lateral view of voiding cystourethrogram in male with high lesion. Fistula between distal rectal pouch and urethra is outlined (arrow) along with contrast medium in rectum. (From Kelalis, P. P., King, L. R., and Belman, A. B.: Clinical Pediatric Urology, Vol. 2. Philadelphia, W. B. Saunders Co., 1976, p. 606.)

In males a fistulous communication invariably exists between the blind-ending rectal pouch and the prostatic urethra. This is not considered a separate urinary tract abnormality but is part of the basic underlying intestinal pathologic anatomy. Rarely this fistula may communicate with the bladder rather than the urethra.

In girls the distal rectum communicates with the vagina or posterior fourchette (Fig. 13–15). Supralevator imperforate anus in the female is often a more severe abnormality frequently presenting as a single perineal opening (cloaca) joining the urinary, vaginal, and rectal tracts (Chap. 10). However, the vast majority of girls with imperforate anus present with an infralevator lesion.

CLINICAL COURSE

The initial care of these children rests in the hands of the pediatric surgeon. In view of the known high incidence of urinary tract anomalies, evaluation of the urinary tract is recommended in all but is essential in those with supralevator lesions (Belman and King, 1972). Unilateral renal agenesis is the most common urinary tract abnormality seen in this group; however, in itself it constitutes no risk to life if the other kidney is normal. Vesicoureteral reflux also appears to occur more frequently than in normal children. In a group in whom the incidence of neurogenic bladder is increased because of sacral pathologic development and in whom there is often a communication between a stump of rectum and the urethra, the risk of urinary tract infection is increased during an age when the effects of renal infection may be markedly worsened (Chap. 4). We would recommend an excretory urogram or renal scan in the newborn period to evaluate the status of the kidneys and a voiding cystourethrogram as a means of outlining the lower urinary tract and screening for reflux. Often the fistulous communication between the bladder and rectal pouch can also be seen on these films (Fig. 13–16).

UROLOGIC CARE

In view of the complexity of the overall problem, it is advisable to maintain long-term "guardian maintenance" care in this group of patients. Neurogenic bladder can be anticipated in about 10 per cent of this group owing either to the associated sacral abnormalities or as a rare consequence of the rectal pull-through operation. One must be aware of the increased incidence of urinary tract infection secondary to a poorly functioning (emptying) bladder in that group and the ultimate risks to renal function. Those with frequent recurrent or continuous infection not associated with an obvious reversible cause may require long-term antibacterial prophylaxis. Stone disease, stasis in a remnant of blind-ending colon, and urethral stricture are all uncommon but highly likely problems that may occur in this complicated group of children.

REFERENCES

Belman, A. B., and King, L. R.: Urinary tract abnormalities associated with imperforate anus. J. Urol., *108*:823, 1972.

Crissey, M. M., Steele, G., and Gittes, R. F.: Rat model for carcinogenesis in ureterosigmoidostomy. Science, *207*:1079, 1980.

Duhamel, B.: From the mermaid to anal imperforation: The syndrome of caudal regression. Arch. Dis. Child., *36*:152, 1961.

Ladd, W. E., and Gross, R. E.: Congenital malformation of anus and rectum: Report of 162 cases. Am. J. Surg., *23*:167, 1934.

Chapter Fourteen

PRUNE BELLY
SYNDROME

Congenital absence of the abdominal musculature is but one manifestation of a syndrome that has fascinated physicians for years. The major components of this association comprise a triad: absence of the abdominal musculature, hydronephrosis, and cryptorchidism (Nunn and Stephens, 1961). The earliest description of this problem was Frohlich's, but the entire triad was first described by Parker (Silverman and Huang, 1950). Several terms have been utilized to describe this problem, the most descriptive being that of prune belly, which describes the outward appearance of the child's abdomen at birth (Spence and Allen, 1964). Although often ascribed to Osler, the origin of this term is apparently lost in medical antiquity. Other names that are frequently used include the Eagle-Barrett syndrome, the triad syndrome, absent abdominal muscular syndrome, and the mesenchymal dysplasia syndrome.

The incidence of this syndrome is unknown but is presumed by some to be about 1 in 40,000. Only 45 cases had been reported by 1950, but many more have been reported in the last 30 years as the problem is more frequently recognized. Males are affected approximately 20 times more frequently than females. More importantly, females, when affected, usually have no other involvement than the abdominal wall defect (Williams, 1968).

There is no question that the prune belly syndrome is represented by a wide spectrum ranging from patients very mildly affected to those quite severely so. The natural history is not well documented, but until recently it had been estimated that 20 per cent died in infancy and 50 per cent died within the first two years of life (Williams and Parker, 1974). However, there are some reports of patients living into old age with this syndrome (Silverman and Huang, 1950), and more recent advances have markedly altered the prognosis. A recent article appeared pointing out that many internists would not recognize this syndrome, and yet it must be kept in mind as a cause for renal failure in adults (Lee, 1977).

ETIOLOGY

The etiology is unknown. It is probably not a sex-linked problem as it occurs in both sexes, although the marked disparity in distribution is unexplained. There is no familial tendency toward this problem, but it has been, on occasion, reported in twins. More importantly, there also has been discordance in twins with the problem. Prune belly syndrome does occur spontaneously in other animals and has been reported in horses (Miller et al., 1966).

There are three prevalent theories of pathogenesis (Spence and Allen, 1964). One states that there is primary urethral obstruction, which leads to an abdominal wall defect and cryptorchidism. This seems untenable as (1) there are many cases of severe urinary tract obstruction without such changes or cryptorchidism, such as posterior urethral valves and (2) the abdominal wall is formed before urine secretion begins, and the histology of the abdominal wall in the prune belly syndrome is that of embryologic (primitive) muscle rather than atrophy.

A second theory is just the reverse, that is, that the abdominal wall defect is primary and that, because intra-abdominal pressure is decreased, there is decreased ureteral peristalsis and poor vesical emptying. The cryptorchidism is thought to be mechanical in both of these theories; that is, the full bladder prevents descent. This theory also seems unlikely as patients with omphalocele or gastroschisis do not have associated hydronephrosis.

The third and most plausible theory states that all the major and minor changes of the syndrome are due to an arrest of mesenchymal development during the sixth to tenth week of embryogenesis. This would also explain the intestinal malrotation so frequently seen in these children. It does not, however, satisfactorily explain the cryptorchidism.

PATHOPHYSIOLOGY

Perhaps the easiest way to view the problems manifest in this syndrome is in terms of its effect on organ systems. The abdominal wall defect is the most obvious of the abnormalities. There is a patchy deficiency in the number of skeletal muscle cells present. Additionally, many of these cells have an embryonic appearance. The deficient muscles are replaced by connective tissue. In infants, because there is very little subcutaneous tissue, the skin has a characteristic wrinkled appearance, hence the name prune belly syndrome (Fig. 14–1). However, as the child grows and gains sub-

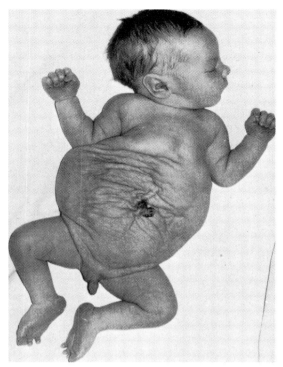

Figure 14–1. Newborn infant with the prune belly syndrome, showing the characteristic appearance of the abdominal wall, the empty scrotum, and talipes equinovarus. (From Harrison, J. H., Gittes, R. F., Perlmutter, A. D., et al.: Campbell's Urology, Vol. 2, 4th ed. Philadelphia, W. B. Saunders Co., 1979, p. 1744.)

cutaneous fat, the abdominal wall tends to smooth out somewhat, and the appearance is better characterized by the term "potbellied syndrome" (Fig. 14–2). There have been attempts in the past to increase the support of the abdominal musculature either by operative procedures such as plication of the abdominal muscle or by the use of protective devices. By and large, the results of these operative procedures have not as yet been proved to be of functional benefit, although they may produce some cosmetic improvement. In some infants, because of the weak abdominal wall there is an increased predisposition to pneumonia because of an inability to cough well. It also needs to be pointed out that despite the deficiency in abdominal wall musculature, surgical wounds in patients with prune belly syndrome heal just as well as in patients with normal musculature.

The kidneys are usually affected, and the patient's prognosis depends largely on

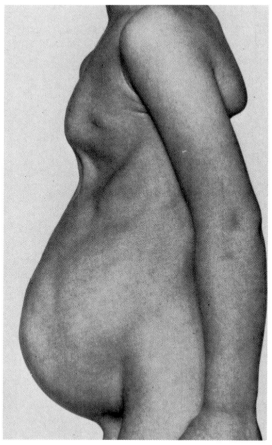

Figure 14–2. Older child with the prune belly syndrome, showing the absence of wrinkling, the "pot-belly" appearance, and the consequent deformity of the lower ribs. (From Harrison, J. H., Gittes, R. F., Perlmutter, A. D., et al.: Campbell's Urology, Vol. 2, 4th ed. Philadelphia, W. B. Saunders Co., 1979, p. 1744.)

the degree of renal dysplasia present. Even in those kidneys that are not affected with gross or microscopic evidence of dysplasia, there certainly is dysmorphism of the calyces and infundibula. Frequently the calyces are ballooned, and the infundibula are narrowed and spider-like (Fig. 14–3). Despite the fact that the upper urinary tract is dilated, there is generally no increase in intrarenal pressure. Whether there is obstruction present or whether this is a steady state must be ascertained in each patient.

The ureters are dilated, elongated, and tortuous and tend to follow a rather characteristic course that can be diagnostic on radiographs (Fig. 14–4). Ureteral peristalsis is poor. The ureters do tend to straighten

somewhat with growth (Fig. 14–5). Histologic studies have shown that there is an increase in the amount of fibrous tissue in the distal ureters (Palmer and Tesluk, 1974). This may explain the rather uniformly poor results that have been achieved with conventional types of remodeling and reimplantation procedures.

The bladder is invariably large (Fig. 14–6). There is often a large urachal remnant in the form of a diverticulum at the dome, and the bladder tends to be attached to the umbilicus. The urachus is sometimes patent. The trigone is poorly developed, and the bladder neck is widened. Some patients, especially prior to puberty, will have problems with incontinence. Interestingly, these tend to respond somewhat to imipramine. Although these patients often have impressively large amounts of residual urine following voiding, urodynamic assessment of their voiding demonstrates that they have low intravesical pressures and void with normal voiding pressures and normal urine flows.

The posterior urethra is often quite dilated (Fig. 14–7). Histologically, the prostatic epithelial elements are absent (De Klerk and Scott, 1978). There may be a utricular diverticulum. The radiographic appearance of the posterior urethra resembles that of posterior urethral valves and has led some authors to consider these children to have obstructions (Lattimer, 1958). However, true obstruction as demonstrated by urodynamic studies is indeed rare. There may also be abnormalities of the anterior urethra. Megalourethra, that is, an absence of the corpus spongiosum, segmental or complete, when present acts as a diverticulum of the anterior urethra (Fig. 14–8). Some patients have been reported to have partial or complete stenosis of the membranous or bulbous urethra. Those patients with complete stenosis often have a patent urachus. The prognosis for those children born with urethral stenosis is rather poor.

In males, intra-abdominal testes are the rule. They are often located near the iliac vessels. Histologically, the testes are no different from those in other cryptorchid patients. The testes are notably difficult to bring down surgically, and often one must

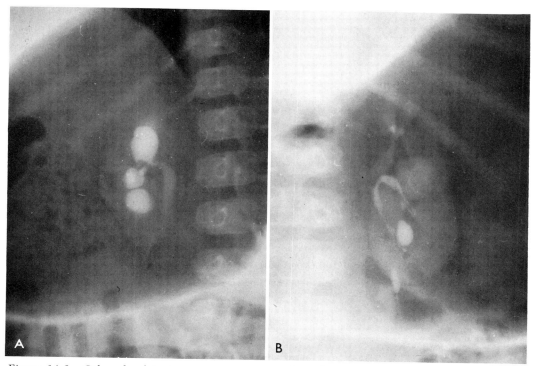

Figure 14–3. Calyceal architecture on excretory urography in the prune belly syndrome. (From Kelalis, P. P., King, L. R., and Belman, A. B.: Clinical Pediatric Urology, Vol. 2. Philadelphia, W. B. Saunders Co., 1976, p. 622.)

Figure 14–4. Characteristic course of the ureters in a patient with the prune belly syndrome. (From Kelalis, P. P., King, L. R., and Belman, A. B.: Clinical Pediatric Urology, Vol. 2. Philadelphia, W. B. Saunders Co., 1976, p. 630.)

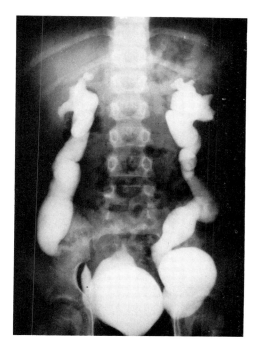

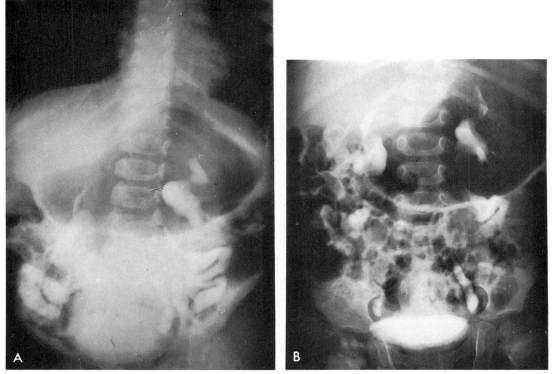

Figure 14–5. Intravenous urograms. *A,* At one year, and *B,* At two and one half years, demonstrating significant ureteral straightening. From Kelalis, P. P., King, L. R., and Belman, A. B.: Clinical Pediatric Urology, Vol. 2. Philadelphia, W. B. Saunders Co., 1976, p. 616.)

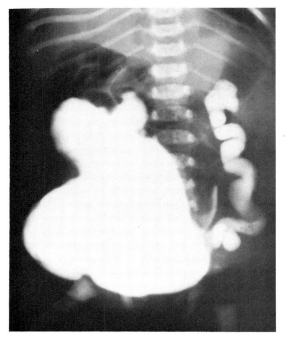

Figure 14–6. Large bladder in a patient with the prune belly syndrome. (From Kelalis, P. P., King, L. R., and Belman, A. B.: Clinical Pediatric Urology, Vol. 2. Philadelphia, W. B. Saunders Co., 1976, p. 625.)

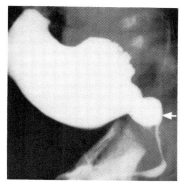

Figure 14–7. Dilated posterior urethra (arrow) in the prune belly syndrome. (From Kelalis, P. P., King, L. R., and Belman, A. B.: Clinical Pediatric Urology, Vol. 2. Philadelphia, W. B. Saunders Co., 1976, p. 624.)

malities, such as malrotation and imperforate anus, have also been noted. Congenital heart disease is occasionally seen in the form of either ventriculoseptal defects or atrial septal defects. Some patients have pectus carinatum or pectus excavatum.

MANAGEMENT

Because of the alarming radiographic picture and the relatively poor prognosis in infancy reported in the past, there was a move to use somewhat aggressive surgical measures in these children in an attempt to improve urinary drainage and influence survival. Many of these have ended disastrously. Consequently, most pediatric urologists today have adopted a surgically conservative attitude toward these patients. If the patients can be kept infection-free using continuous antibacterial prophylaxis, many will do quite well, and their radiographic appearance will improve with growth. A significant number of these children have renal dysplasia, making them more susceptible to problems associated with infection. Some develop frank renal insufficiency. In these instances, nonintubated diversionary procedures and reconstruction of the urinary tract as a means of reducing stasis have been employed with some limited success.

resort to the Fowler-Stephens maneuver of cutting the spermatic vessels in order to place the testes in the scrotum. Perfusion is then supplied by the vessels of the vas deferens. When this maneuver is employed in these cases, the testes can often be successfully placed in the scrotum. Nevertheless fertility in males affected by the prune belly syndrome has not been demonstrated.

There are other anomalies that have been reported with the syndrome. These include limb anomalies, such as talipes equinovarus, absence of limbs, congenital hip dislocation, polydactyly, syndactyly, and arthrogryposis. Gastrointestinal abnor-

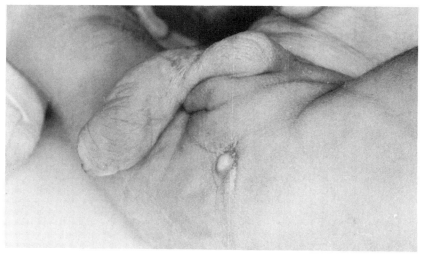

Figure 14–8. Megalourethra in a boy with prune belly syndrome. (From Kelalis, P. P., King, L. R., and Belman, A. B.: Clinical Pediatric Urology, Vol. 2. Philadelphia, W. B. Saunders Co., 1976, p. 625.)

Perhaps as many as three fourths of these patients have some degree of vesicoureteral reflux. Attempts to repair this problem have resulted in failure in many instances. For this reason, there is now a tendency to postpone reimplantation in such patients when possible.

As we stated earlier, we are not convinced that a surgical procedure is indicated for the abdominal wall defect. Early orchidopexy is desirable, although it may be a cosmetic procedure. None of the patients with prune belly syndrome to date have been reported to be fertile. There are a few reasons for this. Firstly, the bladder neck may be incompetent and the prostate itself may be abnormal so that ejaculatory incapability might exist. Also, the fertility potential of intra-abdominal testes, even if brought down at an early age, may be decreased. Finally, early orchidopexy has not been practiced long enough to determine if the effects will be beneficial.

Woodard (1978) has recently presented an alternate means of management of these patients. Complete reconstruction of the urinary tract was performed in infancy in a single stage through a long transabdominal incision. Ureteral reconstruction involved largely the use of the upper portions of the ureter where musculature is better, and the lower portions of the ureter were discarded. After the ureters were straightened and tapered, they were reimplanted into the bladder. A large portion of the bladder was excised, and the dome of the bladder was freed from its urachal tethering. In the course of this reconstruction, the testes were brought down relatively easily. The results have been successful anatomically and functionally. If the long-term results prove as good as the short-term ones, this would certainly warrant a new look at the treatment of this problem.

REFERENCES

DeKlerk, D. P., and Scott, W. W.: Prostatic maldevelopment in the prune belly syndrome: A defect in prostatic stromal-epithelial interaction. J. Urol., *120*:341, 1978.

Lattimer, J. K.: Congenital deficiency of the abdominal musculature and associated genitourinary anomalies. J. Urol., 79:343, 1958.

Lee, S. M.: Prune belly syndrome in a 54-year-old man. J.A.M.A., *237*:2216, 1977.

Miller, R. M., Kind, R. E., and Rich, R. W.: Congenital anomalies of the abdominal musculature and urogenital tract in a foal. Vet. Med., *15*:652, 1966.

Nunn, N., and Stephens, F. D.: The triad syndrome. J. Urol., *86*:782, 1961.

Palmer, J. M., and Tesluk, H.: Ureteral pathology in the prune belly syndrome. J. Urol., *111*:701, 1974.

Silverman, F. N., and Huang, N.: Congenital absence of the abdominal muscles. Am. J. Dis. Child., *80*:91, 1950.

Spence, H. M., and Allen, T.: Congenital absence of the abdominal musculature. J.A.M.A., *187*:814, 1964.

Williams, D. I.: Pediatric Urology. New York, Appleton-Century-Crofts, 1968, pp. 282–286.

Williams, D. I., and Parker, .R. M.: The role of surgery in the prune belly syndrome. *In* Johnston, J. H., and Goodwin, W.: Reviews in Pediatric Urology. Amsterdam, Excerpta Medica, 1974.

Woodard, J. R.: The prune belly syndrome. Urol. Clin. North Am., 5:75, 1978.

Chapter Fifteen

TUMORS OF THE GENITOURINARY TRACT

Tumors of the Kidney, Renal Pelvis and Ureter

Renal tumors are not often seen in children, and yet malignancy is the second most common cause of childhood death prior to age 14 (Case, 1965). Malignant renal tumors are one of the more frequently encountered neoplasms in this age group. Despite this, it must be emphasized that most renal masses in children are not neoplastic and actually represent hydronephrosis (Melicow and Uson, 1954).

CLINICAL PRESENTATION

The usual presentation of a child with a renal neoplasm is that of the child with a palpable abdominal mass. Such masses are frequently detected by one of the parents while bathing the child but are sometimes detected by the physician in the course of a routine examination. Gross hematuria is occasionally a cause for presentation (Westra et al., 1967). Microscopic hematuria, although a more frequent occurrence with renal tumors in children than is gross hematuria, is rarely the factor that brings the problem to attention (Aron, 1974). Occasionally a renal tumor may come to light after trauma because an abnormal kidney is more prone to injury than is a normal kidney. Abdominal pain, however, is not a frequent presentation of children with renal tumors, although admittedly it can occur. Pain may be provoked in such patients by bleeding either because of hemorrhage directly into the tumor or by the passage of clots that stimulate ureteral colic. Ureteral tumors may also cause urinary tract obstruction and hydronephrosis, which can be painful. In rare instances, renal failure may be a cause for presentation; this is especially true in some patients with lymphomatous infiltrations.

Hypertension may be associated with renal tumors in childhood (Aron, 1974). Approximately 10 per cent of all Wilms' tumor patients will be hypertensive. A certain percentage of children with renal cell carcinoma will be hypertensive. Hemangiopericytomas, benign renin-producing tumors of the juxtaglomerular apparatus, commonly present with hypertension as the initial problem.

261

DIAGNOSTIC EVALUATION

The diagnosis of most renal tumors is made on excretory urography. Plain films of the abdomen may suggest a mass, and the mass may be localized to the kidney by virtue of displacement of other organs (Fig. 15–1). However, after the injection of contrast agents, it is usually distortion of the renal outline or of the collecting system that indicates the presence of an intrarenal tumor (Fig. 15–2). Complete nonvisualization of the kidney rarely is the result of tumor and usually indicates renal agenesis, obstruction, or cystic disease (Lalli et al., 1966). Ultrasound examination of the abdomen has in recent years proved quite helpful in distinguishing solid masses from cystic masses (including hydronephrosis) (Hunig and Kinser, 1973).

When a renal tumor is suspected, it has been our practice to inject contrast agents through a leg vein so that an inferior vena cavagram can be obtained prior to the pyelogram. Admittedly, this method is not as

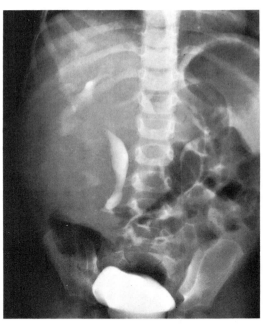

Figure 15–2. Excretory urogram showing displacement and distortion of the right collecting system by a renal tumor. (From Kelalis, P. P., King, L. R., and Belman, A. B.: Clinical Pediatric Urology, Vol. 2. Philadelphia, W. B. Saunders Co., 1976, p. 902.)

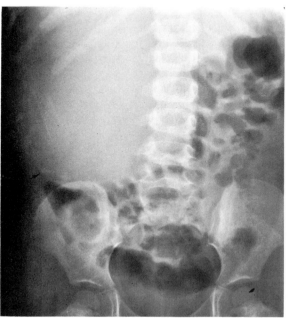

Figure 15–1. Plain film showing huge right abdominal mass with calcification (arrows) displacing bowel. (From Kelalis, P. P., King, L. R., and Belman, A. B.: Clinical Pediatric Urology, Vol. 2. Philadelphia, W. B. Saunders Co., 1976, p. 902.)

reliable as a formal cavagram but when normal allows some prediction of the resectability of the tumor. Formal venography is reserved for those suspected of having caval extension (Fig. 15–3).

Arteriography is a modality that is rarely utilized in the evaluation of tumors of the kidney in childhood. If the diagnosis is not clear-cut after excretory urography and ultrasonography, aortography may sometimes be of value (Fig. 15–4). The same may be said for computed tomography. Nuclear renal imaging has little place in the evaluation of most renal tumors of childhood, although renal cortical scanning agents (glucoheptinate and DMSA) are useful in the differentiation of functioning renal masses (so-called pseudotumors) from nonfunctioning neoplasms (Pollack et al., 1974).

If a renal tumor has been identified, chest radiographs should be performed to seek pulmonary metastases. Bone marrow examinations and skeletal surveys are also helpful in the search for evidence of metastases. Liver function studies are rarely enlightening but are routinely performed.

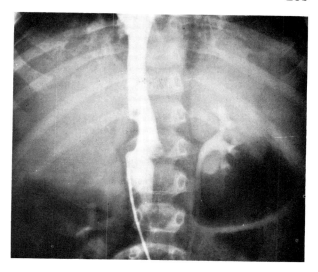

Figure 15–3. Inferior venacavagram showing occlusion of the right renal vein and a tumor thrombus projecting into the inferior vena cava. (From Kelalis, P. P., King, L. R., and Belman, A. B.: Clinical Pediatric Urology, Vol. 2. Philadelphia, W. B. Saunders Co., 1976, p. 903.)

Liver scans usually are not performed until a histologic diagnosis is available. Urinary screening for excretion products of catecholamines, specifically homovanillic and vanillylmandelic acid, may be beneficial in distinguishing renal tumors from neural crest tumors.

WILMS' TUMOR (NEPHROBLASTOMA)

Wilms' tumor is unequivocally the most common of the renal tumors of childhood.

Its incidence is estimated to be one new tumor per 200,000 to 250,000 children per year (Innis, 1972). This incidence is relatively constant worldwide and translates into 150 new cases occurring in the United States annually. The peak age incidence of Wilms' tumor is during the third year of life (Ledlie et al., 1970). There are certain congenital abnormalities that seem to carry an increased risk for the development of Wilms' tumor. The magnitude of this increased risk in any of these abnormalities is unknown. These include hemihypertrophy

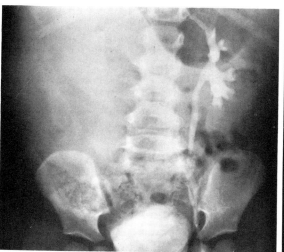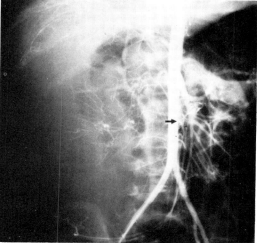

Figure 15–4. Left, Excretory urogram, showing a huge, functionless, right renal mass. *Right,* Arteriogram, showing a malignant neoplasm (Wilms' tumor) supplied by the main renal artery and also by a vessel arising from the anterior portion of the aorta about 3 cm below the renal artery, probably a capsular vessel (arrow). (From Kelalis, P. P., King, L. R., and Belman, A. B.: Clinical Pediatric Urology, Vol. 2. Philadelphia, W. B. Saunders Co., 1976, p. 902.)

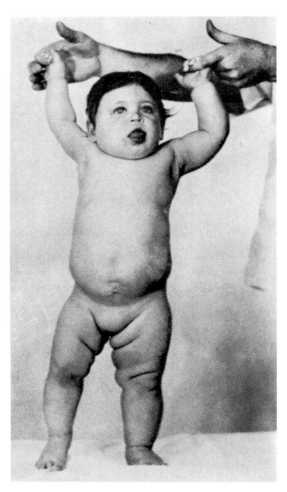

Figure 15–5. A child from whom a Wilms' tumor was removed, showing crossed hemihypertrophy. The left extremities and the right side of the face are involved. (From Wilson, F. C., and Orlin, H.: Crossed congenital hemihypertrophy. J. Bone Joint Surg., *47A*:1609–1614, 1965. Courtesy of Dr. Frank Wilson and the Journal of Bone and Joint Surgery.)

(Fig. 15–5) (Fraumeni et al., 1967), Beckwith-Wiedemann syndrome (Fig. 15–6) (Reddy et al., 1972), sporadic aniridia (Fig. 15–7) (Miller et al., 1964), and geni-

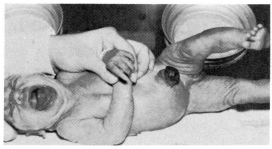

Figure 15–6. Newborn with Beckwith-Wiedemann syndrome. Note macroglossia and omphalocele. (From Smith, D. W.: Recognizable Patterns of Human Malformation, 2nd ed. Philadelphia, W. B. Saunders Co., 1976, p. 95.)

tourinary anomalies. It must be recognized that most patients with Wilms' tumor do not have any other abnormalities. Wilms' tumor is probably not a genetic disease, although there is some evidence to suggest that two sequential mutations may result in these tumors in some cases (Knudson and Strong, 1972).

As was previously stated, most Wilms' tumor patients present because a mass is palpated. These masses usually do not cross the midline in contradistinction to neuroblastoma, in which extension across the midline is frequent. Occasionally, an increase in temperature will be noted in Wilms' tumor patients, leading to some diagnostic confusion with infection. Weight loss is a very unusual mode of presentation for patients with Wilms' tumor unless there is widespread metastatic disease.

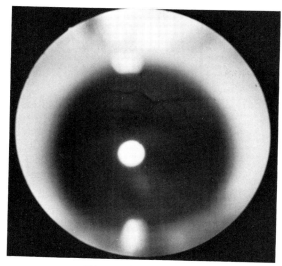

Figure 15-7. Aniridia.

Table 15-1. Staging Scheme Employed by the National Wilms' Tumor Study

Group I — Tumor limited to the kidney. The renal capsule is intact.

Group II — Tumor extends beyond the kidney or into blood vessels but does not involve adjacent organs or regional lymph nodes.

Group III — Residual tumor in the abdomen (not involving the liver) after surgical excision of the lesion

Group IV — Evidence of hematogenous metastases

Group V — Bilateral tumors

(Modified from Penn, I., and Starzl, T. E.: Immunosuppression and cancer. Transplant. Proc.,5:943,1973.)

Wilms' tumor has the capacity to destroy and displace normal kidney tissue. The tumor is usually surrounded by a pseudocapsule and on cut section has a mucinoid or gray-white (fish flesh) appearance. Necrosis, degeneration, and hemorrhage are quite frequently seen. The tumor tends to spread by direct infiltration into the kidney and through the renal capsule into surrounding structures. In addition, there is often invasion of the intrarenal vessels and extension into the renal vein and inferior vena cava. Lymph node metastases can occur, but usually the initial indicator of spread is pulmonary metastases presumably via hematogenous spread. Hepatic metastases are less common. Osseous and cerebral metastases are rare.

Histologically, these tumors consist of undifferentiated renal blastema with varying amounts of loose mesenchyme. Smooth muscle, striated muscle, cartilage, osteoid, and adipose tissue may be present, and there may also be some primitive tubules and glomeruli recognized. Wilms' tumors can be staged pathologically. Prognosis correlates well with such staging. The most helpful staging scheme clinically seems to be that established by the National Wilms' Tumor Study (Penn and Starzl, 1973) (Table 15-1). There also seems to be correlation between an anaplastic histologic appearance of a Wilms' tumor and aggressive behavior (Breslow et al., 1978).

Because Wilms' tumor is the most common renal neoplasm occurring in childhood, evaluation and therapy of all solid renal masses must proceed as if the lesion in question is a Wilms' tumor until proved otherwise. Although it has been conclusively shown that rapid operative intervention does favorably affect prognosis, this does not imply that there is not sufficient time available for adequate work-up. There is no place for "emergency" operations in such patients, for all diagnostic studies can be effectively completed within 24 to 48 hours of the child's presentation. It is strongly recommended that a renal mass highly suggestive of being a neoplasm be extirpated intact, avoiding tumor spill. Biopsy should be reserved only for those in whom there is an overwhelming suspicion of benign disease.

Without nephrectomy, one would not anticipate survival of the child with Wilms' tumor (Ledlie et al., 1970). Surgical excision is considered the cornerstone of therapy for all children with Wilms' tumor. Surgery can prove quite formidable. There may be sizable blood loss, it may be necessary to occlude the inferior vena cava, the pleural cavity may require entry, or there may be difficulty in maintaining the patient's normal body temperature. The usual surgical approach requires wide operative exposure through either a transperitoneal or thoracoabdominal approach. After inspection of the abdominal contents, including careful palpation of the contralateral kidney, the ipsilateral renal artery and then the renal vein are first isolated and ligated, after which the tumor is extirpated. If there is tumor extension into the renal vein or the vena cava, these extensions are removed at the same time as the primary tumor. In rare instances, the tumor will extend sufficiently cephalad in the vena cava that cardiopulmonary bypass must be utilized for total removal of the caval extension. It has been recommended by some that all lymphatics in the renal area be widely excised; however, data have not been presented to indicate that this in any way affects prognosis (Martin and Reyes, 1969). Occasionally it may be necessary to remove contiguous structures that are invaded by tumor, such as the spleen, colon, tail of the pancreas, diaphragm, psoas muscle, or liver.

When Wilms' tumor is bilateral (Fig. 15–8), the treatment of choice is bilateral partial nephrectomy, if feasible. If not, unilateral nephrectomy and partial nephrectomy on the other side have been utilized. Occasionally, it is possible to enucleate tumor nodules from the renal parenchyma in these bilateral cases. With diffuse bilateral involvement by tumor, initial biopsy, postoperative radiotherapy, chemotherapy, and a second-stage exploration have been advised (Ehrlich and Goodwin, 1973). Although bilateral nephrectomy and delayed renal transplantation have been reported in such patients, data would suggest that this modality should be offered only to those patients who are untreatable by any other means (White et al., 1976).

Radiation therapy would seem to play a definite role in the management of Wilms' tumor. However, in patients with well-encapsulated tumors without demonstrable metastatic spread, radiation is of questionable benefit (D'Angio et al., 1976). Complications of radiation therapy include the scoliotic effect of radiation on skeletal growth when only portions of the spinal cord are irradiated. The incidence of post-treatment scoliosis can be decreased by including the entire width of the vertebral column in the treatment field; however, this does influence total growth potential. Radiation pneumonitis, nephritis, and hepatitis have been well described after treatment of Wilms' tumor (Oliver et al., 1978).

Current data suggest that radiation therapy is not necessary for Stage I disease; however doses varying from 1800 to 4000 rads are still recommended for patients with

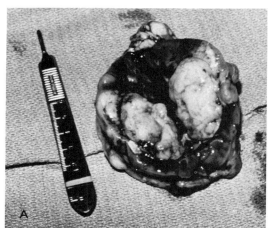

Figure 15–8. A, Right kidney of a two-year-old girl with bilateral Wilms' tumor. *B,* Left kidney. The tumor has been enucleated from the midportion of the kidney.

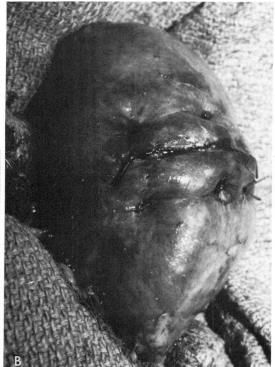

Stage II disease. In Stage IV disease with pulmonary metastases, the lungs can be radiated with a dose of 1400 rads. With such regimens, resolution of these pulmonary tumors has been seen rather consistently. Hepatic metastases should be radiated only if they are nonresectable. The same is true of brain and bone metastases.

Since the advent of actinomycin D, there has been a dramatic improvement in the survival of patients with Wilms' tumor (Burgeat and Glidewell, 1967). This drug is currently administered intravenously in doses of 15 μg per kg per day for five days, the first dose being given within 48 hours of diagnosis. These five-day courses are repeated at six weeks and three, six, nine, and 12 months thereafter. Toxic manifestations include local tissue necrosis and ulceration from extravasation of the drug, nausea and vomiting (especially in older patients), buccal ulcerations, alopecia, anemia, leukopenia, and thrombocytopenia. In addition, actinomycin D may increase the intensity of the skin reactions produced by irradiation.

Another chemotherapeutic agent of benefit is vincristine (Jones et al., 1978). It has been shown that the use of both vincristine and actinomycin D in patients with Stage II and III disease is superior to either drug alone and, consequently, both drugs are now utilized for these patients. Vincristine is administered intravenously in a dose of 0.05 mg per kg up to a total dose of 2 mg. Its major toxic effects are neurologic and include paresthesia, pain, hyporeflexia, muscular atrophy, wrist drop, and foot drop. Paralytic ileus is often a problem, and alopecia is frequent. Adriamycin has recently been released for use and is sometimes effective in these patients (Tan et al., 1973). Its major toxic effect is cardiac. Cyclophosphamide has some activity against Wilms' tumor and has been used in patients who are resistant to the more conventional agents.

PROGNOSIS

The prognosis of patients with Wilms' tumor depends largely on the stage of the tumor at the time of diagnosis (Table 15–2).

Table 15–2. Stage at Presentation

Group I	42%
Group II	26%
Group III	20%
Group IV	9%
Group V	3%

(Modified from Penn, I., and Starzl, T. E.: Immunosuppression and cancer. Transplant. Proc., 5:943, 1973.)

Eighty per cent of patients with Stage I disease can be expected to be tumor-free three years later; the same survival rates are currently being seen in patients with Stage II and III disease. Roughly sixty per cent of patients with Stage IV disease survive two years. About 40 per cent survival of patients with Stage V disease has also been reported at two years (D'Angio et al., 1976). Another significant factor in prognosis is the patient's age. Patients under two years of age at the time of diagnosis have a significantly higher rate of survival than do older patients. It is also true that younger patients have a significantly higher rate of localized disease at presentation than older children.

MESOBLASTIC NEPHROMA

There is an apparently benign variant of Wilms' tumor seen predominantly in early infancy (Bolande et al., 1967). Synonymous terms for this variant include congenital mesoblastic nephroma, fetal renal hamartoma, leiomyomatous hamartoma, and fetal mesenchymal hamartoma. It is the commonest of the renal neoplasms seen within the first few weeks of life. Clinical presentation is usually that of an asymptomatic abdominal mass detected on routine neonatal examination. On gross examination of the excised lesion, the tumors are firm and rubbery (Fig. 15–9) (as opposed to the mucoid appearance of the conventional Wilms' tumor). Hemorrhage and necrosis are generally absent. Histologically, these tumors are composed largely of fibrous or mesenchymal stroma with spindle-shaped cells of fibrous and leiomyomatous types. These tumors are almost always cured by nephrectomy alone and neither radiation nor che-

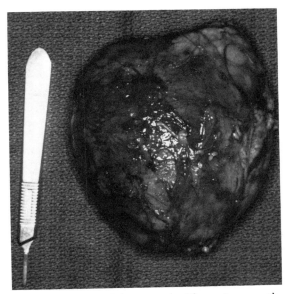

Figure 15–9. Kidney removed from a two-month-old infant. The histologic diagnosis was mesoblastic nephroma.

tanephric epithelium resembling Wilms' tumor and are usually found in both kidneys. These nodules may be microscopic in size; they also often are an incidental autopsy finding in very young children. Rarely, the nodules may be so large that they replace the entire outer portion of the renal cortex and present as bilateral renal enlargement. If arteriography is performed in such cases, the neoplasm appears relatively avascular and seems symmetrically to compress the pyelocalyceal system. Smaller lesions are referred to as nodular renal blastema, whereas the more diffuse forms are called nephroblastomatosis.

The possibility exists that in some instances, classic Wilms' tumors may arise from foci of nodular renal blastema. Nephroblastomatosis seems to respond to actinomycin D alone or in combination with radiation. It would seem that the surgeon's only role in the treatment of these disorders is to obtain a biopsy specimen for diagnosis.

motherapy is indicated in the treatment of mesoblastic nephroma. Local recurrence or distant metastasis has been reported in a few instances, however (Fu and Kay, 1973; Walker and Richard, 1973).

EPITHELIAL NEPHROBLASTOMATOSIS

Another variant includes tumors that have been called well-differentiated epithelial nephroblastomas (Datnow and Daniel, 1976). These tumors are composed largely of well-differentiated nephronal epithelium and lack much connective tissue. Tumors that fall into this group are benign multilocular cystic nephroma, tubular Wilms' tumor, and papillary adenomas. These tumors similarly tend to be benign in behavior.

DIFFUSE NEPHROBLASTOMATOSIS

Diffuse nephroblastomatosis and nodular renal blastema are another group of rare tumors that are present at birth (Liban and Kozenitzky, 1970). These present as discrete subcapsular nodules of primitive me-

RENAL CELL CARCINOMA

Renal adenocarcinoma (clear-cell carcinoma) is primarily an adult tumor but has been reported in children as young as three months of age (Castellanos et al., 1974). The mean reported age of children with renal cell carcinoma, however, is nine years, in contrast to Wilms' tumor, which peaks in incidence between three and four years. The presentation of renal cell carcinoma patients is virtually identical to that of patients with Wilms' tumor; the tumors can be differentiated only on histologic examination. Radical nephrectomy with retroperitoneal node dissection is the recommended treatment. There is no evidence that either radiation therapy or chemotherapy is of particular benefit in these patients, and the prognosis tends to be related entirely to the stage of the tumor at the time of diagnosis. Additionally, the prognosis for renal cell carcinoma in children seems no different from that observed in adults; roughly 50 per cent of patients with renal cell carcinoma survive five years.

RENAL SARCOMA

Primary rhabdomyosarcomas or primary leiomyosarcomas of the kidney have been reported (Loomis, 1972). The prognosis for these tumors has historically been poor; in light of the recent success seen with the chemotherapy of sarcomas arising from other sites in children, it is hoped that similar results will be seen with these renal sarcomas. The presentation of these tumors is no different from that of any other renal tumor.

SECONDARY RENAL TUMORS

Lymphosarcomas may occasionally arise in the kidney primarily and will then present either as a discrete renal mass or as diffuse involvement (Jaffe and Tefft, 1973). In Hodgkin's disease or leukemia, the initial presentation may rarely be renal failure due to diffuse infiltration of the kidney. In both of these states, the renal failure is often ameliorated by appropriate chemotherapy of the tumor. The kidney can be involved by metastatic tumors, especially tumors of the liver, but usually such a diagnosis is obvious.

BENIGN RENAL TUMORS

There are several benign tumors that can affect the kidney in childhood. The most important of these is angiomyolipoma (hamartoma) (McCullough et al., 1971). This tumor is composed of tissue normally present in the organ but is present in the tumor in abnormal quantities. Hence, the lesion has angiomatous, myomatous, and lipomatous elements. This tumor occurs sporadically in the general population but has been reported in as many as 80 per cent of patients with tuberous sclerosis. In this latter instance, the tumors may be bilateral and multiple and can sometimes simulate infantile or adult polycystic renal disease. The angiographic features of this tumor include increased abnormal vessels similar to those seen with renal adenocarcinoma. Seldom do these tumors cause symptoms, although occasionally they may bleed spontaneously and massively into the retroperitoneum. Bleeding is not a usual childhood presentation, however.

HEMANGIOMAS

Renal hemangiomas are frequently considered as a diagnostic possibility in children with gross hematuria (Wallach et al., 1959). However, very few have actually been reported in children, and when such hemangiomas present, they are usually seen in children with hemangiomas elsewhere in the body. Lymphangiomas and fibromas are quite rare but have been reported. Hemangiopericytoma has also been reported in a child (Conn et al., 1973).

TUMORS OF THE RENAL PELVIS AND URETER

Tumors of the renal pelvis are also rare in children. Usually when renal pelvic tumors are suspected urographically, one is actually dealing with a Wilms' tumor that has invaded the renal pelvis. Nonetheless, transitional and squamous cell epitheliomas of the renal pelvis have been reported in children as young as three months of age. When these latter tumors are discovered, the treatment of choice is nephroureterectomy.

Tumors of the ureter are seen quite infrequently in childhood. Most such tumors have proved to be benign fibrous polyps, which caused intermittent ureteral obstruction and pain (Colgan et al., 1973). Because of their benign nature, the treatment of choice is simply local removal of the polyp and the small area of ureter from which it arises and ureteral reanastomosis by either ureteropyelostomy or ureteroureterostomy, whichever technique seems more appropriate.

REFERENCES

Aron, B. S.: Wilms' tumor. A clinical study of 81 patients. Cancer, 33:637, 1974.

Bolande, R. P., Brough, A. J., and Izant, R. J., Jr.: Congenital mesoblastic nephroma of infancy. Pediatrics, 40:272, 1967.

Breslow, N. E., Palmer, N. F., Hill, L. R., Buring, J., and D'Angio, G. J.: Wilms' tumor. Cancer, 41:1577, 1978.

Burgeat, E. D., Jr., and Glidewell, O.: Dactinomycin in Wilms' tumor. J.A.M.A., 199:464, 1967.

Case, R. A. M.: Mortalities from cancers in childhood. Proc. R. Soc. Med., 58:607, 1965.

Castellanos, R. D., Aron, B. S., and Evans, A. T.: Renal adenocarcinoma in children. J. Urol., 111:534, 1974.

Colgan, J. R., Skaist, L., and Morrow, J. W.: Benign ureteral tumors in childhood. J. Urol., 109:308, 1973.

Conn, J. W., Bookstein, J. J., and Cohen, E.: Renin-secreting juxtaglomerular-cell adenoma. Radiology, 106:543, 1973.

D'Angio, G. J., Evans, A. E., Breslow, N., et al.: The treatment of Wilms' tumor. Cancer, 38:633, 1976.

Datnow, B., and Daniel, W. W., Jr.: Polycystic nephroblastoma. J.A.M.A., 236:2528, 1976.

Ehrlich, R. M., and Goodwin, W. E.: The surgical treatment of nephroblastoma. Cancer, 37:1145, 1973.

Fraumeni, J. F., Geiser, C. F., and Manning, M. D.: Wilms' tumor and congenital hemihypertrophy. Pediatrics, 40:886, 1967.

Fu, Y., and Kay, S.: Congenital mesoblastic nephroma and its recurrence: An ultrastructural observation. Arch. Pathol., 96:66, 1973.

Hunig, R., and Kinser, J.: Ultrasonic diagnosis of Wilms' tumors. Am. J. Roentgenol., 117:119, 1973.

Innis, M. D.: Neophroblastoma. Med. J. Aust., 1:18, 1972.

Jaffe, N., and Tefft, M.: Unsuspected lymphosarcoma of the kidneys diagnosed as bilateral Wilms' tumor. J. Urol., 105:593, 1973.

Jones, P. H. M., Illingsworth, R. S., Pearson, D., et al.: Management of neuroblastoma in childhood. Arch. Dis. Child., 53:112, 1978.

Knudson, A. G., Jr., and Strong, L. C.: Mutation and cancer. J. Natl. Cancer Inst., 48:313, 1972.

Lalli, A. F., Ahstrom, L., and Ericsson, N. D.: Nephroblastoma (Wilms' tumor). Radiology, 87:495, 1966.

Ledlie, E. M., Mynors, L. S., Draper, G. J., and Gorbach, P. D.: Natural history and treatment of Wilms' tumor. Br. Med. J., 4:195, 1970.

Liban, E., and Kozenitzky, I. L.: Metanephric hamartomas and nephroblastomatosis in siblings. Cancer, 25:885, 1970.

Loomis, R. C.: Primary leiomyosarcoma of the kidney. J. Urol., 107:557, 1972.

Martin, L. W., and Reyes, P. M.: An evaluation of 10 years with retroperitoneal lymph node dissection for Wilms' tumor. J. Pediatr. Surg., 4:684, 1969.

McCullough, D. L., Scott, R., Jr., and Seybold, H. M.: Renal angiomyolipoma. J. Urol., 105:32, 1971.

Melicow, M. M., and Uson, A. C.: Palpable abdominal masses in infants and children. J. Urol., 81:705, 1954.

Miller, R. W., Fraumeni, J. F., and Manning, M. D.: Association of Wilms' tumor with aniridia, hemihypertrophy, and other congenital malformations. N. Engl. J. Med., 270:922, 1964.

Oliver, J. H., Gluck, G., Gledhill, R. B., and Chevalier, L.: Musculoskeletal deformities following treatment of Wilms' tumor. Can. Med. Assoc., 119:459, 1978.

Penn, I., and Starzl, T. E.: Immunosuppression and cancer. Transplant. Proc., 5:943, 1973.

Pollack, H. M., Edell, S., and Morales, J. O.: Radionuclide imaging in renal pseudotumors. Radiology, 111:639, 1974.

Reddy, J. K., Schimke, R. N., and Chang, C. H., Jr.: Beckwith-Wiedemann syndrome. Arch. Pathol., 94:523, 1972.

Tan, C., Etcubanas, E., and Wollner, N.: Adriamycin. Cancer, 32:9, 1973.

Walker, D., and Richard, G. A.: Fetal hamartoma of the kidney. Recurrence and death of a patient. J. Urol., 110:352, 1973.

Wallach, J. B., Sutton, A. P., and Claman, M.: Hemangioma of the kidney. J. Urol., 81:515, 1959.

Westra, P., Kieffer, S. A., and Mosser, D. G.: Wilms' tumor. Am. J. Roentgenol., 100:214, 1967.

White, J. J., Galladay, E. S., Kaizer, H., Pinney, J. D., and Haller, J. A., Jr.: Conservatively aggressive management with bilateral Wilms' tumor. J. Pediatr. Surg., 11:859, 1976.

Tumors of the Adrenal and Retroperitoneum

NEUROBLASTOMA

Tumors of the adrenal medulla are among the most common of the malignant solid tumors of children. Neuroblastoma is the most frequently occurring of these and accounts for approximately seven per cent of all cancer deaths in children (Miller, 1969). Neuroblastoma has a higher incidence than either Wilms' tumor or rhabdomyosarcoma. Approximately one third of the neuroblastomas occur within the first year of life (Peterson, 1968). They do not seem to be an inherited problem (Miller et al., 1968).

PRESENTATION

Presentation depends almost entirely upon the site of origin of the primary tumor as well as the extent of any metastatic disease that may be present. One half to two thirds are discovered because of an abdominal mass, and 34 per cent will present with fever, weight loss, or anemia. Twenty-two per cent have neurologic abnormalities, and 23 per cent have gastrointestinal complaints, such as diarrhea. Only five per cent of the total are hypertensive (Donahue et al., 1974).

Metastatic disease is already present in approximately 70 per cent of patients with neuroblastoma at the time of diagnosis (Evans et al., 1971). The most common site of metastasis is to the bone marrow; however, actual bony metastases are demonstrable radiographically in approximately 50 per cent. The next most common site for metastases is the liver, followed by lymph nodes, skin, brain, and lung. Thirty-two per cent of patients with neuroblastoma will have calcification at the site of the primary tumor that is detectable on plain radiographs of the abdomen (Fig. 15–10). The upper pole of the kidney itself is usually displaced caudally and laterally if a tumor arises in the adrenal gland (Fig. 15–11). The lower pole of the kidney may be displaced laterally and possibly cranially if a tumor arises in the retroperitoneal sympathetic ganglia. These changes in renal position are usually detected on excretory urography.

Because neuroblastomas produce catecholamine and increased amounts of vanillylmandelic acid (VMA) or homovanillic acid (HVA), breakdown products of catecholamine metabolism can be found in the urine of approximately 90 per cent of neuroblastoma patients (Williams and Greer, 1963). Seventy per cent will already have a tumor invading bone marrow at the time of diagnosis. This is the reason for the high incidence of thrombocytopenia in this group. If thrombocytopenia is identified,

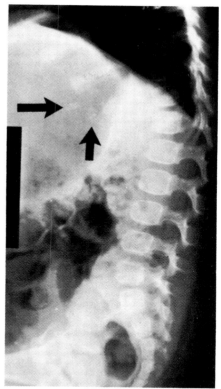

Figure 15–10. Suprarenal calcification in a neuroblastoma. (From Kelalis, P. P., King, L. R., and Belman, A. B.: Clinical Pediatric Urology, Vol. 2. Philadelphia, W. B. Saunders Co., 1976, p. 978.)

coagulation studies should also be performed (Finkelstein et al., 1970).

Neuroblastoma is a fascinating tumor because there is a high incidence of spontaneous regression, especially in infancy (Bolande, 1971). Additionally, neuroblastomas may mature into ganglioneuromas or neurofibromas. The reasons for these spontaneous regressions and maturations are unknown; however, they have been well documented in a number of patients.

TUMOR STAGING

Neuroblastomas can be staged pathologically, and the stage at diagnosis has some definite bearing on the prognosis

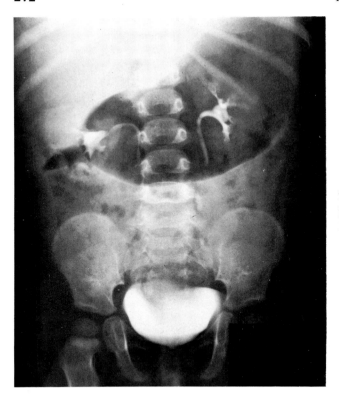

Figure 15–11. Right kidney displaced by a neuroblastoma. (From Kelalis, P. P., King, L. R., and Belman, A. B.: Clinical Pediatric Urology, Vol. 2. Philadelphia, W. B. Saunders Co., 1976, p. 978.)

(Evans, 1971). The staging system most widely employed is summarized in Table 15–3.

TREATMENT

Surgery. Surgery is usually employed in the treatment of neuroblastoma. It is, unfortunately, not always possible to remove the entire tumor. Despite this, it is important to excise as much tumor as is surgically possible so that adjunctive therapy may be more effective (Koop and John-

Table 15–3. Staging Scheme for Neuroblastoma

Stage	0	— Neuroblastoma in situ
Stage	I	— Tumor confined to the organ of origin
Stage	II	— Tumors that extend beyond the organ of origin but that do not cross the midline
Stage	III	— Tumors that cross the abdominal midline
Stage	IV	— Remote metastases
Stage	IV-S	— Tumors that would be a Stage I or II were it not for the presence of metastases in the liver, skin, or bone marrow

(Modified from Evans, A. E., D'Angio, G. J., and Randolph, J. A.: Proposed staging for children with neuroblastoma. Cancer, 27:374, 1971.)

son, 1971). Sometimes it can be quite difficult to excise even a majority of the tumor because vital structures such as the aorta, vena cava, or superior mesenteric artery have been surrounded by the tumor. However, those tumor masses that have surrounded the great vessels can often be "split" so that the great vessels can be identified. Once the vital structures are identified, these tumor masses then can often be "peeled away" from them.

Radiotherapy. Although neuroblastomas are radiosensitive, radiotherapy has not proved of great utility. Despite this, radiotherapy is routinely employed in patients over one year of age (D'Angio, 1968).

Chemotherapy. There are many chemotherapeutic agents that are effective in neuroblastoma, and yet these agents have not affected the overall survival rate of patients with neuroblastoma. Cyclophosphamide (Cytoxan) and vincristine are the agents most commonly employed for therapy (James et al., 1965), but daunorubicin (Samuels et al., 1971) and Adriamycin (Protocol #7141) have both produced tumor remission in some patients.

Surgery alone is generally recommended as the treatment necessary for Stage I tumors (Gilchrist and Tank, 1976). In patients with Stage II and III tumors, radiation therapy to the tumor bed and chemotherapy with vincristine and cyclophosphamide are also employed as adjunctive measures. It is also recommended that a "second-look" operation be performed approximately 12 to 15 months following diagnosis of a Stage II or III lesion to further remove tumor that might have been rendered resec- table by treatment. Patients with Stage IV disease are usually treated with chemotherapy and surgery; radiation may be employed for palliation as indicated. Patients with Stage IV-S disease are managed primarily with surgery and chemotherapy. Despite the remarkable advances made in the salvage of children with widespread Wilms' tumor and rhabdomyosarcomas, the survival rates for children with neuroblastoma remain unaffected (Sutow et al., 1970) (Fig. 15–12).

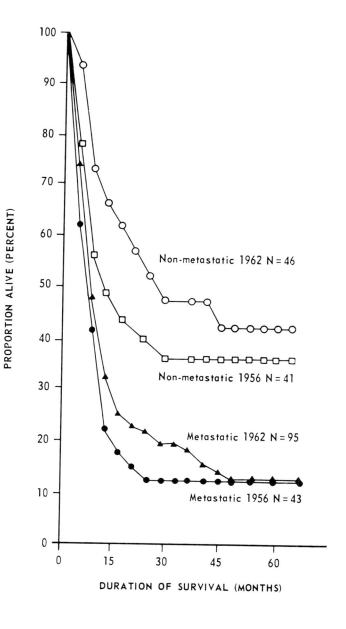

Figure 15–12. Survival curves of children with neuroblastoma diagnosed in 1956 and 1962. Survival curves today are unfortunately similar. (From Sutow, W. W., Gehan, E. A., Heyn, R. M., et al.: Comparison of survival curves, 1956 versus 1962, in children with Wilms' tumor and neuroblastoma. Report of the Subcommittee on Childhood Solid Tumors, Solid Tumor Task Force, National Cancer Institute. Pediatrics, *45*:800–811, 1970. Copyright © American Academy of Pediatrics, 1970.)

Table 15–4. Children with Neuroblastoma Surviving 2 Years Free of Disease

| | CLINICAL STAGE | | | | | |
AGE AT DIAGNOSIS	I	II	III	IV	IV–S	All Stages
0 to 11 months	11 of 12 (92%)	15 of 16 (94%)	2 of 4 (50%)	5 of 18 (28%)	18 of 19 (95%)	51 of 69 (74%)
12 to 23 months	3 of 4 (75%)	3 of 7 (43%)	5 of 8 (62.5%)	0 of 25 (0%)	1 of 3 (33%)	12 of 47 (25%)
24 months and over	4 of 5 (80%)	4 of 12 (33%)	3 of 15 (20%)	3 of 93 (3%)	2 of 5 (40%)	16 of 130 (12%)
All ages	18 of 21 (86%)	22 of 35 (63%)	10 of 27 (37%)	8 of 136 (6%)	21 of 27 (78%)	79 of 246 (32%)

(Modified from Breslow, N., and McCann, B.: Statistical estimation of prognosis for children with neuroblastoma. Cancer Res., *31*:2098–2103, 1971. Used by permission.)

PROGNOSIS

A number of variables have been shown to affect prognosis; age at diagnosis is certainly one of the more prominent factors.

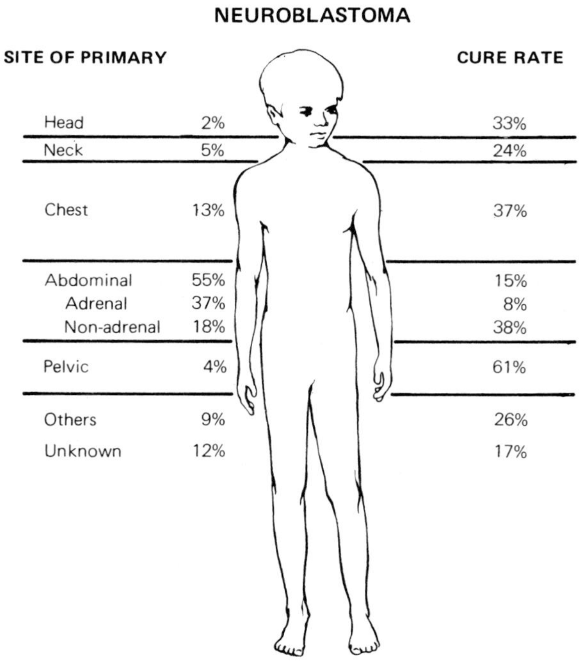

Figure 15–13. Analysis of composite data from the literature. The cure rate is the percentage of children with neuroblastoma of the corresponding primary site who are said by the authors to be alive and free of neuroblastoma at least 14 months and usually longer than two years after diagnosis. (From Sutow, W. W., Vietti, T. J., and Fernbach, D. J.: Clinical Pediatric Oncology. St. Louis, the C. V. Mosby Co., 1973. Used by permission.)

Treatment of neuroblastoma in patients who present at less than one year of age will result in cure in 60 to 74 per cent (Bolande, 1971). Only 25 per cent of children who present between one and two years of age will be cured by treatment, and after two years of age only 13 per cent of patients will be salvaged. The stage of the tumor at the time of presentation is another important factor in prognosis (Breslow and McCann, 1971) (Table 15–4). Eight-six per cent of patients with Stage I disease and 63 per cent of those with Stage II disease can be expected to survive; however, only 37 per cent of patients with Stage III disease and six per cent of those with Stage IV disease survive. Patients with Stage IV-S disease, on the other hand, have a 78 per cent survival rate. Prognosis is also affected by the site of origin (Sutow et al., 1973) (Fig. 15–13). Pelvic neuroblastomas carry a much better prognosis than do intra-abdominal neuroblastomas. Additionally, neuroblastomas that arise from extra-adrenal sites carry a better prognosis than do those that arise in the adrenal.

GANGLIONEUROMAS

Ganglioneuromas are benign tumors that may in fact be mature neuroblastomas (Willis, 1967). Patients with ganglioneuroma present with a mass, although occasionally a patient will present with diarrhea presumably produced by circulating cate-cholamines. Elevated levels of urinary cate-cholamines have been found in a number of patients with ganglioneuroma. The treatment of children with ganglioneuroma is surgical removal of the tumor.

PARAGANGLIONEUROMAS

Paraganglioneuromas are rare tumors that are most often benign in nature. However, when paraganglioneuromas arise in the retroperitoneum they can obstruct the urinary tract; rarely they will metastasize. The treatment for paraganglioneuromas is the same as that suggested for metastatic neuroblastoma.

PHEOCHROMOCYTOMA

Pheochromocytoma is a tumor of neural crest origin. It accounts for one per cent of all cases of hypertension in children (Freier et al., 1973). The youngest case reported to date presented at one year of age. The average age of children presenting with pheochromocytoma has been 12 years. Pheochromocytomas may arise anywhere neural crest tissue is found, most commonly in the adrenal gland but also anywhere else along the sympathetic ganglionic chain. They have also been reported to arise in the wall of the bladder (Perry and Scott, 1961).

In children, boys will be affected twice as frequently as girls, whereas in adults the reverse is true. Multiple pheochromocytomas are more common in children than in adults and have been seen in 32 per cent of the children with this tumor. Additionally, extra-adrenal pheochromocytomas are more common in children than in adults; these account for approximately 25 per cent of all childhood cases of pheochromocytoma. Five per cent of the patients with pheochromocytoma will have a family history of other affected individuals. When familial, this lesion is inherited as an autosomal dominant trait. A subgroup of the familial patients are those with the Sipple syndrome (medullary carcinoma of the thyroid, pheochromocytoma, and hyperparathyroidism). Pheochromocytomas will develop in approximately six per cent of the children with neurofibromatosis. Most children with pheochromocytoma present with sustained rather than episodic hypertension, as opposed to adults, in whom the reverse is true.

Pheochromocytomas are usually discovered because they are suspected. When pheochromocytoma is suspected, urinary levels of vanillylmandelic acid, other cate-cholamines, and metanephrine should be determined. If these levels prove to be abnormal, studies for localization of the suspected tumor can be performed. An excretory urogram is often helpful, as it may demonstrate displacement of the ipsilateral kidney by the tumor. Aortography is currently the single most useful study for localization of pheochromocytomas, but in the future, CAT scanning or ultrasonography may prove equally effective.

Aortography can be quite hazardous in patients with pheochromocytoma, provoking a hypertensive crisis. Since the advent of the alpha-adrenergic blocking agents, aortography in those with pheochromocytomas has become much safer (Harrison et al., 1969). It is currently recommended that alpha-blockade with phenoxybenzamine (Dibenzyline) in a dose of 1 mg per kg per day be utilized prior to the performance of aortography in this group.

Once a pheochromocytoma is localized, it should be surgically removed. This had also been a very hazardous undertaking, but it has become much safer owing to the advent of preoperative alpha-blockade. Along with preoperative blockade, the patient's blood volume must be expanded so that problems with intraoperative hypotension following anesthesia induction and the removal of the tumor can be reduced. Anesthetic agents like halothane and cyclopropane, both of which sensitize the myocardium to catecholamines, are best avoided in these patients. Currently, methoxyflurane (Penthrane) or droperidol and fentanylcitrate (Innovar) are recommended by many authors for the anesthetic management of pheochromocytoma patients (Crout and Brown, 1969). The surgical approach should be transabdominal when dealing with pheochromocytoma so that there can be a careful search of the entire retroperitoneum for other tumor sites.

ADRENAL CORTICAL TUMORS

Adrenal cortical tumors are rare in childhood (Hayles et al., 1966). There is a female preponderance of children with adrenal cortical tumors of 3 to 1. The usual symptoms of these tumors are those of virilization, but symptoms of Cushing's syndrome have also been noted. Rarely, these tumors can cause feminization (Bacon and Lowrey, 1965). Aldosterone-producing tumors of the adrenal cortex are the rarest of the adrenal cortical tumors seen during childhood.

When an adrenal cortical tumor is suspected, its presence can be further established by the dexamethasone suppression test (Wilkins, 1965). Dexamethasone will suppress the hormone production of a normal adrenal gland but will not suppress the hormone production of a tumor. Localization of the tumor site may be accomplished by excretory urography looking for a suprarenal mass or by selective adrenal venography. Aortography is of little help because adrenal cortical tumors are rarely vascular. Adrenal venography, on the other hand, is often quite helpful because the normal adrenal venous pattern is often altered by the tumor. If an adrenal cortical tumor has been well localized to one side or the other and is producing Cushing's syndrome, it is quite appropriate to approach the tumor surgically through the flank. If there is any question of location, it probably is preferable to use a transabdominal approach. Patients with functioning adrenal cortical tumors need to receive exogenous cortisone preoperatively as well as postoperatively. In children with adrenal cortical carcinoma in whom metastases are present or in whom the local disease proves inoperable, ortho-para-DDD is of some limited utility as a chemotherapeutic agent.

TERATOMAS

Teratomas can arise in the retroperitoneum (Gross et al., 1951). Most are benign, but occasionally a malignant teratoma will be seen. Most teratomas arise in ovarian or testicular tissue; another frequent site of origin in childhood is the presacral area (Fig. 15–14). Presacral or sacrococcygeal teratomas occur in females four times more commonly than in males. Infants with presacral teratomas at birth will often present with a mass protruding from the buttocks (Gwinn et al., 1955). Rarely, however, the mass is confined entirely between the rectum and sacrum with the infant presenting with severe constipation. Recognition of its presence revolves around adequate and early rectal examination. The surgical extirpation of presacral teratomas can sometimes prove a formidable undertaking, but in most instances the end result is good. Those that present at birth are usually benign, whereas those presenting later are more frequently malignant. In those with benign disease, it is important to excise the coccyx to prevent local recurrence. These children often have a secondary neuropathic bladder and require long-term urologic follow-up to prevent renal damage.

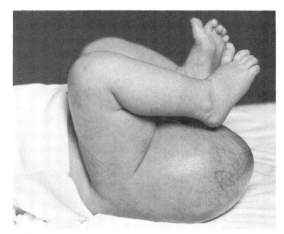

Figure 15–14. Sacrococcygeal teratoma. (From Kelalis, P. P., King, L. R., and Belman, A. B.: Clinical Pediatric Urology, Vol. 2. Philadelphia, W. B. Saunders Co., 1976, p. 993.)

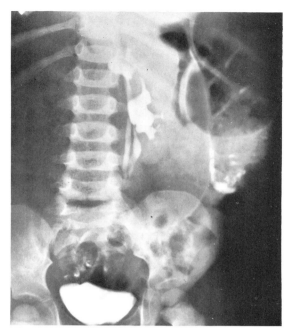

Figure 15–15. Retroperitoneal lipoma. Note relative lucency over left kidney and displacement of colon. (From Kelalis, P. P., King, L. R., and Belman, A. B.: Clinical Pediatric Urology, Vol. 2. Philadelphia, W. B. Saunders Co., 1976, p. 992.)

OTHER RETROPERITONEAL TUMORS

There are many other retroperitoneal tumors occasionally encountered during childhood. These usually present as a palpable mass, and most are benign. Lipomas of the retroperitoneum are the most frequently seen of these tumors (Harvard, 1953) (Fig. 15–15). They are usually well encapsulated and can therefore be easily excised. A clue to the presence of a lipoma can be the observation of an area of relative radiolucency on a plain radiograph of the abdomen or during the total body opacification phase of an excretory urogram. Sarcomas may also arise in the retroperitoneum; when encountered they are best treated by extensive resection (Soule et al., 1968). Unfortunately, the results of therapy of these retroperitoneal sarcomas are poor. Lymphangiomas, hemangiomas, and hemangiopericytomas have all been reported

to arise in the retroperitoneum. Occasionally neurofibromas are found in the retroperitoneum, but these are usually a local manifestation of von Recklinghausen's disease rather than an isolated occurrence. Retroperitoneal lymphomas are not infrequently the initial presentation of any of the lymphomatous diseases.

REFERENCES

Acute leukemia group B. Protocol #7141. Unpublished data.

Bacon, G. E., and Lowrey, G. H.: Feminizing adrenal tumor in a six-year-old boy. J. Clin. Endocrinol. Metab., 25:1403, 1965.

Bolande, R.: Benignity of neonatal tumors and concept of cancer repression in early life. Am. J. Dis. Child., 122:12, 1971.

Breslow, I. N., and McCann, B.: Statistical estimation of prognosis for children with neuroblastoma. Cancer Res., 31:2098, 1971.

Crout, J. R., and Brown, B. R., Jr.: Anesthetic management of pheochromocytoma. Anesthesiology, 30:29, 1969.

D'Angio, G. J.: Effects of radiation on the neuroblastoma. J. Pediatr. Surg., 3:179, 1968.

Donahue, J. P., Garrett, R. A., Baehner, R. L., and Thomas, M. H.: The multiple manifestations of neuroblastoma. J. Urol., 111:260, 1974.

Evans, A. E., D'Angio, G. J., and Randolph, J. A.: Proposed staging for children with neuroblastoma. Cancer, 27:374, 1971.

Finkelstein, J. Z., Ekert, H., and Isaacs, H., Jr.: Bone marrow metastases in children with solid tumors. Am. J. Dis. Child., 119:49, 1970.

Freier, D. T., Tank, E. S., and Harrison, T. S.: Pediatric and adult pheochromocytomas. Arch. Surg., 107:252, 1973.

Gilchrist, G. S., and Tank, E. S.: Tumors of the adrenal medulla and sympathetic chain. *In* Kelalis, P. P., King, L. R., and Belman, A. B. (Eds.): Clinical Pediatric Urology. Philadelphia, W. B. Saunders Co., 1976.

Gross, R. E., Clatworthy, H. W., Jr., and Meeker, I. A., Jr.: Sacrococcygeal teratomas in infants and children. Surg. Gynecol. Obstet., 92:341, 1951.

Gwinn, J. L., Dockerty, M. G., and Kennedy, R. L. J.: Presacral teratomas in infancy and childhood. Pediatrics, 16:239, 1955.

Harrison, T. S., Dagher, F. J., and Beck, L.: Rationale and indications for preoperative adrenergic receptor blockade in pheochromocytoma. Med. Clin. North Am., 53:1349, 1969.

Harvard, B. M.: Retroperitoneal lipoma in children. J. Urol., 70:159, 1953.

Hayles, A. B., Hahn, H. B., Jr., and Sprague, R. G.: Hormone-secreting tumors of the adrenal cortex in children. Pediatrics, 37:19, 1966.

James, D. H., Husto, W., Wrenn, E. L., and Pinkel, D.: Combination chemotherapy of childhood neuroblastoma. J.A.M.A., 194:123, 1965.

Koop, C. E., and Johnson, D. L.: Neuroblastoma: An assessment of therapy in reference to staging. J. Pediatr. Surg., 6:595, 1971.

Miller, R. W.: Fifty-two forms of childhood cancer: United States mortality experience 1960–1966. J. Pediatr., 75:685, 1969.

Miller, R. W., Fraumeni, J. F., Jr., and Hill, J. A.: Neuroblastoma: Epidemiologic approach to its origin. Am. J. Dis. Child., 115:253, 1968.

Perry, K. W., Jr., and Scott, E. V. Z.: Pheochromocytoma of the bladder. J. Urol., 85:156, 1961.

Peterson, D. R.: The epidemiology of neuroblastoma. J. Pediatr. Surg., 3:135, 1968.

Samuels, L. D., Newton, W. A., and Heyn, R.: Daunorubicin therapy in advanced neuroblastoma. Cancer, 27:831, 1971.

Soule, E. W., Mahour, G. W., and Mills, S. D.: Soft tissue sarcomas of infants and children. Mayo Clin. Proc., 43:313, 1968.

Sutow, W., Gehan, E., and Heyn, R.: Comparison of survival curves, 1956 vs. 1962, in children with Wilms' tumor and neuroblastoma. Pediatrics, 45:800, 1970.

Sutow, W. W., Vietti, T. J., and Fernbach, D. J.: Clinical Pediatric Oncology. St. Louis, The C. V. Mosby Co., 1973.

Wilkins, L.: The Diagnosis and Treatment of Endocrine Disorders in Childhood and Adolescence, 3rd ed. Springfield, Ill., Charles C Thomas, 1965, p. 359.

Williams, C. M., and Greer, M.: Homovanillic acid and vanillylmandelic acid in diagnosis of neuroblastoma. J.A.M.A., 183:836, 1963.

Willis, R. A.: Pathology of Tumours, 4th ed. New York, Appleton-Century-Crofts, 1967, pp. 857–885.

Tumors of the Lower Genitourinary Tract

Tumors of the bladder, prostate, and vagina are rare in children. Unfortunately, the majority of those that do occur can be highly malignant.

BENIGN TUMORS

Fibromas of various types, including neurofibromas associated with von Recklinghausen's disease, have been found in the urinary bladder (Carlson and Wilkinson, 1972; Ray et al., 1973). These are generally of no clinical significance, although occasionally they can cause bladder outlet symptoms by virtue of their location.

Hemangiomas and lymphangiomas may also rarely be found in the urinary bladder. Hemangiomas are often associated with similar lesions in other areas and have been reported in the Klippel-Trenaunay-Weber syndrome (Klein and Kaplan, 1975). Endoscopic biopsy of an hemangioma may result in life-threatening hemorrhage — the treatment of choice is wide, open excision. Preoperative angiographic evaluation is suggested to ascertain the extent of the lesion.

There have been a few cases reported of obstructive benign fibrous enlargement (fibroelastosis) of the prostate in children (Presman et al., 1972; Pagano and Passerini, 1976). This abnormality appears to be quite rare, however, and has not been seen clinically by either of the authors. Diagnosis is made histologically from a biopsy specimen.

Congenital fibroepithelial polyps of the prostatic urethra-verumontanum are rare obstructive lesions seen in young boys. Patients present with a history of acute urinary retention and may occasionally report that the urinary stream stops abruptly without warning. Although the polyp may originate above the external sphincter, it can prolapse into the distal urethra (Fig. 15–16).

MALIGNANT TUMORS

Approximately 15 per cent of rhabdomyosarcomas in children originate in the true pelvis (Jaffe et al., 1973; Kilman et al., 1973). Included are those of the bladder, prostate, and vagina. Depending on the primary site, patients may present with hematuria, vaginal bleeding, passage of cyst-like material, obstructive symptoms, or even urinary retention. Occasionally, grape-like clusters may be seen protruding from the urethra or vagina (Fig. 15–17). Although rhabdomyosarcoma does present in older

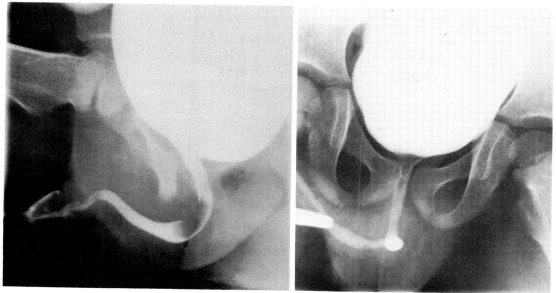

Figure 15–16. Congenital polyp of prostatic urethra as shown on voiding cystourethrograms. *Left,* Lateral view. *Right,* Anteroposterior view demonstrates pedunculated polyp as a filling defect in the posterior urethra. Note change of position. (From Stadaas, J. O.: Pedunculated polyp of posterior urethra in children causing reflux and hydronephrosis. J. Pediatr. Surg., 8:517–521, 1973. Reproduced by permission of Grune and Stratton.)

children, the majority are under five years of age.

The diagnosis of prostatic sarcoma must be considered in boys with urinary retention or severe voiding difficulties. Digital rectal examination should be performed to rule out a prostatic mass in such patients. Girls with vaginal sarcoma often present

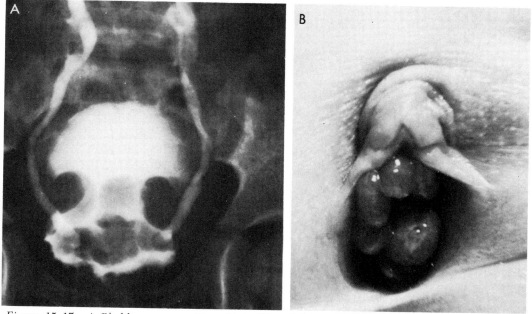

Figure 15–17. *A,* Bladder sarcoma with multiple filling defects evident in the bladder. *B,* Prolapse of typical botryoid tumor. (Reproduced with permission from Colodny, A. H., and Lebowitz, R. L.: Abnormalities of the bladder and prostate. *In* Ravitch, M. M., et al. (Eds.): Pediatric Surgery, 3rd ed. Copyright © 1979 by Year Book Medical Publishers, Inc., Chicago.)

with a blood[4] discharge on their underpants. This should not be confused, however, with urethral prolapse or ectopic ureterocele, both of which have a typical appearance (Chaps. 10 and 12).

DIAGNOSIS

If one suspects a lower urinary tract sarcoma, urographic evaluation should immediately be carried out. If present, an abnormality generally will be seen on the bladder phase of the excretory urogram (Fig. 15–18). However, a separate cystogram may be necessary. Endoscopic confirmation along with transurethral biopsy (bladder) or perineal needle biopsy (prostate) confirms the diagnosis. Vaginal sarcomas are also accessible for endoscopy and local biopsy.

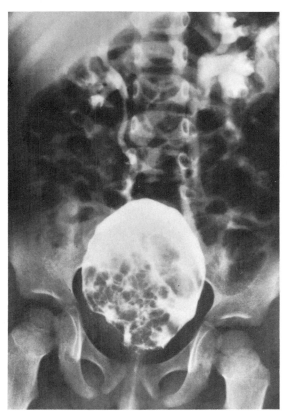

Figure 15–18. Excretory urogram of a three-year-old boy with hematuria. Bladder defects are clearly visible on this study.

TREATMENT

The classic approach to the treatment of solid tumors has been radical surgical extirpation. Until recently, the prognosis was extremely poor for patients with genitourinary rhabdomyosarcoma treated less extensively (Tefft and Jaffe, 1973). The addition of multimodality chemotherapy has raised the expectations of survival significantly (Ghavimi et al., 1975). Unfortunately, even with this spectacular improvement in survival, the removal of major organs of reproduction as well as urinary and occasionally bowel diversion has left many of these children with a life of severe disability.

A few reports have recently been published advocating moderation in the extent of surgical removal (Johnson, 1975; Kilman et al., 1973). Others have questioned the necessity for removal of the primary tumor if it appears responsive to aggressive chemotherapy (Rivard et al., 1975; Belman and Baum, 1976). After definitive tissue diagnosis by biopsy, multimodality chemotherapy is instituted (vincristine, actinomycin, and cyclophosphamide). Careful radiographic monitoring and repeat biopsy in those in whom an ablative surgical approach is not elected is essential. The addition of radiation therapy or exenteration or both may become necessary if it is apparent that a rapid response (six to eight weeks) is not forthcoming (Maurer et al., 1977). Fortunately, bladder, prostatic, and vaginal sarcomas are all readily accessible for repeated biopsy either endoscopically or, in the case of the prostate, percutaneously. Tumor size can also be monitored in those with bladder sarcoma by radiographic means as well as careful bimanual examination.

PHEOCHROMOCYTOMA

There have been a few reports of pheochromocytoma of the urinary bladder, although these are very rare. Meyer and colleagues (1979) recently reported a 12-year-old girl and reviewed the reports of two other children. The distinctive clinical presentation is headache, fainting, and hypertension initiated by voiding. Hematuria may also be present. Pheochromocytoma may be either benign or malignant.

CARCINOMA

Epithelial tumors of the urinary tract, while a leading malignancy in adults, are extremely rare in children (Ray et al., 1973). Whereas gross hematuria or persistent microscopic hematuria must always be investigated endoscopically in adults to insure the absence of bladder tumors, transitional cell carcinoma is virtually never considered in the differential diagnosis of hematuria in children. In the few cases reported, local recurrence has been noted in only one (Li et al., 1972), and we are not aware of any reports of metastatic transitional cell carcinoma in children. The most common presenting symptom has been gross, painless hematuria. The diagnosis is made endoscopically.

Adenocarcinoma appears to be even rarer in children than transitional cell carcinoma, although urachal remnants and unclosed exstrophic bladders have the potential for developing this malignancy. However, they do so during the second or third decade of life and not during childhood.

INTRASCROTAL TUMORS

CLINICAL PRESENTATION

The finding of a hard, nontender scrotal mass suggests a tumor. Although testis tumors obviously do not occur suddenly, they may be suddenly discovered and present as an "acute" mass. The importance of early diagnosis is obvious.

The differential diagnosis of a scrotal mass includes testicular or paratesticular tumor, testis torsion, epididymitis, hydrocele, hernia, and hematocele. Some clues that aid in diagnosis include the fact that both torsion and epididymitis are painful, torsion and epididymitis occur most commonly in adolescent males, testis tumors are rare in blacks, hydroceles transilluminate, and hernias have an obvious inguinal component (see Table 9–2).

Because of the nature of the sexually self-conscious age of the group in question and the fact that the general public is unaware of the occurrence of testis tumors, these malignancies in adolescents tend to present late. Tumor spread may well have occurred by the time of initial diagnosis.

DIAGNOSIS

The diagnosis of scrotal malignancy can only be made surgically. Tumor exploration should not be delayed when there is a serious question as to its likelihood. To avoid scrotal contamination, exploration for a suspected tumor should be made through an inguinal rather than a scrotal incision. Application of a noncrushing clamp to the spermatic cord prior to delivery of the testis and draping of the wound prior to opening the tunica vaginalis help prevent tumor spread. Because of the accessibility of the organ, it is possible to open the tunica vaginalis and even to biopsy the testis without serious additional risk of tumor spill if the diagnosis is in doubt. However, this is not recommended as a routine procedure. Transcrotal biopsy, on the other hand, is to be strongly condemned.

Testis tumors spread primarily by lymphatic drainage. The extreme care alluded to in the previous paragraph reflects the differing lymphatic drainage between the testis and the scrotum. Testicular lymphatics follow the spermatic cord and vessels to the level of the renal vessels, whereas the scrotum drains to the superficial and deep inguinal nodes. When searching for metastatic disease in an individual suspected of having a testis tumor, the palpating hand should concentrate in the epigastrium at the level of the renal vessels and not the groin. Pulmonary metastases are also common.

TESTIS TUMORS OF GERM CELL ORIGIN

Three fourths of testis tumors in prepubertal boys are of germ cell origin (yolk

sac or embryonal cell carcinoma and teratomas). Non–germ cell tumors (interstitial
cell, Sertoli cell, connective tissue, and metastatic tumors) comprise the remainder
(Brosman, 1979).

Age distribution analysis reveals three
incidence peaks for testis tumors. The first
is at age two years, the second is in early
adulthood, and the last is in older men
(Barzell and Whitmore, 1979). The two
tumor types seen most commonly in
younger children include teratomas and the
infant embryonal carcinoma (yolk sac carcinoma, orchioblastoma, embryonal carcinoma of the infantile or juvenile type, and
endodermal sinus tumor) (Brown, 1976).

In postpubertal males, germ cell tumors
are almost always malignant and are a leading cause of solid tumor cancer death in
young men. These are most commonly either embryonal carcinoma or teratocarcin-
oma. Pure seminoma is rare in this age
group. Choriocarcinoma is rare in all ages.
Well-differentiated adult teratomas are also
uncommon.

The approach and treatment of testis
tumors in adolescents corresponds to that in
adults. This area has been well studied, and
the treatment regimen has been fairly standardized (Barzell and Whitmore, 1979). Since
the age group in question generally falls
outside the range of the pediatric population, the subject will not be dealt with
further. However, the primary physician
must keep this diagnosis in mind when
seeing an adolescent male with a nontender, hard scrotal mass.

INFANT EMBRYONAL CARCINOMA (YOLK SAC CARCINOMA)

This tumor is the most frequently occurring testis tumor in children, representing over half of all reported cases (Jeffs,
1973). The age of presentation appears to
influence survival — the younger the patient, the better the prognosis (Houser et al.,
1965).

Because of the rare occurrence of testis
tumors in children, a standardized therapeutic regimen has not as yet been worked
out. However, based on the information

gained from adult testis tumor patients,
it is best to approach all patients initially
with a suspected tumor through an inguinal incision with the idea of performing a "high" orchiectomy (removal of the
spermatic cord to the level of the internal
inguinal ring) followed by transabdominal
retroperitoneal lymphadenectomy. As previously mentioned, the lymphatic drainage
of the testis follows the testicular blood
supply, which originates at the level of the
renal vessels. Inguinal or iliac node biopsy
is of no value in determining evidence of
distant tumor spread.

The presence of lymphatic metastases
suggests the need for aggressive chemotherapy. The course is unclear when the retroperitoneal node dissection does not reveal
distant spread. However, in the series presented by Jeffs (1973), survival was improved in those with node dissection even
when those nodes were negative for metastases. It would appear that all patients
should have at least one year of intermittent
actinomycin D therapy regardless of the
findings at retroperitoneal node dissection
(Hopkins et al., 1978).

TERATOMAS

Teratomas in children should be considered to be benign lesions (Fig. 15–19).
High inguinal orchiectomy is adequate
treatment, and retroperitoneal node dissection and chemotherapy are not recommended, as metastases have not been reported in
children. Distant metastases have been
noted in adults with apparently benign
teratomas, however.

GONADOBLASTOMA

A mixed tumor of both germinal and
mesenchymal origins has been noted to
occur in dysgenetic testes. The majority of
those in whom this tumor occur have the
mosaic chromosome pattern 45XO/46XY.
The risk of malignancy approaches 25 per
cent in this group with mixed gonadal dysgenesis (Scully, 1970).

The diagnosis should be suspected in

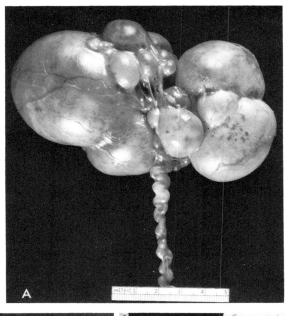

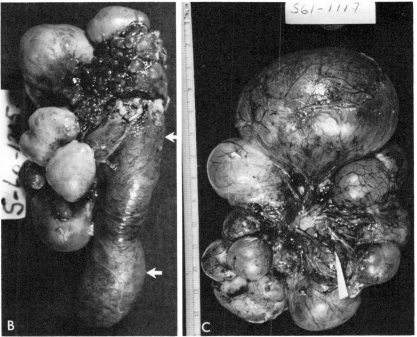

Figure 16–1. Three examples of the variety of multicystic disease. *A*, Multicystic kidney with a tortuous atretic ureter. The cysts vary in size and appear to be held together by fibrous tissue. *B*, Multicystic kidney from a one-month-old girl. The arrows indicate the dilated pelvis and proximal ureter. *C*, Multicystic kidney from a four-day-old female. No ureter was found during the nephrectomy. (From Kelalis, P. P., King, L. R., and Belman, A. B.: Clinical Pediatric Urology, Vol. 2. Philadelphia, W. B. Saunders Co., 1976, p. 710.)

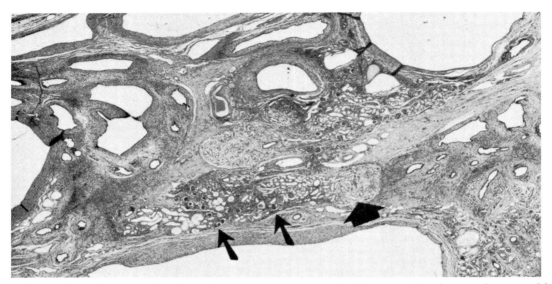

Figure 16–2.   Multicystic dysplasia. Microscopic examination of solid tissue within the central portion of the cystic kidney discloses rudimentary lobules of metanephric tissue in which glomeruli and tubules (arrows) are related to adjacent primitive ducts (broad arrow) in the manner of cortex to medulla. These islands of metanephric tissue may account for opacification of the solid portions and of the septa on high-dose excretory urography. Hematoxylin and eosin staining; × 18. (From Harrison, J. H., Gittes, R. F., Pearlmutter, A. D., et al.: Campbell's Urology, Vol. 2, 4th ed. Philadelphia, W. B. Saunders Co., 1979, p. 1435.)

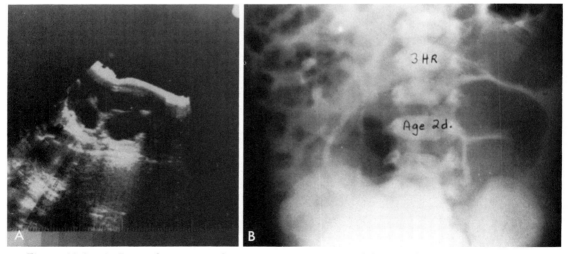

Figure 16–3.   A, Prenatal sonogram demonstrating a cystic renal lesion while the fetus is in utero. B, Excretory urography of the same patient after birth demonstrating a nonfunctioning left kidney. This proved to be a multicystic kidney.

radionuclides. Occasionally, if there is an unusual amount of renal tissue in the septa between the cysts, faint opacification of the septa may be noted on delayed studies. Even less frequently, a cyst may fill with contrast medium (Warshawsky et al., 1977).

Ureteral obstruction may be helpful diagnostically. Retrograde pyelography can demonstrate this finding should the diagnosis be in sufficient doubt to warrant such a study. In the majority, however, this does not become necessary. The diagnosis can be made with a great deal of accuracy when nonvisualization of a palpable flank mass is accompanied by the typical cystic appearance on ultrasonography (Fig. 16–3).

The eventual prognosis of the patient with a multicystic kidney is determined not by the mass itself but by the status of the contralateral kidney. In most instances, the contralateral kidney is normal, but in up to 40 per cent of cases there is some abnormality, usually obstruction (Greene et al., 1971). This contralateral problem is usually remediable, and for that reason, it must be recognized early if the patient is to be helped. Recently it has been shown that in instances of multicystic kidney in which ureteral atresia is proximal, the dysplasia is usually unilateral and the patient's prognosis is good. However, in cases in which the atresia is distal in the ureter, dysplasia may be bilateral and consequently implies a very poor prognosis (De Klerk et al., 1977).

The time-honored treatment for the multicystic kidney has been its extirpation, but this practice has come into question in recent years (Bloom and Brosman, 1978). It has been assumed that neoplasms, infection, and hypertension can result from multicystic kidneys left in situ, but if so, such problems have rarely been documented. The major impetus to approach these lesions surgically has been the desire to avoid misdiagnosing obstructive or malignant disease that could have been corrected with prompt treatment. With modern diagnostic methods, however, the likelihood for diagnostic confusion in this area is very small. Additionally, there does not seem to be any genetic implication to the diagnosis of multicystic kidney; consequently, a tissue diagnosis is not required for genetic counseling.

SEGMENTAL CYSTIC DYSPLASIA

On occasion in patients with renal duplication, there may be cystic dysplasia of only one segment of the duplication. This cystic dysplasia may then present as a mass. The therapy in these instances is usually removal of the involved segment with salvage of the normal portion of the kidney.

INFANTILE POLYCYSTIC DISEASE

Another lesion that is recognized during infancy is infantile polycystic disease (Fig. 16–4) (Lieberman et al., 1971). These kidneys are usually quite large and occupy almost the entire abdomen. Hence, they present as palpable masses. There is a very characteristic appearance seen with excretory urography in which there is a greatly prolonged nephrogram for as long as 48 to 72 hours. The collecting system itself is not well seen. The nephrogram is composed of dilated tubules that appear as streaks or rays of contrast perpendicular to the long axis of the kidney (Fig. 16–5); however, as the child grows older, more calyceal definition is apparent. It has been shown by microdissection that the cysts, all of which are very small, are really made up of dilated collecting tubules (Osathanondh and Potter, 1964).

Infantile polycystic disease is inherited as a true autosomal recessive characteristic. Consequently, it is important to the family that the problem be accurately diagnosed. Because the diagnosis can be made radiographically with great certainty, there is very little role for surgery in these patients, although, on occasion, biopsy material is desirable. It was once thought that infants born with this problem invariably died within the first few months of life, but this impression has recently been shown to be

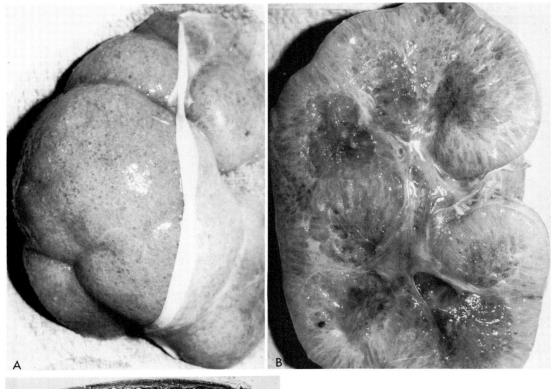

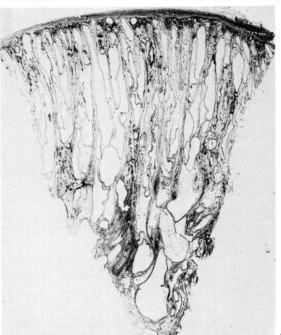

Figure 16–4. *A,* Subcapsular surface of an infantile polycystic kidney from a neonate. Innumerable small cysts can be seen beneath the capsule. *B,* Cross-section of the same kidney. The radial arrangement of the dilated ducts can be seen. *C,* Low-power view of the cortex from an infantile polycystic kidney. Notice the arrangement of dilated ducts, which are perpendicularly oriented to the capsule. (Hematoxylin and eosin; × 18.) (From Kelalis, P. P., King, L. R., and Belman, A. B.: Clinical Pediatric Urology, Vol. 2. Philadelphia, W. B. Saunders Co., 1976, pp. 689–690.)

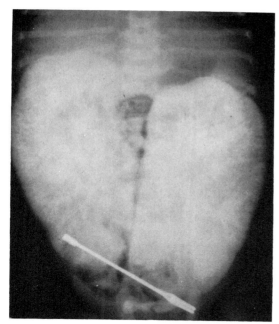

Figure 16–5. Excretory urogram from a two-day-old girl with infantile polycystic kidney disease. Notice the sunray appearance of the contrast material and the enormous renal size. (From Kelalis, P. P., King, L. R., and Belman, A. B.: Clinical Pediatric Urology, Vol. 2. Philadelphia, W. B. Saunders Co., 1976, p. 686.)

and Ockenden, 1971). This lesion is inherited as a true autosomal dominant trait and consequently has profound genetic implications. Once again, these patient will usually present with otherwise asymptomatic palpable masses. However, other modes of presentation include urinary tract infection, hematuria, and hypertension. Urographically, the kidneys will be large and the calyces splayed. The lesion progresses to renal failure usually within a decade of its recognition. Renal transplantation is a therapeutic option. Hypertension is a common component of this entity. Inasmuch as the problem is inherited, those suspected of being affected can be screened with ultrasonography. This is a noninvasive means of early diagnosis.

RENAL PATHOLOGIC CONDITIONS ASSOCIATED WITH TUBEROUS SCLEROSIS

One entity that may be easily confused with adult polycystic disease is the cystic forme fruste of the tuberous sclerosis complex (Stapleton et al., 1980). It may be that most cases of adult polycystic disease seen during childhood are really this entity, but this thought is speculative. The kidneys grossly resemble those of adult polycystic disease. Upon microscopy, however, there are findings that definitely identify the lesion as tuberous sclerosis. This problem can either be familial or can appear as a spontaneous mutation. More commonly, adults with tuberous sclerosis will have hamartomatous renal involvement (angiomyolipomas) (McCullough et al., 1971).

incorrect. Most of the early deaths are from respiratory causes; with improved respiratory care, most affected infants now survive into late childhood, albeit with some compromised renal function or with hypertension. At that time, they usually succumb to problems associated with hypertension unless renal transplantation is employed. However, hepatic fibrosis may be present and may even be a more dominant feature than the renal involvement. Renal transplantation in patients in whom immunosuppression is necessary may be precluded in patients with severe hepatic fibrosis as azathioprine also can be a hepatotoxin.

ADULT POLYCYSTIC DISEASE

Adult polycystic disease (Fig. 16–6) usually does not present in childhood, although rare cases have been reported (Blyth

SIMPLE CYSTS

Simple renal cysts are rarely seen in childhood but do occasionally pose a problem when they present as large asymptomatic or infected abdominal masses (Deweerd and Simon, 1956). Such cysts almost invariably are initially thought to be renal tumors, an error that could lead to a needless nephrectomy. However, proper diagnostic studies should clearly differentiate cysts from tumors. When correctly identified, such cysts can be handled by marsupialization of the cyst alone. There are no known genetic implications to simple cysts.

BENIGN CYSTIC NEPHROMA

Another rare problem that has various names is the multilocular cyst adenoma or benign cystic nephroma (diffuse nephroblastomatosis). This lesion usually presents as a mass. Inasmuch as microscopic ele-

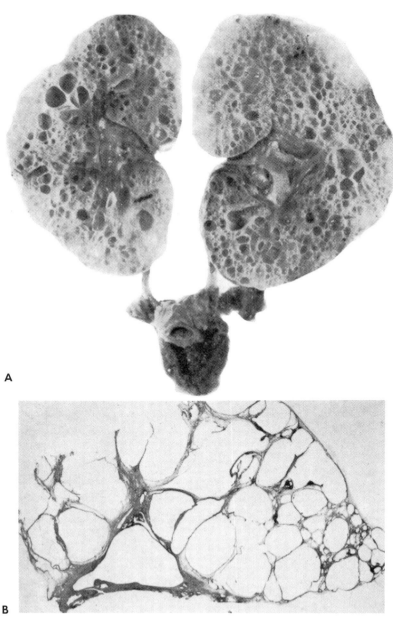

Figure 16–6. A, An example of adult polycystic kidney disease in a three-month-old infant. Notice the rounded cysts of varying size. B, Low-power view from the same kidney. Foci of normal renal tissue are seen between the grossly dilated tubules. (From Blyth, H., and Ockenden, B. G.: Polycystic disease of kidneys and liver presenting in childhood. J. Med. Genet., 8:257–284, 1971. Reproduced by permission.)

ments of Wilms' tumor may be found in the walls of the cysts, they are best treated by nephrectomy of the involved side.

MEDULLARY SPONGE KIDNEY

Medullary sponge kidney is benign and usually is detected incidentally in the course of an excretory urogram obtained for some unrelated reason (Pyrah, 1966). Adults with this problem will rarely form small stones or occasionally will have problems with hematuria or recurring infection. Occasionally, intrarenal cysts of a similar nature will be seen in echinococcal disease or tuberculosis.

RENAL CYSTIC DISEASE PRESENTING AS RENAL FAILURE

Renal cystic disease may be discovered in the evaluation of infants or children with renal failure. These patients usually present with nondescript symptoms, such as failure to thrive, vomiting, or diarrhea. In most such cases, the kidneys are either of normal size or hypoplastic. The diagnosis is usually made urographically, but occasionally it is made at the time of surgical biopsy. An example of this type of problem is dysplastic hypoplasia (Habib, 1974). Dysplastic hypoplastic kidneys are small and fibrotic; often there are small cortical cysts on the renal surface. Microscopically, elements of dysplasia, such as mesonephric tubules and cartilage, are present.

HEREDITARY SYNDROMES

Several hereditary syndromes in which cystic disease can be present include Meck-el's syndrome, Zellweger's cerebrohepatorenal syndrome, Jeune's asphyxiating thoracic dystrophy, and von Hippel-Lindau's disease. Cortical renal cysts are sometimes seen in syndromes of multiple congenital malformations. Renal cysts also occur in the renal medulla and are seen most often in familial juvenile nephrophthisis, medullary cystic disease, and renal retinal dysplasia. All these problems carry a grave prognosis (Bernstein, 1973).

REFERENCES

Bernstein, J.: The classification of renal cysts. Nephron, 11:91, 1973.

Bloom, D. A., and Brosman, S.: The multicystic kidney. J. Urol., 120:211, 1978.

Blyth, H., and Ockenden, B. G.: Polycystic disease of kidneys and liver presenting in childhood. J. Med. Genet., 8:257, 1971.

De Klerk, D. P., Marshall, F. F., and Jeffs, R. D.: Multicystic dysplastic kidney. J. Urol., 118:306, 1977.

Deweerd, J. H., and Simon, H. B.: Simple renal cysts in children. J. Urol., 75:912, 1956.

Greene, L. F., Feinzaig, W., and Dahlin, D. C.: Multicystic dysplasia of the kidney. J. Urol., 105:482, 1971.

Habib, R.: Renal dysplasia, hypoplasia, and cysts. In Strauss, J. (Ed.): Nephrology: Current Concepts in Diagnosis and Management. New York, Intercontinental Medical Book Corp., 1974, p. 1209.

Lieberman, E., Salinas-Madrigal, L., Gwinn, J. L., Brennan, L. P., Fine, R. N., and Landing, B. H.: Infantile polycystic disease of the kidneys and liver. Medicine, 50:277, 1971.

McCullough, D. L., Scott, R., Jr., and Seybold, H. M.: Renal angiomyolipoma (hamartoma). J. Urol., 105:32, 1971.

Osathanondh, V., and Potter, E. L.: Pathogenesis of polycystic kidneys. Survey of results of microdissection. Arch. Pathol., 77:510, 1964.

Pyrah, L. N.: Medullary sponge kidney. J. Urol., 95:274, 1966.

Spence, H. M.: Congenital unilateral multicystic kidney. J. Urol., 74:693, 1955.

Stapleton, F. B., Johnson D. L., Kaplan, G. W., and Griswold, R.: The cystic renal lesion in tuberous sclerosis. J. Pediatr., 97:574, 1980.

Warshawsky, A. B., Miller, H. E., and Kaplan, G. W.: Urographic visualization of multicystic kidneys. J. Urol., 117:94, 1977.

Chapter Seventeen

RENAL AND ADRENAL VENOUS THROMBOSIS; ADRENAL HEMORRHAGE

RENAL VENOUS THROMBOSIS

The problem of renal venous thrombosis in the newborn is occurring less frequently than formerly as greater attention is paid to hydration during the neonatal period. The two recognized forms of renal venous thrombosis include one associated with frank dehydration secondary to diarrhea and an idiopathic variety most often related to maternal diabetes mellitus. Idiopathic renal venous thrombosis has been seen in association with hydramnios, toxemia, cytomegalovirus infection, and prenatal maternal treatment with thiazides for hypertension. Frequently, however, no predisposing cause for renal venous thrombosis can be identified.

PATHOGENESIS

Both diarrhea and maternal diabetes mellitus cause hemoconcentration, which appears to play a significant role in pathogenesis by leading to circulatory sludging in the small intrarenal venules. Thrombosis is

initiated in these venules and may then propagate to involve secondarily the larger venous tributaries and ultimately the main renal veins and vena cava. Although it appears likely that renal venous thrombosis rarely may arise primarily in the main renal veins or the vena cava itself, it would seem that this is a less common occurrence.

An association between renal venous thrombosis and the nephrotic syndrome has been recognized in adults; recently, renal venous thrombosis has also been observed to follow congenital nephrosis (Roy et al., 1964; Alexander and Campbell, 1971). Renal venous thrombosis may also precede the nephrotic state (Lewy and Jao, 1974). The significance of this latter observation in terms of the long-term renal survival of infants with renal venous thrombosis is as yet unclear. An autoimmune state could theoretically be initiated by the thrombotic episode, which may at a later date manifest itself as significant renal disease, such as the nephrotic syndrome. However, Kaplan (1978) suggests that when both entities are seen in the same patient, the nephrotic syndrome always is the primary event.

CLINICAL PRESENTATION

There are no other clinical situations that mimic the presentation of renal venous thrombosis. One or more flank masses, hematuria, thrombocytopenia, and renal nonvisualization on urography or poor visualization on renal scan need confirmation only by inferior venacavography definitely noting thrombosis.

The differential diagnosis includes other causes of flank masses in the neonate, but these rarely are associated with hematuria and virtually never with thrombocytopenia. The septic infant may also present with thrombocytopenia and anuria but will not have an associated flank mass unless the cause is obstructive urinary sepsis.

EVALUATION

The accompanying thrombocytopenia in these cases is most likely the result of a consumptive-type coagulopathy, which can be confirmed by obtaining a coagulation profile. One finds a prolonged partial thromboplastin time, depressed fibrinogen level, increased fibrin split product levels, fragmented red cells, and burr cells. Bilirubin concentration elevation is not part of this syndrome (Renfield and Kraybill, 1973). Significant azotemia is not generally seen in unilateral cases.

In the neonate, radiographic evaluation is best carried out using the more sensitive renal scan rather than the standard excretory urogram. Interference with urographic visualization by increased intraintestinal gas as well as the diminished renal concentrating ability in the neonate both tend to render the renal scan superior to standard urography for this purpose (Fig. 17–1A). Additionally, newer scanning techniques can also demonstrate renal vascular perfusion, the definition of which may have significant prognostic implications.

Little is to be gained by performing cystoscopy and retrograde pyelography in these patients except when obstruction is a significant consideration in the differential diagnosis. Ultrasonography, however, can generally rule out obstruction without the necessity of resorting to invasive diagnostic modalities.

The definitive diagnosis is made by

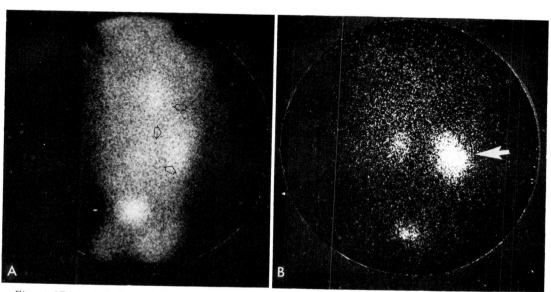

Figure 17–1. A, Radionuclide scan during the acute phase of left renal vein thrombosis in a neonate. The right kidney is functioning (arrows); however, no radioactive pickup is noted on the left side. B, Radionuclide scan in the same patient four months later. There is excellent function on the right (arrow) with poor function on the left. This result was to be anticipated in view of the poor pickup on the study done during the acute phase *(A).* (Courtesy of Dr. James Conway.) (From Kelalis, P. P., King, L. R., and Belman, A. B.: Clinical Pediatric Urology, Vol. 2. Philadelphia, W. B. Saunders Co., 1976, p. 855.)

inferior venacavography. When both kidneys are severely involved, the entire cava may also be obstructed. Venous drainage from the inferior extremities is then carried through the azygos and hemiazygos systems (Fig. 17–2). In less severe cases, the cava itself may be free of thrombus; however, a small intrusion at the ostium of the involved renal vein may be seen on the cavogram. Another presumptive finding includes decreased renal venous outflow as determined by selective renal vein catheterization.

Arteriography is also a means by which vascularization may be evaluated. McDonald and associates (1974) suggest that the presence of adequate arterial perfusion may predict ultimate renal functional survival. Renal death is not the result of poor venous drainage alone but rather occurs because the renal tissue is not perfused when edema compresses the intrarenal arteries. Renal scanning during the early phases of renal venous thrombosis may be an equally effective but less invasive method of making the same determination (Fig. 17–1A).

MANAGEMENT

The most vital step in treatment is correction of the underlying hemoconcentration. Standard treatment for correction of fluid and electrolyte imbalance is recommended.

Nephrectomy in unilateral cases was once thought to be life-saving (Campbell and Matthews, 1942). It became apparent with experience, however, that children survived in spite of rather than because of nephrectomy (Stark, 1964). It is now obvious even to the most stalwart advocates of surgery that removal of the involved kidney in the child with clinically evident unilateral involvement becomes necessary only when supervening renal infection jeopardizes the patient's chances for survival. Currently, because of the availability of potent antibiotics, this is a rare occurrence.

The main reason to avoid nephrectomy is that up to 50 per cent of affected kidneys will regain function (Belman et al., 1970). Although those kidneys that become contracted have the potential for producing renin-mediated hypertension on an ischemic basis, this is an unlikely complication and does not justify preventive nephrectomy.

Controversy persists, however, when there is clinically apparent bilateral involvement. There are reports in which caval thrombectomy and aspiration of a clot from the renal vessels have been associated with patient survival (Lowry et al., 1970; Mauer et al., 1971; Thompson et al., 1975; Verhagen et al., 1965). The conclusion followed, therefore, that the surgical procedure was responsible for the favorable end result. However, an equal number of cases of bilateral renal venous thrombosis have also been reported in which the patient survived without benefit of surgery. Return of func-

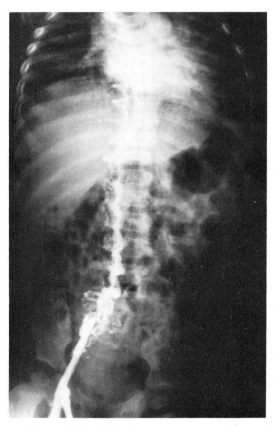

Figure 17–2. Inferior venacavagram. There is complete occlusion of the vena cava with collateral drainage through the azygous, hemiazygous, and vertebral systems. (Courtesy of Dr. Ruth A. Seeler.) (From Kelalis, P. P., King, L. R., and Belman, A. B.: Clinical Pediatric Urology, Vol. 2. Philadelphia, W. B. Saunders Co., 1976, p. 854.)

tion was noted in both kidneys in some of these children (McDonald et al., 1974; Seeler, 1970).

If surgery is not to be employed, there is the additional question of the necessity for anticoagulation therapy in these patients. Heparinization has been advocated (Renfield and Krayhill, 1973) and has been thought to influence the dissolution of the caval thrombosis (McDonald et al., 1974), which appears to persist if otherwise untreated (Fig. 17–3). Although the most significant step in the treatment of renal venous thrombosis continues to be control of the underlying hemoconcentration, a 10- to 14-day course of systemic heparin therapy should be seriously considered in those situations in which persistent platelet depression leads one to suspect that the thrombotic process is progressing. Otherwise, it is our conviction that in the majority of patients this is a self-limiting disease and therefore does not require further therapeutic measures. Dialysis may be necessary in those patients with severe bilateral involvement; death may still occur when renal necrosis results from thrombosis. Whether thrombectomy would improve survival in this small subgroup is unknown.

ADRENAL VENOUS THROMBOSIS

Incidental adrenal venous thrombosis may accompany renal venous thrombosis

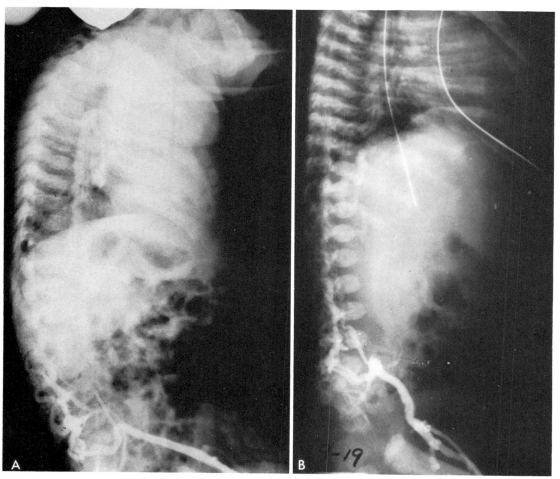

Figure 17–3.   A, Lateral view inferior venacavagram in a neonate with bilateral renal vein thrombosis and thrombosis of the vena cava. B, Same patient as A, several months later. Caval obstruction persists; clinically the child is thriving. (Courtesy of Dr. Ruth A. Seeler.) (From Kelalis, P. P., King, L. R., and Belman, A. B.: Clinical Pediatric Urology, Vol. 2. Philadelphia, W. B. Saunders Co., 1976, p. 857.)

more commonly in infants born to diabetic mothers (Oppenheimer and Esterly, 1965). Since the primary illness revolves around the renal manifestations, little is known about the adrenal aspects. Adrenal venous thrombosis would appear to be of minor significance.

ADRENAL HEMORRHAGE

PATHOGENESIS

Massive adrenal hemorrhage in the neonate is a rare vascular accident of unknown etiology. There appears to be a relationship between adrenal hemorrhage and traumatic delivery, particularly with the breech presentation. Compression of the relatively large adrenals by the delivering physician, increased pressure in the vena cava transmitted to the adrenals, and compression of the right adrenal gland between the liver and kidney have all been suggested, without validation, to explain its occurrence. The greater frequency of right-sided involvement (70 per cent) has been offered as an argument in favor of hepatic compression as a significant cause of this phenomenon.

CLINICAL PRESENTATION

Five to 10 per cent of neonatal adrenal hemorrhages are bilateral. The majority occur in males. The patient presents at three to four days of age with one or more flank masses and jaundice. The jaundice may be prolonged and is a consequence of the breakdown and absorption of the retroperitoneal hematoma (Rose et al., 1971). Clinically, the patient is usually asymptomatic; however, massive bleeding occasionally produces signs of anemia and even circulatory collapse. Adrenal insufficiency per se does not develop even in those infants with bilateral involvement.

The masses may not be recognized or may not be present in the immediate postnatal period. If uncomplicated, the problem may never come to attention. Failure to gain weight, anemia, unexplained leukocytosis, or a suprarenal mass may lead to the diagnosis of a secondarily infected adrenal hemorrhage (Favara et al., 1970; Carty and Stanley, 1973). The proposed pathogenic scheme was offered by Favara and colleagues (Fig. 17–4).

Infrequently, adrenal bleeding is not confined to a fixed suprarenal area. The hematoma capsule may rupture so that there is extension to the groin or, more importantly, into the peritoneal cavity.

Adrenal hemorrhage and renal venous thrombosis may occur simultaneously. This presents a diagnostic dilemma, particularly if opposite sides are affected.

EVALUATION

The presumptive diagnosis of adrenal hemorrhage is made radiographically with rapid high-dose excretory urography (3 to 4 ml per kg). During the very early total body opacification phase, the contrast medium perfuses all vascular spaces. Any avascular space, such as a large hematoma or a large hydronephrotic renal pelvis, appears as a negative shadow. Films must be taken at one and two minutes to detect this finding.

In adrenal hemorrhage the ipsilateral kidney is displaced inferiorly by the hematoma (Fig. 17–5). The peritoneal contents may also be pushed anteriorly by the large retroperitoneal mass. Ultrasonography is helpful in demonstrating whether this avascular mass is fluid-filled (hydronephrosis), whether it has some internal echoes (blood clot), or whether it is solid (tumor) (Lawson and Teele, 1978).

The differential diagnosis includes duplication of the renal collecting system in which a dilated, obstructed upper renal segment pushes the normal segment inferiorly (Fig. 17–6). A hydronephrotic duplicated upper segment should particularly be considered when a filling defect is noted in the bladder, suggesting the presence of a ureterocele. Delayed radiographic visualization of a poorly functioning upper segment should also be sought (see Chap. 12).

Adrenal hemorrhage may be confused

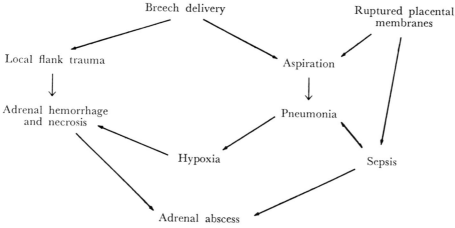

Figure 17–4. Proposed pathogenic scheme for adrenal abscess in the neonate. (From Favara, B. E., Akers, D. R., and Franciosi, R. A.: Adrenal abscess in a neonate. J. Pediatr., 77:682–685, 1970.)

with neuroblastoma because both appear as suprarenal masses. Histologic evidence of neuroblastoma has been noted in a surgically removed adrenal hemorrhage (Sober and Hirsch, 1965); however, this was most likely "neuroblastoma in situ" without clinical significance (Beckwith and Perrin, 1963).

Renal tumors in the neonate are also rare and when present are generally benign mesoblastic nephromas. However, since adrenal hemorrhage is not really intrarenal but extrinsic to the kidney, the various radiographic studies should effectively rule out an intrarenal pathologic condition.

Finally, one must be aware that adrenal hemorrhage may be a manifestation of the Waterhouse-Friderichsen syndrome. A child with this syndrome will be in shock secondary to fulminating meningococce-

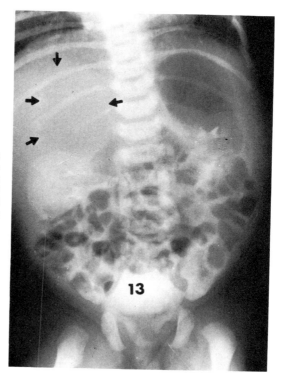

Figure 17–5. Excretory urogram of a newborn with neonatal adrenal hemorrhage. Note the radiolucent suprarenal mass on the right (arrows), not to be confused with stomach gas on the left. (Courtesy of Dr. Harvey White.) (From Kelalis, P. P., King, L. R., and Belman, A. B.: Clinical Pediatric Urology, Vol. 2. Philadelphia, W. B. Saunders Co., 1976, p. 858.)

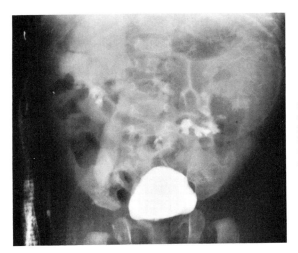

Figure 17–6. Left collecting system inferiorly displaced. Right collecting system is obviously duplicated with normal configuration of the lower system and massively enlarged upper collecting system and ureter. Conclusion: There is probably bilateral duplication with obstruction of both upper segments, resulting in displacement of the lower segments.

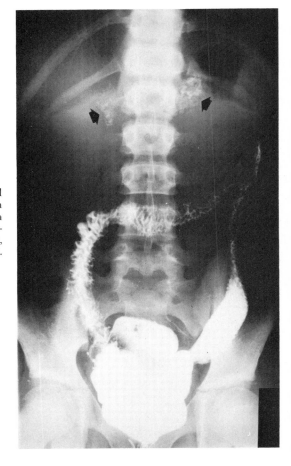

Figure 17–7. Thirteen-year-old girl with bilateral adrenal calcification picked up incidentally on barium enema. Changes are typical of triangular stippling seen after neonatal adrenal hemorrhage. (Courtesy of Dr. Harvey White.) (From Kelalis, P. P., King, L. R., and Belman, A. B.: Clinical Pediatric Urology, Vol. 2. Philadelphia, W. B. Saunders Co., 1976, p. 859.)

mia; adrenal hemorrhage is a secondary manifestation. It is unlikely that the Waterhouse-Friderichsen syndrome will be confused with the relatively benign idiopathic adrenal hemorrhage.

MANAGEMENT

The course is generally self-limiting, and the hematoma resolves within a few weeks, leaving only triangular-shaped calcifications in the suprarenal areas. These may be noted as incidental radiographic findings (Fig. 17–7). The classic crescent shape should prevent its being confused with more serious causes for calcification in this area. Adrenal insufficiency is not a part of this picture, neither acutely nor on a long-term basis.

Occasionally, as previously mentioned, bleeding may be severe, requiring transfusion and even surgical exploration. Additionally, the necrotic hemorrhagic focus is a perfect location for abscess formation, producing an indolent illness difficult to diagnose until a mass is palpable.

REFERENCES

Alexander, F., and Campbell, W. A. B.: Congenital nephrotic syndrome and renal vein thrombosis. J. Clin. Pathol., 24:27, 1971.

Beckwith, J. B., and Perrin, E. V.: In situ neuroblastomas: A contribution to the natural history of neural crest tumors. Am. J. Pathol., 43:1089, 1963.

Belman, A. B., Susmano, D. F., Burden, J. J., and Kaplan, G. W.: Nonoperative treatment of unilateral renal vein thrombosis in the newborn. J.A.M.A., 211:1165, 1970.

Campbell, M. F., and Matthews, W. F.: Renal thrombosis in infancy. J. Pediatr., 20:604, 1942.

Carty, A., and Stanley, P.: Bilateral adrenal abscesses in a neonate. Pediatr. Radiol., 1:63, 1973.

Favara, B. E., Akers, D. R., and Franciosi, R. A.: Adrenal abscess in a neonate. J. Pediatr., 77:682, 1970.

Kaplan, B. S.: Nephrotic syndrome in renal vein thrombosis. Am. J. Dis. Child., 132:367, 1978.

Lawson, E. D., and Teele, R. L.: Diagnosis of adrenal hemorrhage by ultrasound. J. Pediatr., 92:423, 1978.

Lewy, P. R., and Jao, W.: Nephrotic syndrome in association with renal vein thrombosis in infancy. Report of a case and review of the literature. J. Pediatr., 85:359, 1974.

Lowry, M. F., Mann, J. R., Abrams, L. D., and Chance, G. W.: Thrombectomy for renal venous thrombosis in infant of diabetic mother. Br. Med. J., 3:687, 1970.

Mauer, S. M., Fraley, E. E., Fish, A. J., and Najarian, J. S.: Bilateral renal vein thrombosis in infancy. Report of a survivor following surgical intervention. J. Pediatr., 78:509, 1971.

McDonald, P., Tarar, R., Gilday, D., and Reilly, B. J.: Some radiologic observations in renal vein thrombosis. Am. J. Roentgen. Rad. Ther., 120:368, 1974.

Oppenheimer, E. H., and Esterly, J. R.: Thrombosis in the newborn: Comparison between infants of diabetic and nondiabetic mothers. J. Pediatr., 68:549, 1965.

Renfield, M. L., and Kraybill, E. N.: Consumptive coagulopathy with renal vein thrombosis. J. Pediatr., 82:1054, 1973.

Rose, J., Berdon, W. E., Sullivan, T., et al.: Prolonged jaundice as presenting sign of massive adrenal hemorrhage in newborn: Radiographic diagnosis by IVP with total-body opacification. Radiology, 98:263, 1971.

Roy, C. C., Bedard, G., Bonenfant, J. C., and Fortin, R.: Congenital nephrosis associated with thrombosis of the inferior vena cava and of the right renal vein in a six week old premature infant. Can. Med. Assoc. J., 90:786, 1964.

Seeler, R. A.: Renal vein thrombosis in the newborn. J.A.M.A., 213:1906, 1970.

Sober, I., and Hirsch, M.: Unilateral massive adrenal hemorrhage in newborn infant. J. Urol., 93:430, 1965.

Stark, H.: Renal vein thrombosis in infancy: Recovery without nephrectomy. Am. J. Dis. Child., 108:430, 1964.

Thompson, I. M., Schneider, R., and Lababidi, Z.: Thrombectomy for neonatal renal vein thrombosis. J. Urol., 113:396, 1975.

Verhagen, A. D., Hamilton, J. P., and Benel, M.: Renal vein thrombosis in infants. Arch. Dis. Child., 40:214, 1965.

Chapter Eighteen

HYPERTENSION

Hypertension is a problem that can occur at any age; there is no question that it is seen in the pediatric age group. The true incidence of hypertension in children is completely unknown but has been estimated at one to two per cent of the population less than 15 years of age (Lieberman, 1974). Hypertension may be defined as a systolic or diastolic blood pressure consistently higher than the 95th percentile of the expected blood pressure for the child's age. Although there have been sufficient measurements to provide good standards for blood pressure levels in children older than two years (Fig. 18–1) (Londe, 1966), there are no good data to indicate what constitutes a normal blood pressure in premature infants, in normal-term infants, and in very young children. It has been determined, however, that the blood pressure as measured directly in the lower aorta of neonates is 70 ± 8 mm Hg systolic and 44 ± 7 mm Hg diastolic (Kitterman et al., 1968). Most children with significant hypertension in infancy or childhood present with such marked elevations of blood pressure that there is little question that the recorded values are abnormal.

One of the major difficulties in detecting hypertension in children is the difficulty associated with measurement of the child's blood pressure. It is unfortunate that

routine measurement of blood pressure is not a standard practice of office pediatrics. Largely owing to efforts of the American Academy of Pediatrics to correct this pattern, assessment of blood pressure may become routine in the not too distant future. Certainly all would agree that the blood pressure of seriously ill children should be monitored.

A major difficulty encountered with measurement of blood pressure in children is the selection of an appropriate-sized cuff. When a cuff too narrow for the child's arm is utilized, falsely high blood pressure may be obtained. It is recommended that the cuff occupy two thirds of the area of the upper arm (Blumenthal et al., 1977). In infants, it is often difficult to hear the Korotkoff sounds, and consequently blood pressures are sometimes determined by palpation or even by flush. Another adjunct, especially useful in the hospital setting, is an instrument that utilizes a Doppler principle for assessment of blood pressure.

If one extrapolates from adult experience, it is presumed that chronic elevation of blood pressure causes significant morbidity and mortality over a period of time. Additionally, in the pediatric age group, there is a higher incidence of "curable" hypertension than is encountered in adults (Loggie, 1969); hence, hypertension in chil-

302

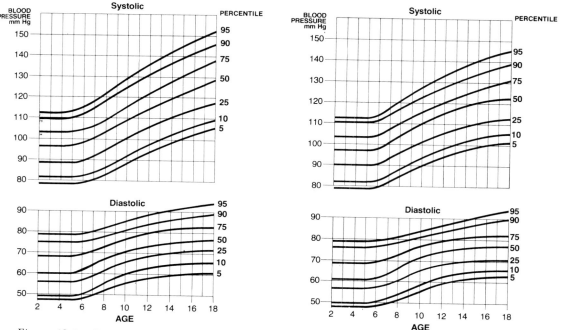

Figure 18–1. Percentiles of blood pressure measurements. *A,* In boys (right arm with the patient seated) and *B,* In girls (right arm with the patient seated). (From Blumenthal, S., et al.: Report of the Task Force on Blood Pressure Control in Children. Pediatrics, 59:803, 1977.)

dren must be viewed as a symptom of an underlying process, and a thorough search must be made for the cause.

sion; it has subsequently been shown that this is due to activation of the renin-angiotensin mechanism.

MECHANISMS OF HYPERTENSION

RENOVASCULAR HYPERTENSION

One of the mechanisms that produces hypertension is an alteration of the renin-angiotensin-aldosterone system (Haber, 1969) (Fig. 18–2). Renin is an enzyme elaborated by the kidneys' juxtaglomerular apparatus; this enzyme acts on renin substrate, which has been formed in the liver to produce the decapeptide angiotensin I. Angiotensin I is then converted to an octapeptide, angiotensin II, by enzymes in the plasma and the lungs. Angiotensin II is a very potent pressor substance that also stimulates the production of aldosterone. Aldosterone acts on the distal renal tubule to produce sodium retention. Goldblatt and colleagues (1934), in their classic experiments in dogs, demonstrated that constriction of the renal artery results in hyperten-

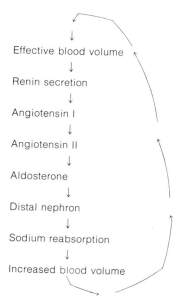

Figure 18–2. The Renin–Angiotensin–Aldosterone System. (From Kelalis, P. P., King, L. R., and Belman, A. B.: Clinical Pediatric Urology, Vol. 2. Philadelphia, W. B. Saunders Co., 1976, p. 823.)

Renal arterial narrowing as a cause for renovascular hypertension occurs in children; three per cent of all instances of renovascular hypertension arise in children less than 16 years of age (Stickler and Kelalis, 1976). Renovascular hypertension has been reported in neonates (Cook et al., 1966) and is occasionally familial (Bloom et al., 1973). It has also been reported to occur in the rubella syndrome (Menser et al., 1966), idiopathic hypercalcemia (Royer et al., 1974), Marfan's syndrome (Loughridge, 1959), and neurofibromatosis (Grad and Rance, 1972). The underlying pathologic condition may be hypoplasia of the renal artery, intimal or fibromuscular hyperplasia, or even arteritis (Coran and Schuster, 1968). The vascular disease is often bilateral or becomes bilateral in this age group (Sinaiko et al., 1973).

Hypertension may also be caused by coarctation of the abdominal aorta (Sealy, 1967). By the same mechanism, hypertension may be seen after radiation therapy, presumably as the result of an arteritis that can involve branches of the renal artery as well as the main renal artery (Colquhoun, 1966).

Renal Parenchymal Disease

Additionally, hypertension may be the result of renal parenchymal disease; this hypertension is also often renin-mediated. Examples include unilateral renal hypoplasia, dysplasia, and severe pyelonephritic scarring (Meares and Gross, 1958). One special variant of this problem is segmental hypoplasia of the kidney, the Ask-Upmark kidney, in which hypoplasia and dysplasia are confined to only one segment of the kidney while the remainder of the kidney is relatively normal (Rosenfeld et al., 1973). Reflux nephropathy commonly presents as hypertension in adolescent girls. A history of urinary tract infection and the demonstration of vesicoureteral reflux in the presence of severe unilateral or bilateral renal scarring confirms the diagnosis (Chap. 4). Hypertension may also be seen as a late complication of renal vein thrombo-

sis due to renal fibrosis and presumed ischemia (Perry and Taylor, 1940).

A rare but definite cause of hypertension is hydronephrosis. In some instances, at least, this is renin-mediated (Belman et al., 1968). Hypertension is occasionally seen in Wilms' tumor patients; it has recently been demonstrated that Wilms' tumors can contain high levels of renin; presumably it is the secretion of this renin that results in this form of hypertension (Mitchell et al., 1970). Tumors of the juxtaglomerular appartus (hemangiopericytomas), which are renin-secreting tumors, have been described in adolescents as young as 13 years (Conn et al., 1973). These patients usually present with hypertension.

Saline-Dependent Hypertension

Another mechanism by which hypertension is produced in children is saline-dependent hypertension, seen especially in advanced renal failure (Merrill et al., 1961). Here, there is expansion of the extracellular fluid compartment. When this mechanism is operative, blood pressure can be controlled by restricting the dietary intake of salt and water, administering diuretics, and, in the most severe circumstances, by dialysis.

Steroidal Causes for Hypertension

Alterations of corticosteroid production will result in high blood pressure. Aldosterone, produced in the zona glomerulosa of the adrenal cortex, enhances sodium-potassium exchange in the distal nephron; its secretion leads to sodium retention and urinary potassium loss. Primary aldosteronism is a syndrome of excessive aldosterone production due to an adrenal cortical adenoma. The youngest reported patient with this syndrome was three years of age (Cavell et al., 1964). Patients with primary aldosteronism will present with mild hypertension, hypokalemic alkalosis, and decreased plasma renin activity. In two varieties of congenital adrenal hyperplasia, the 11-β-hydroxylase deficiency and the 17-

hydroxylase deficiency, hypertension may be a feature, presumably due to aldosterone hypersecretion (Allen, 1976). Glucocorticoid excess, such as Cushing's syndrome or treatment with cortisone or prednisone, similarly can cause hypertension by volume expansion secondary to salt retention (Raiti et al., 1972).

CATECHOLAMINE-PRODUCED HYPERTENSION

Yet another mechanism that produces hypertension is catecholamine excess. Epinephrine and norepinephrine are the principal biologically active catecholamines. Epinephrine is the main hormone produced by the adrenal medulla, whereas norepinephrine is liberated by sympathetic nerve and extra-adrenal chromaffin tissue. Causes of hypertension produced by this mechanism in childhood are tumors such as pheochromocytomas, neuroblastomas, and ganglioneuromas (Stackpole et al., 1963).

TRANSIENT POSTOPERATIVE HYPERTENSION

An unusual form of childhood hypertension sometimes seen in urologic practice is the hypertension that is observed postoperatively, especially after the relief of urinary obstruction. The exact mechanism for this hypertension is unknown. In some instances, at least, this form of hypertension can be renin-mediated (Belman and Lewy, 1974). If it occurs, the hypertension is usually transient, generally lasting less than one week but occasionally for several weeks. It will usually require treatment, as it can be of sufficient degree to produce hypertensive encephalopathy.

ESSENTIAL HYPERTENSION

Essential hypertension is a diagnosis of exclusion and should not be made in children unless all other etiologic possibilities have been considered.

SEQUELAE OF HYPERTENSION

The major consequences of untreated hypertension are cardiac, neurologic, and renal (Lloyd-Still and Cottom, 1967). Persistent hypertension will result in left ventricular hypertrophy, evident on an electrocardiogram before it is detectable clinically; if untreated, it can lead to left ventricular failure. Headaches are common in severe hypertension; convulsions due to hypertensive encephalopathy may occur. When hypertensive encephalopathy is present, there is almost always funduscopic evidence of malignant hypertension. Often papilledema will be seen at this time. Additionally, in the malignant phases of hypertension, renal function may deteriorate.

EVALUATION

The clinical presentation of children with hypertension varies greatly depending on their age. Infants may be completely asymptomatic or, at most, may demonstrate irritability and failure to thrive (Plumer et al., 1975). Young children may not present until convulsions have occurred. The older child may complain of headache or a general lack of well-being. It is obvious that the only real indicator of hypertension is the actual measurement of the blood pressure; it is for this reason that such measurements are so strongly urged.

Once hypertension in a child has been identified and confirmed, evaluation for a possible underlying cause is in our opinion mandatory. An excretory urogram is probably the most rewarding of the initial laboratory studies; however, special attention should be paid to the manner in which this is performed (Maxwell et al., 1964). Films should be obtained sequentially beginning one minute after injection so that differences in the appearance time of the contrast agent, reflecting differences in renal blood flow, may be identified (Fig. 18–3). Additionally, a delayed film at 20 to 30 minutes should be obtained to demon-

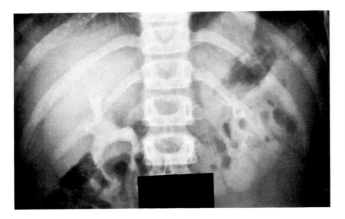

Figure 18–3. Urogram of a nine-year-old girl with renovascular hypertension. There was delayed appearance and decreased concentration of contrast medium on the left. (From Kelalis, P. P., King, L. R., and Belman, A. B.: Clinical Pediatric Urology, Vol. 2. Philadelphia, W. B. Saunders Co., 1976, p. 829.)

strate delayed washout of the contrast agent.

Voiding cystourethrography is probably desirable in most cases but is essential in patients with a contracted kidney to detect underlying vesicoureteral reflux. Appropriate laboratory studies include determinations of serum electrolytes and urinalysis to rule out underlying adrenal or renal diseases. Vanillylmandelic acid and homovanillic acid (VMA and HVA) determinations are useful to detect a catecholamine excess. Adrenal or intra-abdominal calcification on plain abdominal radiographs may similarly indicate the presence of a tumor.

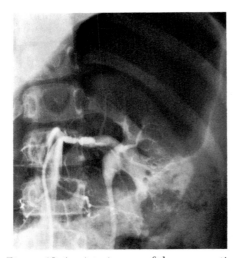

Figure 18–4. Arteriogram of the same patient in Figure 18–3, demonstrating fibromuscular dysplasia of the main renal artery. (From Kelalis, P. P., King, L. R., and Belman, A. B.: Clinical Pediatric Urology, Vol. 2. Philadelphia, W. B. Saunders Co., 1976, p. 829.)

If the foregoing studies are normal and a diagnosis has not been obtained, it is strongly recommended that an arteriogram be performed (Fig. 18–4). Although there is slightly more morbidity noted from arteriography in children as compared to adults, the morbidity of untreated hypertension is sufficient to warrant its use. It is only by this approach that renal vascular hypertension will be uncovered. Additionally, it is suggested that magnification techniques be utilized to outline lesions in the branches of the renal arteries (Fig. 18–5). At the time of arteriography, selective renal vein renin determinations can be obtained. This study is helpful in lateralizing the offending kidney; additionally, it is a good predictor of the potential for success after surgical intervention. However, this study has not proved quite as reliable in children as it has in adults (Marks and Maxwell, 1975).

TREATMENT

The medical management of hypertension will not be discussed, as it is beyond the scope of this presentation. However, philosophically it does need to be emphasized that control of hypertension in a child will probably require lifelong medication. Hence, if one is faced with the possibility of a curative procedure as opposed to lifelong medical management whose consequences are unknown, there is a great deal to be said for definitive surgical treatment.

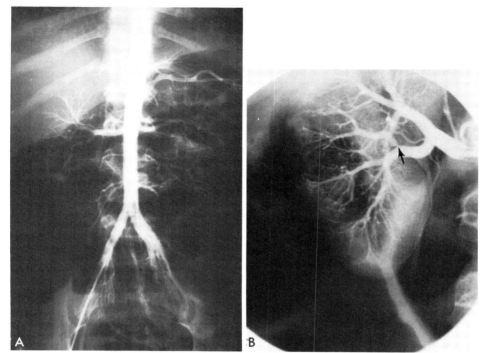

Figure 18–5. A, Aortogram of a six-year-old boy with a lesion of the tertiary branches of the right renal artery. B, Magnification film of the right renal arterial supply demonstrating the lesion (arrow).

In instances of renovascular hypertension, success has been observed with renovascular repair, and this is preferred to nephrectomy whenever feasible (Fry et al., 1973). One special exception, however, is the neonate with a thrombosed renal artery following the use of an inlying umbilical arterial catheter. If this child does not respond promptly to adequate attempts at medical management, nephrectomy is urgently necessary (Plumer et al., 1975). Because these infants are so desperately ill, it is felt completely unjustified to attempt a prolonged procedure for vascular repair. In the majority, however, medical control of the hypertension can be accomplished. Where hydronephrosis has been demonstrated, there often will be resolution of the hypertension following the relief of the obstruction.

When the cause of the hypertension is thought to be secondary to a small and relatively functionless kidney, some serious thought must be given to nephrectomy. Inasmuch as such a kidney usually does not contribute very much to overall renal func-

tion, it can be sacrificed without consequence. When hypertension and reflux coexist, it seems that operations designed to prevent reflux rarely, if ever, have any beneficial effect on the hypertension (Stickler et al., 1971). This special group of patients usually have severe interstitial nephritis. In such patients, if one kidney seems more involved than the other (as determined by differential renin determinations), it would seem appropriate to contemplate nephroureterectomy of the affected side for resolution of the hypertension. Our own attempts at removal of the more severely scarred kidney and partial nephrectomy on the contralateral side where only a renal pole was involved did not meet with success in resolving the hypertension. However, improvement in control with less medication required has been reported (Poutasse et al., 1978). In some patients with chronic renal failure and hypertension in whom the hypertension cannot be controlled by dialysis, bilateral nephrectomy has proved beneficial in the relief of hypertension (Siegler, 1974). If renal tumors are identified as a cause for hypertension, the hypertension will usually respond to the removal of the tumor.

REFERENCES

Allen, T. A.: Disorders of sexual differentiation. Urology, 7(Suppl.), 1, 1976.

Belman, A. B., and Lewy, P. R.: Acute transient renin-mediated hypertension in children following urinary diversion. Urology, 3:693, 1974.

Belman, A. B., Kropp, K. A., and Simon, N. M.: Renal-pressor hypertension secondary to unilateral hydronephrosis. N. Engl. J. Med., 278:1133, 1968.

Blom van Assendelft, P. M., Kooiker, C. J., Dorhout Mees, E. J., and Hameleers, A. J.: Renovascular hypertension in three children from one family. J. Clin. Pathol., 26:359, 1973.

Blumenthal, S., et al.: Methodology and instrumentation for blood pressure measurement in infants and children. Pediatrics, 59:800, 1977.

Cavell, B., Sandegard, E., and Hökfelt, B.: Primary aldosteronism due to an adrenal adenoma in a three year old child. Acta Paediatr. Scand., 53:215, 1964.

Colquhoun, J.: Hypoplasia of the abdominal aorta following therapeutic irradiation in infancy. Radiology, 86:454, 1966.

Conn, J. W., Bookstein, J. J., and Cohen, E. L.: Renin-secreting juxtaglomerular-cell adenoma. Radiology, 106:543, 1971.

Cook, G. T., Marshall, V. F., and Todd, J. E.: Malignant renovascular hypertension in a newborn. J. Urol., 96:863, 1966.

Coran, A. G., and Schuster, S. R.: Renovascular hypertension in childhood. Surgery, 64:672, 1968.

Fry, W. J., Ernst, C. B., Stanley, J. C., and Brink, B.: Renovascular hypertension in the pediatric patient. Arch. Surg., 107:692, 1973.

Goldblatt, H., Lynch, J., Hanzal, R. F., and Summerville, V. W.: Studies in experimental hypertension. J. Exp. Med., 59:347, 1934.

Grad, E., and Rance, C. P.: Bilateral renal artery stenosis in association with neurofibromatosis. J. Pediatr., 80:804, 1972.

Haber, E.: Recent developments in pathophysiologic studies of the renin-angiotensin system. N. Engl. J. Med., 280:148, 1969.

Kitterman, J. A., Phipps, R. H., and Tooley, W. H.: Aortic blood pressure in normal newborn infants during the first 12 hours of life. Pediatrics, 44:959, 1968.

Lieberman, E.: Essential hypertension in children and youth. J. Pediatr., 85:1, 1974.

Lloyd-Still, J. D., and Cottom, D.: Severe hypertension in children. Arch. Dis. Child., 42:34, 1967.

Loggie, J. M. H.: Hypertension in children and adolescents. J. Pediatr., 74:331, 1969.

Londe, S.: Blood pressure in children as determined under office conditions. Clin. Pediatr., 5:71, 1966.

Loughridge, L. W.: Renal abnormalities in the Marfan syndrome. Q. J. Med., 28:531, 1959.

Marks, L. S., and Maxwell, M. H.: Renal vein renin. Urol. Clin. North Am., 2:311, 1975.

Maxwell, M. H., Gonick, H. C., Wilta, R., and Kaufman, J. J.: Use of the rapid sequence intravenous pyelogram in the diagnosis of renovascular hypertension. N. Engl. J. Med., 270:213, 1964.

Meares, E. M., Jr., and Gross, D. M.: Hypertension owing to unilateral renal disease. J. Urol., 39:611, 1958.

Menser, M. A., Dorman, D. C., Reye, R. D. K., and Reid, R. R.: Renal artery stenosis in the rubella syndrome. Lancet, 1:790, 1966.

Merrill, J. P., Giordano, L., and Heetderks, D. R.: The role of the kidney in human hypertension. Am. J. Med., 31:931, 1961.

Mitchell, J. D., Baxter, Z. J., Blairwest, J. R., and McCredie, D. A.: Renin levels in nephroblastoma (Wilms' tumor). Arch. Dis. Child., 45:376, 1970.

Perry, C. B., and Taylor, A. L.: Hypertension following thrombosis of renal veins. J. Pathol. Bacteriol., 51:369, 1940.

Plumer, L. B., Mendoza, S. A., and Kaplan, G. W.: Hypertension in infancy. J. Urol., 113:555, 1975.

Poutasse, E. F., Stecker, J. F., Jr., Ladaga, L. E., and Sperber, E. E.: Malignant hypertension in children secondary to chronic pyelonephritis. J. Urol., 119:264, 1978.

Raiti, S., Grant, D. B., Williams, D. I., and Newns, G. H.: Cushing's syndrome in childhood. Arch. Dis. Child., 47:597, 1972.

Rosenfeld, J. B., Cohen, L., Garty, I., and Ben-Bassat, M.: Unilateral renal hypoplasia with hypertension (Ask-Upmark kidney). Br. Med. J., 2:217, 1973.

Royer, P., Habib, R., Mathieu, H., and Broyer, M.: Pediatric Nephrology. Philadelphia, W. B. Saunders Co., 1974, p. 188.

Sealy, W. C.: Coarction of the aorta and hypertension. Ann. Thorac. Surg., 3:15, 1967.

Siegler, R. L.: Malignant hypertension in children. Am. J. Dis. Child., 128:853, 1974.

Sinaik, O., Najarian, J., and Michael, A. F.: Renal auto-transplantation in the treatment of bilateral renal artery stenosis. J. Pediatr., 83:409, 1973.

Stackpole, R. H., Melicow, M. M., and Uson, A. C.: Pheochromocytoma in children. J. Pediatr., 63:315, 1963.

Stickler, G. B., and Kelalis, P. P.: Hypertension in children. In Kelalis, P. P., King, L. R., and Belman, A. B. (Eds.): Clinical Pediatric Urology. Philadelphia, W. B. Saunders Co., 1976, p. 821.

Stickler, G. B., Kelalis, P. P., and Burke, E. C.: Primary interstitial nephritis with reflux. Am. J. Dis. Child., 122:144, 1971.

Chapter Nineteen

CALCULUS DISEASE

Stone disease in children has been known since antiquity. It seems forgotten in many modern, scientific treatises that "cutting for the stone" is the oldest of the elective surgical procedures performed for the relief of a specific pathologic state and that many such operations were performed in childhood. Indeed, a bladder stone dating back to 4800 B.C. was found in the grave of an Egyptian boy estimated to have been 16 years of age at his demise. Celsus in the first century A.D. described a method of lithotomy and recommended it only for children aged 9 to 14 years.

DEMOGRAPHY

Today calculus disease in children is worldwide in distribution but is quite variable in its incidence. Centers in the United Kingdom report an incidence of 10 to 12 new cases per year (Ghazali et al., 1973), whereas those in the United States report only one to six cases per year (Bass and Emanuel, 1966). Conversely, areas of Southeast Asia report 175 new cases per year (Unakul, 1961). It is suspected that the reported incidence in the United States is falsely low, and one of the authors reports one new case of calculus disease of every 60 new pediatric urologic patients seen (Walther et al., 1980).

In most reported series there is a 2 to 1 male preponderance for reasons that are not clear (Malek and Kelalis, 1975). In our own series there was no prepubertal sex preponderance. Many of the older studies reported a peak incidence in children less than four years of age (Campbell, 1930). Recent studies conversely report an even incidence from birth through 15 years of age (Malek and Kelalis, 1975). Again, the reasons for this discrepancy are unknown. It has been suggested that Negro and Latin American children are affected by stone disease less often than Caucasian children (Raeschner et al., 1960), but this may reflect the population mix of reporting centers more than ethnic differences. Such was indeed our own experience.

COMPOSITION

Human urinary stones are usually composed of one or more of the following crystalline substances: calcium oxalate, calcium phosphate (apatite), magnesium ammonium phosphate (struvite), uric acid or other urates, cystine, xanthine, sulfa, or phenazopyridine. Campbell reported in 1930 that 50 per cent of the stones occurring in children in New York City were composed of urates or uric acid. This incidence no longer pertains, as so-called "infection stones" (magnesium ammonium phosphate) have been, in several series, the most common form of stone disease seen (Walther et al., 1980).

CLASSIFICATION

Stone disease may be classified in a number of different ways, all of which are useful in discussion. First, they may be classified by their position in the urinary tract — nephrocalcinosis, renal pelvis, ureter, bladder, or urethra. Second, they may be primary (arising as a result of a metabolic problem or idiopathic) or secondary (to factors such as infection, stasis, or a foreign body). Most primary stones develop in the kidney. An exception, however, is the previously mentioned endemic stone, which arises primarily in the bladder. Stones may also be classified by their chemical composition (although this is only useful as it provides a clue to etiology) or by the etiologic process through which they were generated.

CALCULOGENESIS

Before considering clinical stone disease, it would be germane to review briefly some factors in stone formation. Because stone disease in children seems more common in lower socioeconomic groups, many authors have suggested that dietary factors may play a role in calculogenesis. Certainly, vitamin A deficiency in rats can result in the formation of hydroxyl apatite stones (Hedenberg, 1954), but this does not seem relevant to the endemic stone disease of children once seen in the United Kingdom and currently accounting for most of the childhood stones seen in Southeast Asia. Recent studies from areas of endemic stone disease suggest that diets of breast milk supplemented by polished rice (a low phosphate diet) may be a factor (Thalut et al., 1976).

Urinary calculi in varying degrees all contain a substance called matrix, a mucoprotein not found in normal urine (Boyce, 1968). It is thought that uromucoid, a normal substance in renal urine, is converted to matrix substance by sialidase in the tubular epithelium of stone formers (Malek and Boyce, 1973). Occasionally one will find stones that are composed almost entirely of matrix. In most stones, however, calcium phosphate covers this matrix, and calcium oxalate is laid down over these fibrils. Other substances, such as uric acid, cystine, or struvite may fill the interlamellar gels of the matrix substance.

Factors that directly affect stone formation are urine pH, solute load, stasis, and urinary tract infection. Urine pH directly affects the solubility of substances such as cystine, uric acid, and struvite (Meyer, 1956). Urinary solute load at any given time can also affect stone formation in all forms of stone disease. Urine is best conceptualized as a supersaturated solution of most of the substances that can lead to stone formation (Vermeulen and Lyon, 1968). Hence, any imbalance in this delicate system can lead to crystallization.

There are inhibitors of stone formation that are normally present in urine (Fleisch and Bisaz, 1962). These include magnesium citrate, pyrophosphates, and other polyphosphates. However, these substances account for only 30 to 40 per cent of the known inhibitors of calculi systems, and their amounts do not vary between known stone formers and normal individuals. The rest of the inhibitors suspected to be present are as yet unidentified substances.

Urinary stasis probably does not lead to crystallization per se. However, should crystallization occur behind an obstruction, for example, the microcrystals formed are not washed out of the urinary tract by flow and may act as a nidus for a stone. Because urine is a supersaturated solution, this nidus leads to stone formation just as the introduction of a string into a supersaturated sugar solution leads to rock candy.

Urinary tract infection may lead to stone formation in several ways. First, urinary tract infection by inhibiting ureteral peristalsis may lead to stasis. Second, the urinary pH may be affected by the growth of bacteria. Additionally, if the bacterium is a urea-splitting organism, urine pH may become quite alkaline, and the ammonia formed by the breakdown of urea may be incorporated into a struvite (magnesium ammonium phosphate) stone.

RENAL TUBULAR ACIDOSIS

Although many calculi that form in children are idiopathic, certain recognized metabolic causes of stone formation must be diligently sought to prevent recurrent stone disease and possible urinary tract deterioration. One such disorder is Type I renal tubular acidosis (Fig. 19–1), a metabolic defect in which the distal renal tubule is unable to maintain a pH gradient between the blood and the tubular urine (Royer, 1974). This occurs because the distal tubular cells have an increased permeability to hydrogen ions. Bicarbonate reabsorption,

however, is normal. As a result, there is a hyperchloremic acidosis and an increased urinary loss of sodium, potassium, calcium, and phosphorus. Calcification is thought to be caused by the resultant hypercalciuria combined with a low urinary citrate secondary to systemic acidosis. Most of the stones formed in these patients are composed of calcium phosphate (apatite). However, even after the metabolic disorder is corrected, some of these patients may still form stones.

One form of this disorder can be transient and is usually seen in infant males, who may present with nephrocalcinosis and may recover fully with treatment (Lightwood, 1935). There is also a permanent type, which usually appears in females over age two years. This is rarely a familial disorder and, if so, appears as an autosomal

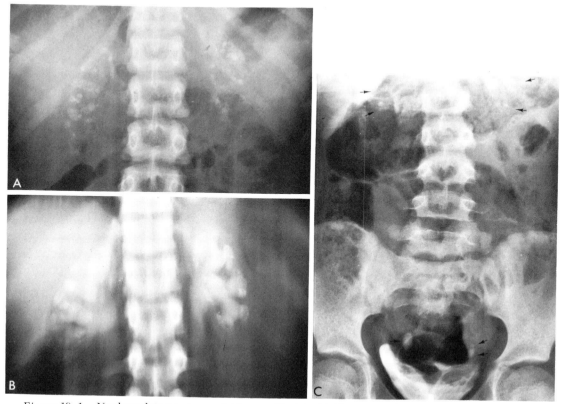

Figure 19–1.   Nephrocalcinosis in an eight-year-old girl with Type I renal tubular acidosis who presented with hematuria. *A*, KUB reveals bilateral nephrocalcinosis. *B*, Excretory urogram distinguishes extensive bilateral renal parenchymal calcification from contrast medium in dilated calyces. *C*, Excretory urogram also shows bilateral nephrocalcinosis (upper arrows) and bilateral lower ureteral calculi (lower arrows). (From Kelalis, P. P., King, L. R., and Belman, A. B.: Clinical Pediatric Urology, Vol. 2. Philadelphia, W. B. Saunders Co., 1976, p. 872.)

dominant trait. Seventy-three per cent of these patients will have nephrocalcinosis or stones (Coe, 1978). Renal tubular acidosis may also be seen as a secondary phenomenon in patients with hypercalcemia, hyperglobulinemia or due to toxins such as amphotericin B. Type II renal tubular acidosis, a proximal tubular disorder of bicarbonate reabsorption, is not associated with renal calculi.

Because the kidney in patients with renal tubular acidosis is unable to acidify urine below a pH of 6, the disorder can easily be identified. If after an overnight fast urine pH is 5.5, this diagnosis is untenable. However, if urine pH is never spontaneously 5.5, the patient can be challenged with ammonium chloride 100 mg per kg given in four divided doses for one day. Patients with renal tubular acidosis will still be unable to acidify their urine maximally despite such a challenge. It is important that the patient's urine be sterile at the time that ammonium chloride is used because in the event of infected urine, urinary acidification still may not occur.

Patients with renal tubular acidosis are treated by replacing bicarbonate, sodium, and potassium, usually in the form of Polycitra, but occasionally as sodium bicarbonate with potassium supplementation. Additionally, oral phosphate is often of benefit. Patients who are given carbonic anhydrase inhibitors, for example, for seizure disorders or glaucoma, can occasionally form stones by the same mechanism as patients with Type I renal tubular acidosis, but stone formation will usually stop after the medication has been discontinued (Parfitt, 1970).

CYSTINURIA

Cystinuria is an inborn error of metabolism associated with urolithiasis in which there are increased amounts of cystine, arginine, and lysine excreted in the urine (Watts, 1976). This disorder is not to be confused with cystinosis, in which no stones are formed (Fig. 19–2). Cystinuria is inherited as an autosomal recessive trait. Homozygotes can be easily identified, as

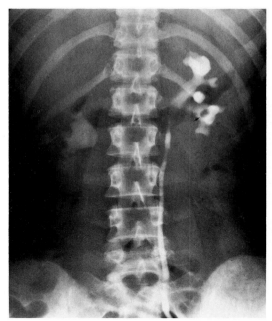

Figure 19–2. Appearance on excretory urogram of cystine stones in a teenager. Note the typical waxy appearance of large staghorn and multiple other cystine stones in the functionless right kidney and the negative filling defect (arrow) produced by another stone in the lower calyx of the left kidney. (From Kelalis, P. P., King, L. R., and Belman, A. B.: Clinical Pediatric Urology, Vol. 2. Philadelphia, W. B. Saunders Co., 1976, p. 874.)

their urinary excretion of cystine is over 500 mg per day. It is only the homozygote who forms stones; the heterozygote does not. When cystine appears in the urine in greatly increased concentrations, it may precipitate out because of its low solubility. The cyanide nitroprusside reaction will qualitatively detect over 75 mg of cystine per gm creatinine in the urine. However, this reaction will also identify heterozygotes. For this reason, in patients suspected of having cystinuria, quantitative determinations of cystine are necessary for both diagnosis and management. It is to be emphasized that cystine crystals can often be identified in urine by an experienced observer, and this simple clue, if followed, may lead to diagnosis (Fig. 19–3).

Cystinuria is best treated by forcing fluids and thereby diluting the urine. To be effective, diuresis must be continual, and patients with cystinuria should be awakened in the middle of the night for addition-

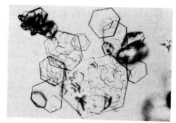

Figure 19–3. Cystine crystals in urinary sediment. (From Kelalis, P. P., King, L. R., and Belman, A. B.: Clinical Pediatric Urology, Vol. 2. Philadelphia, W. B. Saunders Co., 1976, p. 869.)

al fluids to prevent concentration of the urine while sleeping. Additionally, the urine can be alkalinized with Polycitra, for cystine is more soluble in alkaline urine. D-penicillamine is a chelating agent that combines with cystine to form a disulfide that is very soluble. Hence, this medication can be used for either the dissolution or prevention of cystine stones (Fig. 19–4).

However, there is moderate toxicity with this drug, and its use should be somewhat selective.

GLYCINURIA

Glycinuria is a rare genetically determined metabolic disorder of tubular function in which patients may form oxalate stones (DeVries et al., 1957). Such patients are best treated with hydration and urinary alkalinization.

HYPEROXALURIA

Primary hyperoxaluria is another rare disorder, genetically determined as an auto-

Figure 19–4. Effect of chemolysis on cystine stones in a fourteen-year-old boy with recurrent stone disease since right nephrolithotomy at age four. A, Plain tomogram shows large nonobstructive staghorn and several other small cystine stones in the right kidney. B, KUB two years later shows complete lysis of the right renal calculi; treatment included D-penicillamine, fluids, alkalis, and vitamin B₆. (From Kelalis, P. P., King, L. R., and Belman, A. B.: Clinical Pediatric Urology, Vol. 2. Philadelphia, W. B. Saunders Co., 1976, p. 875.)

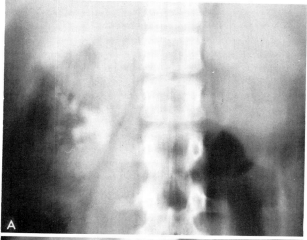

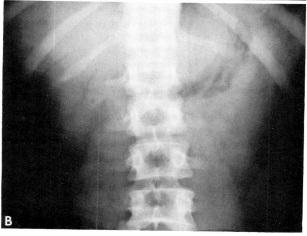

somal recessive trait, which may result in calculogenesis. These patients have both increased synthesis and excretion of oxalate. There are two types of primary hyperoxaluria, both of which can result in stones. In Type I primary hyperoxaluria, there is an increased excretion of oxalate, glyoxalic acid, and glycolic acid secondary to a deficiency of the enzyme alpha-ketoglutarate glyoxalate carboligase. In Type II primary hyperoxuluria, an increased excretion of L-glyceric acid occurs secondary to deficiency of the enzyme D-glyceric dehydrogenase. The clinical picture of both disorders is similar, and symptoms usually start before age five. Both sexes can be affected. Patients present with stones and occasionally with renal insufiency. There is usually growth retardation; some patients may have arthritis or carditis secondary to oxalosis. If untreated, most affected children will die prior to age 20.

Hyperoxaluria can also be an acquired disorder produced by the ingestion of ethylene glycol (antifreeze) or excessive amounts of rhubarb or vitamin C (more than 2 gm daily). Hyperoxaluria may also be manifested in pyridoxine (vitamin B_6) deficiencies, cirrhosis, renal tubular acidosis, and sarcoidosis. Some patients with inflammatory bowel disease may have hyperoxaluria (Smith et al., 1972). About seven per cent of patients with inflammatory bowel disease will have renal calculi. This association is thought to be secondary to disturbances in bile acid metabolism, which lead to an increased absorption of oxalate. Hyperoxaluria, regardless of cause, is documented by an increased urinary excretion of oxalate. Patients with inflammatory bowel disease and hyperoxaluria may be benefited by treatment with cholestyramine or taurine. Vitamin B_6 and inorganic phosphates have also been helpful in patients with hyperoxaluria regardless of etiology.

XANTHINURIA

Xanthinuria is another rare genetic disorder in which an enzyme, xanthine oxidase, is deficient. Because this enzyme converts xanthine to urates, there are increased amounts of xanthine, a relatively insoluble substance, in the urine. Xanthinuria can also be produced by the drug allopurinol, a xanthine oxidase inhibitor. Patients with xanthinuria may form xanthine stones (Seegmiller, 1968). This problem, whether inborn or iatrogenic, can be treated by increased fluid intake and urinary alkalinization.

HYPERCALCEMIA

A number of hypercalcemic states can result in stone formation. However, all these problems are rare in childhood. Chronic hypercalcemia causes renal calcification, which usually starts in the medulla and later spreads to the cortex. The classic example of a hypercalcemic state in adults is primary hyperparathyroidism secondary to a parathyroid adenoma. Sarcoidosis, hypervitaminosis D, the milk alkali syndrome, neoplasms that produce parathormone-like substance, Cushing's syndrome, and prolonged steroid therapy have also been responsible for stones. Prolonged steroid therapy is sometimes a factor in calculogenesis in children. In children receiving chronic steroid therapy, it is thought that there is an abnormal breakdown of protein with a consequent loss of bony matrix. This results in resorption of calcium from bone, hypercalciuria, and stones. Stones can be seen in 4 to 65 per cent of patients with Cushing's syndrome (Pyrah, 1979). Hyperthyroidism may also result in stone formation, as these patients may have osteoporosis with hypercalcemia and resultant hypercalciuria.

Idiopathic infantile hypercalcemia is an inborn error of metabolism that usually becomes apparent during the first year of life (Fellers and Schwartz, 1958). These patients will have hypercalcemia and may also have hypercalciuria and nephrocalcinosis. They usually have characteristic "elfin" facies, are dwarfed, retarded and often have osteosclerosis (Fig. 19–5). Another rare inborn error of metabolism is the blue diaper

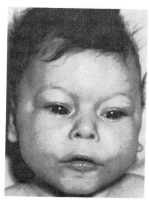

Figure 19–5. Infant with severe hypercalcemia and elfin facies. (From Smith, D. W.: Recognizable Patterns of Human Malformation, 2nd ed. Philadelphia, W. B. Saunders Co., 1976, p. 55.)

syndrome, in which there is a defect in tryptophan metabolism (Drummond et al., 1964). This too is associated with hypercalcemia and nephrocalcinosis. All the hypercalcemic states, regardless of etiology, can be treated by avoidance of Vitamin D and decrease in calcium intake. However, a low dairy diet may increase oxaluria and should not be indiscriminately recommended.

Hypercalcemia can also occur with immobilization. This is especially common in children after femoral fractures treated by prolonged bed rest (Key, 1936). This leads to osteoporosis and hypercalcemia. Hypercalciuria results, and unless fluid volumes are maintained at a high level, stones may form.

URIC ACID STONES

Uric acid or urate stones are relatively rare in children in the Western world but are quite common in developing countries, as they are the major component of endemic bladder stones. Upper urinary tract uric acid stones may be seen in patients with myeloproliferative disorders because of an increased purine turnover (Coe, 1978). Some patients with leukemia may initially present with anuria due to uric acid crystallization obstructing the ureters. This same phenomenon may also be seen in patients with

regional enteritis or after ileostomy presumably secondary to dehydration; this occasionally will occur in childhood. Anuria due to uric acid crystallization has been reported in neonates as well; the etiology of this phenomenon is unclear. Idiopathic uric acid stones do occur in children. There is often a family history of gout, but the serum and urine levels of uric acid in such patients are usually normal; these patients, however, invariably have a very acidic urine. Approximately 25 per cent of patients with gout will form uric acid stones, especially if treated with uricosuric agents without urinary alkalinization. In metabolically normal patients, uric acid bladder stones may form behind bladder neck obstruction.

An inborn error of metabolism that may result in uric acid stone formation is the Lesch-Nyhan syndrome (Lesch and Nyhan, 1964). These patients are severely mentally retarded, have athetoid movements, and are prone to self-mutilation. When treated with allopurinol, such patients may instead form xanthine stones. All uric acid stones, regardless of cause, can be treated by high fluid intake and urinary alkalinization. Additionally, allopurinol can be used to inhibit uric acid formation. Uric acid stones can also be successfully dissolved by this regimen in many patients as long as there is no concomitant urinary tract infection.

ENDEMIC BLADDER STONES

So-called endemic stones are bladder calculi that usually appear in boys under five years of age. Endemic stones were once very common in the United Kingdom; many of the lithotomies of the seventeenth and eighteenth centuries were performed on children for this very disease. However, for reasons that are not at this time clear, it has been well documented in England that at the turn of this century there was a sharp decrease in the incidence of endemic stones (Lett, 1936). Endemic stones, however, are still quite common in Southeast Asia and in other developing countries. These stones are usually composed of ammonium acid urate, and once they are removed, the recurrence rate is quite low.

IDIOPATHIC STONE DISEASE

The idiopathic stones of adults, most of which are calcium stones, are not a common problem in childhood, although in a Mayo Clinic series they accounted for 45 per cent of the stones seen in children (Malek and Kelalis, 1975). Patients with idiopathic stone disease may have hypercalciuria, but most do not. The problem, when recognized, is best treated by a high fluid intake. If hypercalciuria is present the following may also aid in preventing recurrence of stones: (1) a decrease in dietary calcium, (2) hydrochlorothiazide to decrease urinary calcium levels, (3) magnesium oxide (orally), with or without pyridoxine, to reduce calcium absorption, and (4) increased amounts of inorganic phosphates, which also reduce calcium absorption.

Stones can form secondary to stasis, either with or without urinary tract infection. Such stones are usually struvite in composition, especially if infection is present. It must be remembered that the stones are secondary to the primary obstructive process, and the obstruction must be relieved for effective therapy. Additionally, although infection must be treated to prevent recurrence, it is impossible to eradicate infection permanently without removal of the stone (Nemoy and Stamey, 1971). In the presence of foreign bodies in the urinary tract, stones may form at alarming rates. Although it is true that some children have placed foreign bodies in their bladders inadvertently, most of the problems associated with foreign bodies are iatrogenic and result from indwelling catheters, retained fragments of catheters, or occasionally from nonabsorbable suture material in the lumen of the urinary tract.

DIAGNOSIS

The most important factor in the diagnosis of stone disease in children is to consider it in the differential diagnosis. Many stones in children, especially small calculi, pass spontaneously; they are not diagnosed because the problem was not considered and appropriate diagnostic measures undertaken for confirmation. Most adult patients with stone disease will present with classic renal colic, that is, flank pain radiating to the groin or genitalia. However, most children do not localize the pain produced by their stones well and complain only of abdominal pain (Myers, 1957). Appendectomies have been performed on children with stones who presented with only abdominal pain and vomiting. Many renal calculi are silent (painless) and may present as hematuria or urinary tract infection without other symptoms. Bilateral upper urinary tract calculi may obstruct the urinary tract and present as anuria or azotemia. Bladder calculi, on the other hand, are often quite irritating, and these patients have marked dysuria and strangury.

Physical examination may reveal stigmata of underlying problems but is usually unrewarding in pinpointing the diagnosis except in those rare instances of impacted urethral calculi. Urinalysis will often demonstrate hematuria, pyuria, or bacteriuria. Urinary pH may yield a clue to stone composition. Fresh urine should be examined for the presence of crystals, which may suggest the type of stone present. The definitive diagnosis will be made by the demonstration of calculi in appropriate radiographs. Calcium phosphate, calcium oxalate, struvite, and cystine are all radiopaque substances and can be detected in plain films of the abdomen. On the other hand, uric acid, urates, matrix, and xanthine are all radiolucent and will be detected only after contrast medium has been injected and then only by virtue of obstruction or radiolucent filling defects. Excretory urography will confirm the diagnosis of calculi in most instances if appropriate films are obtained. Oblique views are often essential to demonstrate that any given calcific density lies within the urinary tract.

Although it is true that metabolic sources of stone formation must be sought in most children with stone disease, the evaluation of such problems can be somewhat individualized if the composition of the stone present is known. Rather than embarking on a lengthy and expensive search for metabolic causes for stone formation at the outset, after screening for hypercalcemia, hyperuricemia, cystinuria, and infection, crystalographic analysis of a recovered stone is the most rewarding type of procedure that will further direct evaluation. Struvite stones form almost entirely as a result of infection, and no metabolic workup is indicated in these patients. Cystine stones form only in the presence of cystinuria. Patients with calcium phosphate, calcium oxalate, or uric acid stones must be studied for the various causes of stones of these types.

TREATMENT

The treatment of stone disease in children has two facets, the acute problem and chronic management. Acutely, management considerations include pain relief, hydration, treatment of infection, relief of urinary obstruction, and recovery of the calculus for analysis. The pain of renal colic is severe and often requires potent narcotics for relief. Although theoretically undesirable, morphine provides better analgesia than meperidine and, therefore, is preferred when severe renal colic is present. Many patients with ureteral calculi will have vomiting on a reflex basis, and, hence, may become dehydrated. Diuresis can assist in the spontaneous passage of small calculi; therefore, if the patient is unable to drink large quantities of fluids, intravenous hydration may be of benefit.

If urinary tract infection is present, antibiotics should be administered. If the patient has systemic signs of sepsis with an obstructing stone, urgent intervention may be necessary for adequate therapy. Obstruction without infection can be managed expectantly for short periods (weeks) without renal damage, but prolonged obstruction demands relief for maximal preservation of renal function. Additionally, the combination of obstruction and infection can rapidly damage the kidney and necessitates prompt

action for maximal preservation of renal tissue. If one expects that a stone may be passed spontaneously, the urine should be strained so that the stone may be recovered for analysis.

As was stated earlier, small stones (less than 5 mm diameter) often pass spontaneously, and this is the preferred resolution of the problem when possible. Indications for early surgical intervention include high-grade obstruction, severe pain uncontrolled by narcotics, and unresponsive urinary tract infection. Although a discussion of the various surgical modalities is beyond the scope of this presentation, it must be noted that most forms of endoscopic manipulation of stones that are of such great utility in adults have very little place in children for technical reasons.

Often the surgical removal of stones from the kidney or bladder is incomplete in that small fragments may remain behind. This is especially true when dealing with struvite stones. In such a situation, Renacidin or Subey's Solution G are of utility in the dissolution of such residual struvite fragments by direct irrigation through indwelling nephrostomy or cystotomy tubes. The chronic management of stones is designed entirely to prevent recurrence and embodies all the items previously discussed.

REFERENCES

Bass, H. N., and Emanual, B.: Nephrolithiasis in childhood. Clin. Pediatr., 5:79, 1966.
Boyce, W. H.: Organic matrix of human urinary concretions. Am. J. Med., 45:673, 1968.
Campbell, M. F.: Urinary calculi in infancy and childhood. J.A.M.A., 94:1753, 1930.
Coe, F. L.: Nephrolithiasis. Pathogenesis and Treatment. Chicago, Year Book Medical Publishers, 1978.
DeVries, A., Kochwa, S., Lazebink, J., Frank, M., and Djaldetti, M.: Glycinuria, a hereditary disorder associated with nephrolithiasis. Am. J. Med., 23:408, 1957.
Drummond, K. N., Michael, H. F., and Ulstrom, R. A.: The blue diaper syndrome. Am. J. Med., 37:928, 1964.
Fellers, F. Y., and Schwartz, R.: Etiology of the severe form of hypercalcemia of infancy. N. Engl. J. Med., 259:1050, 1958.
Fleisch, H., and Bisaz, S.: Mechanism of calcification. Am. J. Physiol., 200:1296, 1962.
Ghazali, S., Barrett, T. M., and Williams, D. I.: Child-

hood urolithiasis in Britain. Arch. Dis. Child., *48*:291, 1973.

Hedenberg, I.: Macroscopic and microscopic changes and stone formation in the urinary tract in experimentally produced vitamin A deficiency in rats. Acta. Chir. Scand. (Suppl.), 192, 1954.

Key, L. A.: Urinary tract complications in the prolonged immobilization of children. Br. Med. J., *1*:1150, 1936.

Lesch, M., and Nyhan, W. L.: A familial disorder of uric acid metabolism and central nervous system function. Am. J. Med., *36*:561, 1964.

Lett, H.: Urinary calculus with special reference to stone in the bladder. Br. J. Urol., *8*:205, 1936.

Lightwood, E.: Calcium infarction of kidneys in infants. Arch. Dis. Child., *18*:205, 1935.

Malek, R. S., and Boyce, W. H.: Intranephronic calculosis. J. Urol., *109*:551, 1973.

Malek, R. S., and Kelalis, P. P.: Pediatric urolithiasis. J. Urol., *113*:545, 1975.

Meyer, J. Quoted in Butt, A. J.: Etiologic factors in renal lithiasis. Springfield, Ill., Charles C Thomas, 1956.

Myers, N. A.: Urolithiasis in childhood. Arch. Dis. Child., *32*:48, 1957.

Nemoy, N. J., and Stamey, T. A.: Surgical, bacteriological, and biochemical management of infection stones. J.A.M.A., *215*:1470, 1971.

Parfitt, A. M.: Acetazolamide and renal stone formation. Lancet, *2*:153, 1970.

Pyrah, L. N.: Renal calculus. New York, Springer-Verlag, 1979.

Raeschner, C. W., Singleton, E. B., and Curts, J. C.: Urinary tract calculi and nephrocalcinosis in infants and children. J. Pediatr., *57*:721, 1960.

Royer, P., Habib, R., Mathieu, H., and Broyer, M.: Pediatric Nephrology. Philadelphia, W. B. Saunders Co., 1974, pp. 69–77, 107–108.

Seegmiller, J. E.: Xanthine stone formation. Am. J. Med., *45*:780, 1968.

Smith, L. H., Fromm, H., and Hoffman, H. F.: Acquired hyperoxaluria, nephrolithiasis, and intestinal disease. N. Engl. J. Med., *286*:1371, 1972.

Thalut, K., Rizal, A., Brockis, J. G., Bowyer, R. L., Taylor, T. I., and Wisniewsky, Z. S.: The endemic bladder stones of Indonesia: Epidemiology and clinical features. Br. J. Urol., *48*:617, 1976.

Unakul, S.: Urinary stones in Thailand, a statistical survey. Siriraj Hosp. Gaz., *13*:199, 1961.

Vermeulen, C. W., and Lyon, E. S.: Mechanisms of genesis and growth of calculi. Am. J. Med., *45*:684, 1968.

Walther, P. C., Lamm, D., and Kaplan, G. W.: Pediatric urolithiasis: A ten-year review. Pediatrics, *65*:1068, 1980.

Watts, R. W. E.: Cystinuria and cystine stone disease. *In* Williams, D. I., and Chisholm, G. D. (Eds.): Scientific Foundations of Urology. London, Heinemann, 1976.

Chapter Twenty

TRAUMA

Accidents are the most common cause of death in American children. Injuries to the urogenital system account for 2.4 to 7 per cent of all childhood injuries (Malek, 1976). Such injuries can occur at any time during childhood and may even occur during intrauterine life or during the process of delivery itself. Obviously, although the fetus is indeed quite well protected, severe injury to the mother can also result in injury to the intrauterine fetus. Modern technology has provided a new form of injury. During the course of intrauterine transfusion, the abdominal wall of the fetus may be lacerated. Dissection of blood may result in a hematocele or hematoma of the scrotal wall; when present at the time of birth these may be confused with neonatal testicular torsion (Fig. 20–1). Although vaginal delivery of breech presentations is allowed less commonly today than in former years, infants delivered in this presentation are particularly susceptible to adrenal hemorrhage in the course of the obstetric maneuvers necessary for delivery (Chap. 17).

There are multiple modalities that can result in blunt trauma, including the usual bumps and falls sustained by any child. Another form of trauma more frequently recognized than previously is child abuse (Kempe, 1975). In addition, affluence and modern technology have provided us with the automobile, skateboard, motorcycle, and hang gliders, all of which have contributed to the number of injuries in children.

Children can also be injured by missiles (gunshot wounds) or punctures (stab wounds) just as adults are, albeit with reduced frequency.

Trauma resulting in significant renal injury accounts for approximately one of every 860 pediatric hospital admissions (Smith et al., 1966). Another way to look at this is that the kidney is injured in 1.2 to 7 per cent of all traumatized children. Again, because of the lifestyles invoked by our

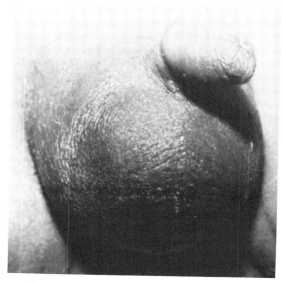

Figure 20–1. Newborn male with scrotal wall hematoma produced by blood dissecting down anterior abdominal wall following intrauterine exchange transfusion. He was explored as a neonatal torsion.

society, boys are involved in trauma three times more often than girls. Renal injuries alone account for between 34 and 68 per cent of all injuries sustained in trauma involving the urogenital system (Malek, 1976). Twenty to 25 per cent of all instances of renal trauma occur in children; more renal trauma is seen in the second decade of life than in the first by a factor of three (Smith et al., 1966).

RENAL TRAUMA

Children as a group are injured less frequently than adults, and yet there are certain anatomic features that predispose the child to renal injury. The kidney is relatively larger in the child than it is in the adult. There is less perirenal fat about the kidney to protect it, and this situation exists until approximately age 10. Additionally, the eleventh and twelfth ribs do not ossify secondarily until approximately age 25.

Blunt renal trauma is approximately 55 times more common than penetrating injuries of the kidney, whereas blunt trauma involves other organs of the urinary system only twice as often as does penetrating injury (Javadpour et al., 1973). The mechanism of injury in blunt renal trauma is thought to be secondary to a sudden deceleration of the body while the kidney itself keeps moving (Fig. 20–2). The kidney then is suddenly arrested by its vessels and other perirenal attachments. This results in both cortical lacerations of the kidney and intimal tears of the renal vessels. Vascular thrombosis may also occur because of high-voltage electroshock injuries. As is true with other organs, the kidney can be injured iatrogenically; it also can occasionally be penetrated by ingested foreign bodies that erode through the gastrointestinal tract.

It is somewhat axiomatic that the abnormal kidney is more predisposed to injury than the normal kidney, and, indeed, abnormal kidneys account for 20 per cent of all instances of renal trauma. Abnormalities that have been associated with this increased propensity are hydronephrosis, a solitary compensatorily hypertrophied kid-

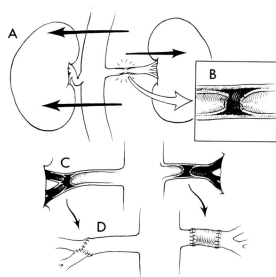

Figure 20–2. Mechanism of renal injury. (From Harrison, J. H., Gittes, R. F., Perlmutter, A. D., et al.: Campbell's Urology, Vol. 1. Philadelphia, W. B. Saunders Co., 1978, p. 895.)

ney, ectopic kidneys, fused kidneys, and renal tumors.

When one is confronted with a patient with renal trauma, there are often associated injuries that may dictate the early, emergency management. This occurs in up to 40 per cent of all patients with renal trauma and includes cerebral trauma, spinal trauma, bony trauma, pulmonary trauma, other abdominal visceral trauma, and vascular trauma (Morse et al., 1967). Approximately 25 per cent of all patients who sustain left renal injury have an associated splenic injury. The mortality rate in patients with renal trauma and associated chest or head injury is approximately 7 per cent (Javadpour et al., 1973).

URETERAL TRAUMA

Ureteral injuries occur, but because the ureter is well protected, blunt injuries of the ureter itself are rare. They occur in only four per cent of all children with some form of urogenital trauma. The mechanism of injury in blunt trauma is felt to be exaggerated hyperextension of the body resulting in avulsion at the ureteropelvic junction. This injury appears unique to childhood (Beckly and Waters, 1972). Obviously, penetrating wounds can result in ureteral injury should the ureter lie within the pathway of the penetrating object.

BLADDER TRAUMA

In spite of the bladder essentially being an abdominal organ in children, it is injured in only three per cent sustaining urogenital trauma (Mertz et al., 1963). Injuries of the bladder are especially common in patients with pelvic fractures. Roughly 10 per cent of patients with fractured pelves will have an associated bladder rupture. In 80 per cent of these bladder ruptures, the rupture itself will be an extraperitoneal one. The distended bladder, with its increased intravesical pressure, is more likely to rupture than is the empty bladder. A sudden marked increase in internal pressure due to the force of injury results in excessive stress to the bladder wall (Fig. 20–3).

On occasion, the bladder can actually be penetrated by a bony spicule in the course of a pelvic fracture. Fortunately, approximately one third of the bladder injuries are merely contusions. In addition, there can be iatrogenic injuries to the bladder during the course of pelvic operations, including simple hernia repair.

URETHRAL TRAUMA

Urethral injuries occur in children just as in adults (Waterhouse and Gross, 1969). Because the urogenital diaphragm is a relatively fixed structure, the urethra may be transected at this point in the course of a pelvic fracture (Fig. 20–4). In straddle injuries, the urethra may also be transected partially or completely by the force of blunt trauma to the perineum (Fig. 20–5). These injuries occur more frequently in males than females. The urethra can also be injured iatrogenically in the course of instrumentation or by the insertion of foreign bodies.

TRAUMA TO THE EXTERNAL GENITALIA

The external genitalia can be injured in the course of breech delivery. Other modes of injury to the external genitalia of children include direct blows during the course of play. Bites, be they animal, insect, or human, do occur. Especially in uncircumcised males, one injury of particular note is

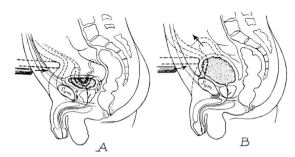

Figure 20–3. Mechanism of vesical rupture. *A,* In a slightly filled bladder, extraperitoneal rupture occurs more frequently. An empty bladder may be lacerated but usually does not rupture. *B,* When the bladder is full and trauma is in the anteroposterior direction, the rupture is usually intraperitoneal. (From Kelalis, P. P., King, L. R., and Belman, A. B.: Clinical Pediatric Urology, Vol. 2. Philadelphia, W. B. Saunders Co., 1976, p. 1047.)

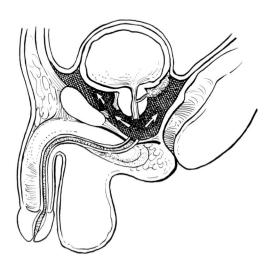

Figure 20–4. Ruptured prostatomembranous urethra. Note ruptured puboprostatic ligaments and collection of blood above the urogenital diaphragm (arrows). (From Kelalis, P. P., King, L. R., and Belman, A. B.: Clinical Pediatric Urology, Vol. 2. Philadelphia, W. B. Saunders Co., 1976, p. 1049.)

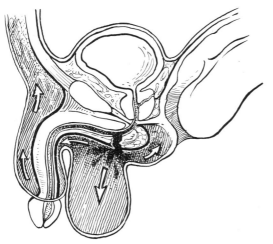

Figure 20–5. Bulbous urethral injury. Note extravasation through ruptured Buck's fascia (heavy solid line) with dissemination underneath Colles' and Scarpa's fasciae (arrows). Voiding will exaggerate the extravasation. (From Kelalis, P. P., King, L. R., and Belman, A. B.: Clinical Pediatric Urology, Vol. 2. Philadelphia, W. B. Saunders Co., 1976, p. 1050.)

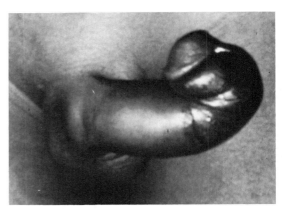

Figure 20–7. Rupture of right corpus cavernosum (penile fracture) in a 10-year-old boy.

the zipper injury, in which a redundant foreskin is caught within the zipper itself. Another injury of similar type, especially prevalent during the toilet-training years, is the injury in which the penis is contused by

a blow from the falling toilet seat as the small child is leaning over the toilet bowl to urinate.

The penis can be strangulated or lacerated by the application of a tourniquet. This may occur accidentally in male infants who are held nude by mothers with long hair (Fig. 20–6) and can also occur when a ligature is tied about the penis to prevent a child from wetting his bed. Urethral fistulae may result. Penile fractures (that is, fractures of the corpora cavernosum) also occur in children if there is a sudden blow to the erect phallus (Fig. 20–7). Scrotal and vulvar lacerations are not infrequent and usually are relatively minor. Testicular injury itself is a most unusual event in the child.

CLASSIFICATION

Injuries of the urogenital system in general can be classified into blunt or penetrating trauma. The management of each differs in that operative intervention is the rule in penetrating trauma yet is often not required with blunt trauma. Renal injuries can be further subdivided into renal contusion, cortical lacerations, urinary extravasation, and pedicle injury (Fig. 20–8). The management of each differs. Bladder injuries with bladder rupture are subdivided into intraperitoneal rupture and extraperitoneal rupture. Injuries of the male urethra are subdivided as to whether the injury is

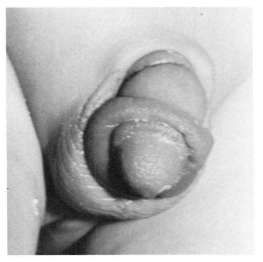

Figure 20–6. Penile tourniquet syndrome caused by a hair. Note the circumferential indentation at the base of the penis (site of the hair).

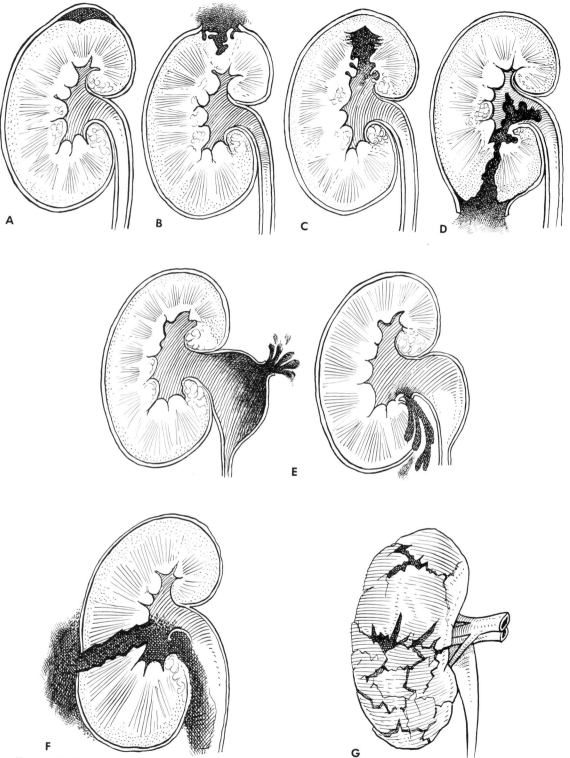

Figure 20–8. *A,* Renal contusion. *B,* Renal cortical laceration causing perirenal bleeding. *C,* Renal calyceal rupture causing intrarenal bleeding. *D,* Rupture of capsule, parenchyma, and calyx causing perirenal and intrarenal bleeding and urinary extravasation. *E,* Rupture of renal pelvis. *F,* Polar rupture. *G,* Shattered kidney. (From Kelalis, P. P., King, L. R., and Belman, A. B.: Clinical Pediatric Urology, Vol. 2. Philadelphia, W. B. Saunders Co., 1976, pp. 1031–1032.)

above or below the urogenital diaphgram in addition to classification of severity.

INITIAL EVALUATION

The initial assessment of the patient with urogenital trauma involves assessment of all other injuries identifying those that must take precedence with regard to survival. Major chest injuries, vascular injuries, and central nervous system injuries overshadow the entire management of the injured child. However, as one begins to focus on the urinary system itself, the mechanism of injury can provide some clues as to what may have transpired. For example, a moderate amount of bleeding into the urinary tract after a rather minimal injury suggests the presence of an abnormal kidney prior to injury. Inspection should include notation of any obvious lacerations, abrasions, or hematomata. The presence of blood at or dripping from the external urethral meatus is virtually pathognomonic of urethral injury. Palpation of the abdomen may reveal the presence of retroperitoneal masses suggesting perirenal hematomata. Auscultation of the abdomen may demonstrate adynamic ileus, which, in the absence of intraperitoneal injury, strongly suggests retroperitoneal bleeding. On rectal examination in the male, one may note that the bladder and prostate are much higher than normal and that the normal area of the prostate is replaced by a boggy fullness suggesting transection of the membranous urethra. It must be emphasized that although hematuria is often present in urinary tract injuries, its absence does not exclude injury to the urogenital system.

RADIOGRAPHIC EVALUATION

The radiograph is the major diagnostic modality for most internal urinary injuries. A plain film of the abdomen is obtained, and notation is made of any fractures. Additionally, one should note the presence or absence of the psoas muscle shadow and the lateral fat stripes. Excretory urography is performed (Figs. 20–9 and 20–10), and it must be emphasized that a large dose of contrast medium should be employed. The doses that are commonly employed for trauma are 2 to 4 ml of a 60 per cent contrast solution per kg body weight. The renal outlines are evaluated, and notation is made of visualization and extravasation. Tomography is often helpful at this stage. Ureteral injuries are especially difficult to diagnose on excretory urography and consequently often present late as a urinoma or ureteral fistula. However, if there is visualization of the involved ureter, one can state with relative certainty that there is no ureteral injury.

Excretory urography itself is of little value in the diagnosis or exclusion of injuries to the bladder or urethra. If one suspects urethral injury because of either urethral bleeding or urinary retention, it is desirable to perform a retrograde urethrogram by placing a small catheter at the urethral meatus and filling the urethra with water-soluble contrast agent (Fig. 20–11). This should be done prior to the performance of the excretory urogram. If urethral injury is strongly suspected, attempts to pass a urethral catheter *should not be made*. If urinary extravasation is identified, this is excellent evidence of urethral injury. If there is no evidence of urethral injury and one is suspicious that a bladder injury may have occurred, a catheter can then be passed into the bladder and the bladder filled with a water-soluble contrast agent. Once again, this is best performed prior to excretory urography, if at all possible. Once the bladder has been filled with contrast material and films have been obtained, the bladder is completely drained of the contrast agent and another film is obtained to be sure that extravasation was not hidden by the contrast agent filling the bladder (Fig. 20–12). Retrograde pyelograms are rarely necessary for the diagnosis of urinary tract injuries in children.

If there is poor visualization of one or both kidneys and if renal injury is suspected, aortography is performed to delineate the vascular and cortical integrity. In some centers, renal scans are used for this pur-

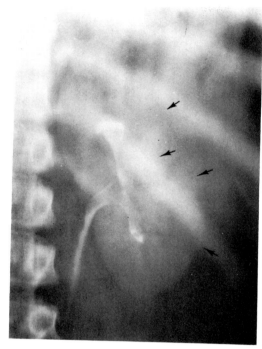

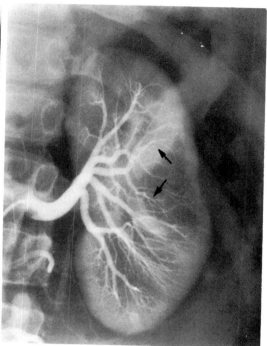

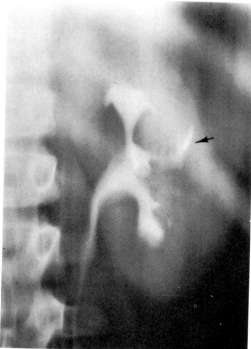

Figure 20–9. Renal contusion in an eight-year-old boy after blunt trauma to left side while sledding; patient presented with gross hematuria. *Upper left,* Excretory urogram (tomogram) showing intact capsule (outer three arrows) and nonvisualization of middle calyx (inner arrow) of left kidney. Note blood clot in renal pelvis. *Upper right,* Selective left renal angiogram, showing location of parenchymal swelling (arrows point to displaced arterial branches). *Lower left,* Excretory urogram (tomogram) two weeks after conservative management, showing left kidney with contrast medium in somewhat deformed middle calyx (arrow).

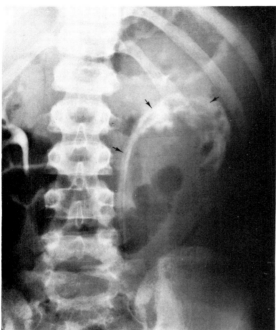

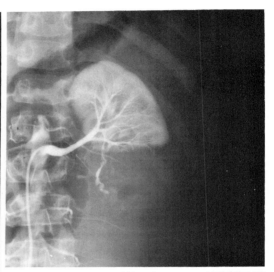

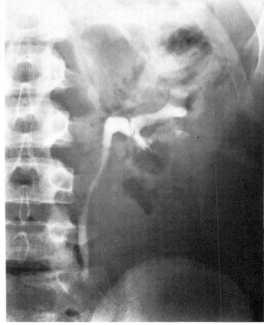

Figure 20–10. Parenchymal rupture (through-and-through) in a nine-year-old boy who fell off his bicycle; patient presented with left-sided abdominal pain, guarding, and gross hematuria. *Upper left,* Excretory urogram, showing extravasation around lower half of left kidney and upper ureter (arrows). *Upper right,* Selective left renal angiogram, showing through-and-through rupture of kidney. Note nonvisualization of lower half of kidney, ground-glass appearance of perineal hematoma, contrast medium escaping from a ruptured artery, and medial displacement of descending colon. *Lower right,* Excretory urogram five months after left lower heminephrectomy. (From Kelalis, P. P., King, L. R., and Belman, A. B.: Clinical Pediatric Urology, Vol. 2. Philadelphia, W. B. Saunders Co., 1976, pp. 1034, 1036.)

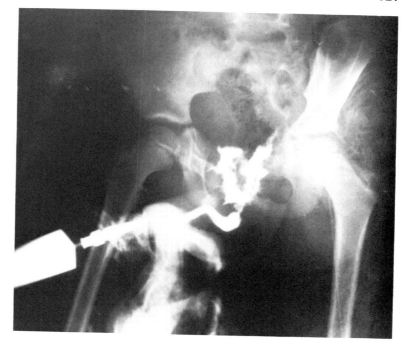

Figure 20–11. Retrograde urethrogram in a four-year-old with a pelvic fracture and complete membranous urethral disruption.

pose. Delayed studies with isotopes may be helpful in following the child after surgery or if an operative approach is immediately elected.

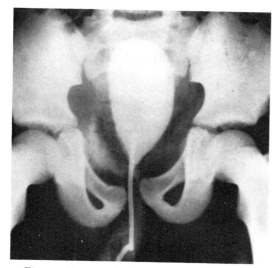

Figure 20–12. Bladder injury in traumatized eight-year-old boy. Cystogram discloses "inverted" teardrop shape of bladder. Note extravasated contrast medium on right side. (Courtesy of Dr. G. C. Prather and Dr. T. F. Kaiser.) (From Kelalis, P. P., King, L. R., and Belman, A. B.: Clinical Pediatric Urology, Vol. 2. Philadelphia, W. B. Saunders Co., 1976, p. 1048.)

MANAGEMENT

RENAL

Many renal injuries can be treated expectantly. The approach to a patient with trauma is usually multidisciplinary. It is essential that only one physician be in charge of the team, however. Approximately 90 per cent of patients with blunt renal injuries treated nonoperatively will stabilize within 24 hours. It is generally agreed that nonpenetrating injuries of the upper urinary tract in the absence of urinary extravasation or extensive hemorrhage should be treated conservatively with bed rest until gross hematuria ceases.

There is some controversy regarding treatment of major nonpenetrating injuries, however. Most authors would agree that if vascular thrombosis has occurred, an attempt to repair this injury should be carried out even up to 18 hours after injury (Skinner, 1973). Approximately five to seven per cent of all blunt renal injuries will result in nephrectomy or some loss of renal substance. It is in this area that controversy exists as to whether the best results are obtained by an aggressive early surgical approach (Scott et al., 1963) or by a nonoperative expectant approach (Thompson et al., 1977). In many patients initially managed nonoperatively, persistent bleeding or, more commonly, extensive urinary extravasation may necessitate delayed exploration and drainage. Most authors agree that patients with penetrating renal trauma should undergo exploratory procedures.

Complications of renal injuries, whether treated operatively or expectantly, include secondary hemorrhage, urinary extravasation, perinephric abscess, and renal failure. Late complications include hypertension secondary to either segmental ischemia of the kidney or a "Page" kidney. Renal stones occur following trauma in rare instances. Hydronephrosis and urinoma can occur; renal scarring very frequently occurs after major injury. Arteriovenous fistulae are seen, especially after percutaneous renal biopsy. Renal atrophy is often the sequel to a major renal injury.

URETERS

Ureteral injuries should be repaired when they are diagnosed regardless of whether they are the result of blunt or penetrating trauma (Beckly and Waters, 1972). The complications of ureteral injury include urinary tract infection, ureteral stricture, ureterocutaneous fistulae, and urinary calculi.

BLADDER

The management of bladder injuries is mildly controversial and is partly dictated by the location of the extravasated urine (Fig. 20–13). If urine is extravasating extraperitoneally, there are many who feel that catheter drainage alone will suffice provided that the urine is sterile. Others feel that the bladder wound must be repaired and the area drained. Additionally, although most

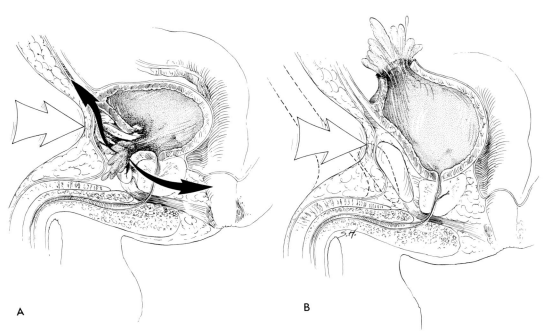

A   B

Figure 20–13. A, Mechanism of extraperitoneal urinary bladder rupture. The pubic rami are fractured, and the bladder is perforated by a bony fragment. B, Mechanism of intraperitoneal vesical rupture. A sharp blow is delivered to the lower abdomen of a patient with a distended urinary bladder. The distensive force is exerted equally on all surfaces of the bladder, and it ruptures at its weakest point, usually the dome. (From Harrison, J. H., Gittes, R. F., Perlmutter, A. D., et al.: Campbell's Urology, 4th ed., Vol. 1. Philadelphia, W. B. Saunders Co., 1978, p. 907.)

authors would feel that intraperitoneal rupture is best repaired surgically, there are those who would feel that in patients with sterile urine these, too, can be handled by catheter drainage alone (Mulkey and Witherington, 1974). Complications that can arise from bladder injury include urinary tract infection, bladder calculus, persistent hematuria, and vesicocutaneous fistulae.

URETHRA

Urethral injuries, once again, are an area of current controversy. Some authors feel that urethral injuries are best treated by suprapubic vesical drainage alone at the time of injury, secondarily repairing the stricture should one develop (Morehouse et al., 1972). Others feel that the urethra should be aligned over a splinting catheter (Malek et al., 1977). Complications that can arise from urethral injuries include urethral strictures and resultant hydronephrosis, urethrocutaneous fistulae, urinary tract infection, and impotence.

GENITALIA

Lesions of the external genitalia in small children may pose an additional problem in that it may require anesthesia merely to determine the extent of the injury alone. Many girls with relatively minor vulvar injury will develop urinary retention because of dysuria and the fear of voiding. Sitz baths rather than urethral catheterization are recommended. Testicular injuries are best treated by surgical debridement and repair.

Penile amputation is a peculiar form of genital injury that is occasionally seen in children. If the amputated member is available, it is best cleansed and packed on ice so that it can be replanted. There has been some success with microsurgical techniques in this regard. If such is not the case, secondary reconstruction of the amputated penis will be required. Parenthetically, this is a formidable undertaking, and the results are never as good as the original organ.

ADRENALS

Adrenal injuries do occur in neonates and often present as a suprarenal mass. If the diagnosis can be established with reasonable certainty, these lesions are best left alone, as the hematoma remains confined, bleeding does not progress, and the hematoma eventually resolves with adrenal calcification (Chap. 17).

REFERENCES

Beckly, D. E., and Waters, E. A.: Avulsion of the pelvi-ureteric junction. Br. J. Radiol., 45:423, 1972.

Javadpour, N., Guinan, P., and Bush, I. M.: Renal trauma in children. Surg. Gynecol. Obstet., 136:237, 1973.

Kempe, C. H.: Uncommon manifestations of the battered child syndrome. Am. J. Dis. Child., 129:1265, 1975.

Malek, R. S.: Genitourinary trauma. In Kelalis, P. P., King, L. R., and Belman, A. B. (Eds.): Clinical Pediatric Urology. Philadelphia, W. B. Saunders Co., 1976, p. 1029.

Malek, R. S., O'Dea, M. J., and Kelalis, P. P.: Management of ruptured posterior urethra in childhood. J. Urol., 117:105, 1977.

Mertz, J. H. D., Wishard, W. N., Jr., and Nourse, M. H.: Injury of the kidney in children. J.A.M.A., 183:730, 1963.

Morehouse, A. D., Belitsky, P., and MacKinnon, K. J.: Rupture of the posterior urethra. J. Urol., 107:255, 1972.

Morse, T. S., Smith, J. P., Howard, W. H. R., and Rowe, M. I.: Kidney injuries in children. J. Urol., 98:539, 1967.

Mulkey, A. P., and Witherington, R.: Conservative management of vesical rupture. Urology, 4:426, 1974.

Scott, R., Jr., Carlton, C. E., Ashmore, A. J., and Duke, H. H.: Initial management of non-penetrating renal injuries. J. Urol., 90:535, 1963.

Skinner, D. G.: Traumatic renal artery thrombosis. Ann. Surg., 177:264, 1973.

Smith, M. J. V., Seidel, R. F., and Bonacarti, A. F.: Accident trauma to the kidneys in children. J. Urol., 96:845, 1966.

Thompson, I. M., LaTourette, H., Montie, J. E., and Ross, G., Jr.: Results of non-operative management of blunt renal trauma. J. Urol., 118:522, 1977.

Waterhouse, K., and Gross, M.: Trauma of the genitourinary tract. J. Urol., 101:241, 1969.

Index

Numbers in *italics* refer to illustrations; (t) following a number refers to a table.